VOLUME ONE HUNDRED AND THIRTEEN

ADVANCES IN
PARASITOLOGY

Current research on naturally
transmitted *Plasmodium knowlesi*

SERIES EDITOR

D. ROLLINSON
Life Sciences Department
The Natural History Museum,
London, United Kingdom
d.rollinson@nhm.ac.uk

J. R. STOTHARD
Department of Tropical
Disease Biology
Liverpool School of Tropical
Medicine, Liverpool, United Kingdom
russell.stothard@lstmed.ac.uk

EDITORIAL BOARD

T. J. C. ANDERSON
Department of Genetics, Texas
Biomedical Research Institute,
San Antonio, TX, United States

M. G. BASÁÑEZ
Professor of Neglected Tropical
Diseases, Department of Infectious
Disease Epidemiology, Faculty of
Medicine (St Mary's Campus),
Imperial College London,
London, United Kingdom

D. D. BOWMAN
Director Cornell CVM MPS—Veterinary
Parasitology, Professor of Parasitology,
C4-119 VMC, Dept Micro & Immunol,
CVM Cornell University, Ithaca,
NY, United States

R. B. GASSER
Faculty of Veterinary and Agricultural
Sciences, The University of Melbourne,
Parkville, VIC, Australia

A. L. GRAHAM
Professor of Ecology & Evolutionary Biology,
Co-Director of the Global Health Program,
Princeton University, Princeton,
NJ, United States

J. KEISER
Head, Helminth Drug Development Unit,
Department of Medical Parasitology and
Infection Biology, Swiss Tropical and Public
Health Institute, Basel, Switzerland

K. KING
Department of Zoology,
University of Oxford,
Oxford, United Kingdom

M. G. ORTEGA-PIERRES
Professor of the Department of Genetics
and Molecular Biology,
Centro de Investigación y de
Estudios Avanzados IPN,
Mexico City, México

D. L. SMITH
Johns Hopkins Malaria Research
Institute & Department of Epidemiology,
Johns Hopkins Bloomberg School
of Public Health, Baltimore,
MD, United States

R. C. A. THOMPSON
Head, WHO Collaborating Centre
for the Molecular Epidemiology
of Parasitic Infections, Principal
Investigator, Environmental
Biotechnology CRC (EBCRC),
School of Veterinary and Biomedical
Sciences, Murdoch University,
Murdoch, WA, Australia

X.-N. ZHOU
Professor, Director, National Institute of
Parasitic Diseases,
Chinese Center for Disease Control
and Prevention, Shanghai,
People's Republic of China

VOLUME ONE HUNDRED AND THIRTEEN

ADVANCES IN
PARASITOLOGY

Current research on naturally transmitted *Plasmodium knowlesi*

Edited by

CHRIS DRAKELEY
*Faculty of Infectious and Tropical Diseases
London School of Hygiene and Tropical Medicine
London, United Kingdom*

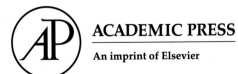

Academic Press is an imprint of Elsevier
125 London Wall, London EC2Y 5AS, United Kingdom
The Boulevard, Langford Lane, Kidlington, Oxford OX5 1GB, United Kingdom
50 Hampshire Street, 5th Floor, Cambridge, MA 02139, United States
525 B Street, Suite 1650, San Diego, CA 92101, United States

First edition 2021

Copyright © 2021 Elsevier Ltd. All rights reserved.

No part of this publication may be reproduced or transmitted in any form or by any means, electronic or mechanical, including photocopying, recording, or any information storage and retrieval system, without permission in writing from the publisher. Details on how to seek permission, further information about the Publisher's permissions policies and our arrangements with organizations such as the Copyright Clearance Center and the Copyright Licensing Agency, can be found at our website: www.elsevier.com/permissions.

This book and the individual contributions contained in it are protected under copyright by the Publisher (other than as may be noted herein).

Notices
Knowledge and best practice in this field are constantly changing. As new research and experience broaden our understanding, changes in research methods, professional practices, or medical treatment may become necessary.

Practitioners and researchers must always rely on their own experience and knowledge in evaluating and using any information, methods, compounds, or experiments described herein. In using such information or methods they should be mindful of their own safety and the safety of others, including parties for whom they have a professional responsibility.

To the fullest extent of the law, neither the Publisher nor the authors, contributors, or editors, assume any liability for any injury and/or damage to persons or property as a matter of products liability, negligence or otherwise, or from any use or operation of any methods, products, instructions, or ideas contained in the material herein.

ISBN: 978-0-323-90727-9
ISSN: 0065-308X

For information on all Academic Press publications
visit our website at https://www.elsevier.com/books-and-journals

Publisher: Zoe Kruze
Acquisitions Editor: Ashlie M. Jackman
Developmental Editor: Tara Nadera
Production Project Manager: Abdulla Sait
Cover Designer: Mark Rogers

Typeset by STRAIVE, India

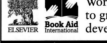

Contents

Contributors ix

Preface xiii

1. Knowlesi malaria: Human risk factors, clinical spectrum, and pathophysiology 1

Nicholas M. Anstey, Matthew J. Grigg, Giri S. Rajahram, Daniel J. Cooper, Timothy William, Steven Kho, and Bridget E. Barber

1. Introduction 2
2. Transmission in humans 3
3. Life cycle in humans 4
4. Human risk factors for symptomatic infection 5
5. Prepatent and incubation periods 6
6. Clinical spectrum in malariotherapy and experimental human infection 7
7. Clinical spectrum in natural infection 8
8. Genetic risk factors 23
9. Pathophysiology 24
10. Conclusion 32
Acknowledgements 32
References 33

2. Clinical management of *Plasmodium knowlesi* malaria 45

Bridget E. Barber, Matthew J. Grigg, Daniel J. Cooper, Donelly A. van Schalkwyk, Timothy William, Giri S. Rajahram, and Nicholas M. Anstey

1. Introduction 46
2. Diagnosis of *Plasmodium knowlesi* 46
3. *In vitro* susceptibility of *P. knowlesi* to antimalarial agents 47
4. Drug resistance mutations 55
5. Treatment of uncomplicated knowlesi malaria 56
6. Clinical management of severe knowlesi malaria 63
7. Treatment of knowlesi malaria in children 67
8. Treatment of knowlesi malaria in pregnancy 68
9. Conclusions 69
Acknowledgements 70
References 70

v

3. *Plasmodium knowlesi* detection methods for human infections— Diagnosis and surveillance 77

Matthew J. Grigg, Inke N. Lubis, Kevin K.A. Tetteh, Bridget E. Barber, Timothy William, Giri S. Rajahram, Angelica F. Tan, Colin J. Sutherland, Rintis Noviyanti, Chris J. Drakeley, Sumudu Britton, and Nicholas M. Anstey

1. Introduction	78
2. Point-of-care diagnosis	81
3. Molecular detection	94
4. Serology	110
5. Conclusion	117
Acknowledgements	117
References	117

4. The vectors of *Plasmodium knowlesi* and other simian malarias Southeast Asia: challenges in malaria elimination 131

Indra Vythilingam, Tock Hing Chua, Jonathan Wee Kent Liew, Benny O. Manin, and Heather M. Ferguson

1. Introduction	132
2. Simian malaria parasites in natural vector mosquitoes	134
3. Vectors of *Plasmodium knowlesi*—Leucosphyrus Group of *Anopheles*	139
4. Bionomics of natural vectors of *Plasmodium kowlesi* in the Leucosphyrus Group of *Anopheles*	144
5. Suspected vectors of knowlesi malaria in other *Anopheles* Groups	148
6. Experimental transmissions of *Plasmodium knowlesi* and other simian malaria parasites in mosquitoes	149
7. Control of vectors of *P. knowlesi* and other simian malarias	167
8. Challenges	172
9. Conclusions and the way forward	174
Acknowledgement	174
References	174

5. Molecular epidemiology and population genomics of *Plasmodium knowlesi* 191

Paul C.S. Divis, Balbir Singh, and David J. Conway

1. Molecular detection in discovery of *Plasmodium knowlesi* as a significant zoonosis	192
2. Molecular surveys of the distribution of *P. knowlesi* infections in humans	193
3. Early utility of a few genetic loci for analysis of *P. knowlesi* polymorphism	198

Contents   **vii**

   4. Multi-locus microsatellite analyses of *P. knowlesi* uncovers population structure   205

   5. Whole-genome sequence analysis of *P. knowlesi* subpopulation divergence   208

   6. Loci under positive natural selection in the *P. knowlesi* genome   211

   7. Assays for efficient surveillance of different *P. knowlesi* subpopulations   213

   8. Adaptation and the future of *P. knowlesi* emerging from local zoonoses   215

   References   217

6. Epidemiology of the zoonotic malaria *Plasmodium knowlesi* in changing landscapes   **225**

Pablo Ruiz Cuenca, Stephanie Key, Amaziasizamoria Jumail,

Henry Surendra, Heather M. Ferguson, Chris J. Drakeley, and

Kimberly Fornace

   1. Introduction   226

   2. Ecological change and mechanisms of disease emergence and transmission   228

   3. Distribution and burden of *Plasmodium knowlesi*   236

   4. Landscape impacts on *P. knowlesi* disease dynamics   244

   5. Transmission dynamics and potential for human to human transmission   257

   6. Designing surveillance and control measures for changing environments   259

   7. Conclusions and future research priorities   266

   References   267

Contributors

Nicholas M. Anstey
Menzies School of Health Research, Charles Darwin University, Darwin, NT, Australia; Infectious Diseases Society Sabah-Menzies School of Health Research Clinical Research Unit, Kota Kinabalu, Sabah, Malaysia

Bridget E. Barber
Menzies School of Health Research, Charles Darwin University, Darwin, NT; QIMR Berghofer Medical Research Institute, Brisbane, QLD, Australia; Infectious Diseases Society Sabah-Menzies School of Health Research Clinical Research Unit, Kota Kinabalu, Sabah, Malaysia

Sumudu Britton
QIMR Berghofer Medical Research Institute, Brisbane, QLD, Australia

Tock Hing Chua
Department of Pathobiology and Microbiology, Faculty of Medicine and Health Sciences, Universiti Sabah Malaysia, Kota Kinabalu, Sabah, Malaysia

David J. Conway
Malaria Research Centre, Universiti Malaysia Sarawak, Kota Samarahan, Sarawak, Malaysia; Department of Infection Biology, London School of Hygiene and Tropical Medicine, London, United Kingdom

Daniel J. Cooper
Menzies School of Health Research, Charles Darwin University, Darwin, NT, Australia; Department of Medicine, University of Cambridge School of Medicine, Cambridge, United Kingdom

Pablo Ruiz Cuenca
Faculty of Infectious and Tropical Diseases, London School of Hygiene and Tropical Medicine, London, United Kingdom

Paul C.S. Divis
Malaria Research Centre, Universiti Malaysia Sarawak, Kota Samarahan, Sarawak, Malaysia

Chris J. Drakeley
Faculty of Infectious and Tropical Diseases, London School of Hygiene and Tropical Medicine, London, United Kingdom

Heather M. Ferguson
Institute of Biodiversity, Animal Health and Comparative Medicine, University of Glasgow, Glasgow, Scotland, United Kingdom

Kimberly Fornace
Faculty of Infectious and Tropical Diseases, London School of Hygiene and Tropical Medicine, London; Institute of Biodiversity, Animal Health and Comparative Medicine, University of Glasgow, Glasgow, Scotland, United Kingdom

Matthew J. Grigg
Menzies School of Health Research, Charles Darwin University, Darwin, NT, Australia; Infectious Diseases Society Sabah-Menzies School of Health Research Clinical Research Unit, Kota Kinabalu, Sabah, Malaysia

Amaziasizamoria Jumail
Danau Girang Field Centre, Kota Kinabalu, Malaysia

Stephanie Key
Faculty of Infectious and Tropical Diseases, London School of Hygiene and Tropical Medicine, London, United Kingdom

Steven Kho
Menzies School of Health Research, Charles Darwin University, Darwin, NT, Australia

Jonathan Wee Kent Liew
Department of Parasitology, University of Malaya, Kuala Lumpur, Malaysia; Environmental Health Institute, National Environment Agency, Singapore, Singapore

Inke N. Lubis
Faculty of Medicine, Universitas Sumatera Utara, Medan, Sumatera Utara, Indonesia

Benny O. Manin
Department of Pathobiology and Microbiology, Faculty of Medicine and Health Sciences, Universiti Sabah Malaysia, Kota Kinabalu, Sabah, Malaysia

Rintis Noviyanti
Eijkman Institute for Molecular Biology, Jakarta, Indonesia

Giri S. Rajahram
Clinical Research Centre, Queen Elizabeth Hospital 1; Queen Elizabeth Hospital 2, Kota Kinabalu; Infectious Diseases Society Sabah-Menzies School of Health Research Clinical Research Unit, Kota Kinabalu, Sabah, Malaysia

Balbir Singh
Malaria Research Centre, Universiti Malaysia Sarawak, Kota Samarahan, Sarawak, Malaysia

Henry Surendra
Eijkman-Oxford Clinical Research Unit, Jakarta; Centre for Tropical Medicine, Faculty of Medicine, Public Health and Nursing, Universitas Gadjah Mada, Yogyakarta, Indonesia

Colin J. Sutherland
Faculty of Infectious and Tropical Diseases, London School of Hygiene and Tropical Medicine, London, United Kingdom

Angelica F. Tan
Menzies School of Health Research, Charles Darwin University, Darwin, NT, Australia; Infectious Diseases Society Sabah-Menzies School of Health Research Clinical Research Unit, Kota Kinabalu, Sabah, Malaysia

Kevin K.A. Tetteh
Faculty of Infectious and Tropical Diseases, London School of Hygiene and Tropical Medicine, London, United Kingdom

Donelly A. van Schalkwyk
London School of Hygiene and Tropical Medicine, London, United Kingdom

Indra Vythilingam
Department of Parasitology, University of Malaya, Kuala Lumpur, Malaysia

Timothy William
Clinical Research Centre, Queen Elizabeth Hospital 1; Gleneagles Medical Centre, Kota Kinabalu; Infectious Diseases Society Sabah-Menzies School of Health Research Clinical Research Unit, Kota Kinabalu, Sabah, Malaysia

Plasmodium knowlesi, an infectious disease challenge for our times

Chris Drakeley

Faculty of Infectious and Tropical Diseases, London School of Hygiene and Tropical Medicine, London, United Kingdom

The large foci of human infections with *Plasmodium knowlesi* in Sarawak, Malaysia, described by Singh et al. (2004) raised the profile of zoonoses of malaria parasites significantly. As part of the impressive efforts of the national malaria control programme in Malaysia in controlling conventional malaria in humans, *P. knowlesi* is now the predominant species of malaria infecting humans in the country with the majority of cases on Borneo island. However, the true extent of infection with *P. knowlesi* elsewhere is unknown and the reliance on clinical and health facility-based information highlights the human-centric focus on infectious disease. The current SARS-CoV-2 pandemic has shown how a lack of knowledge of the various biological, sociological and environmental factors that allow infections to persist and be transmitted can seriously hamper treatment and control.

In terms of basic biology, *P. knowlesi* represents a fascinating plasmodial parasite with a rapid 24-h replication cycle and one that can infect various nonhuman primates and humans. Recent culture adaptation and transfection offer a route to investigate and target invasion mechanisms (Mohring et al., 2020) or treatment regimes for other types of malaria such as *P. vivax* (Ndegwa et al., 2021). At the global level there remains much debate as to whether *P. knowlesi* should be classified as a human parasite alongside the conventional or 'classic' human malaria such as *P. falciparum*; such a classification could have major implications for countries seeking certification of elimination of malaria. Perhaps of most concern is the likelihood of human-to-human transmission of *P. knowlesi* and the profound changes in approach that would be required to control the parasite if this was found to occur at any significant level.

In the chapters in this volume, the authors review the clinical and pathophysiological manifestations of *P. knowlesi* (Anstey and colleagues) and the optimal treatment regimes in humans presenting with clinical infection (Barber and colleagues). These are followed by a review of the diagnostic approaches for detecting infection both directly (i.e., in confirming clinical and asymptomatic infections) and indirectly through exposure to infection for epidemiological assessments (Grigg and colleagues). Vythilingam et al. provide a detailed description of the behaviour and bionomics of the *Leucosphyrus* group of mosquitoes responsible for *P. knowlesi* transmission and include a discussion of potential control measures to target mosquitoes and mosquito–human interaction. Divis et al. present the latest understanding of the molecular epidemiology of the parasite in the mosquito vector and both human and nonhuman primate hosts. Finally, the ecological factors that are associated with *P. knowlesi* transmission are discussed by Cuenca, Key, and colleagues and cover how environmental change may affect parasite distribution in the future.

Periodic reassessment of older literature invariably brings new insights. Anstey et al. review early malariotherapy experiments with *P. knowlesi*, which were initially of low parasitaemia and self-resolving (Nicol, 1935) but subsequently virulence was significantly increased with serial passage through humans (Ciuca et al., 1955). This highlights that there is potential for parasite expansion with sufficient human-to-human transmission events. The malariotherapy studies also record how *P. knowlesi* infections were less successfully established in individuals who had had previous infections. This suggests the role of heterologous immunity in limiting the success and duration of infection at an individual level and, perhaps, by extension, an approach to monitor population susceptibility to *P. knowlesi* infection in areas where the incidence of malaria in humans is declining.

P. knowlesi responds well to treatment with artemisinin combination therapies and adjunct therapies such as paracetamol appear to be beneficial in limiting renal complications in clinical cases. However, while treatment appears effective, the same cannot be said for diagnostics. It has been well documented that morphological similarities between *P. knowlesi* and *P. malariae* have led to misdiagnosis from malaria blood smears, the long-standing mainstay of diagnosis. Currently available rapid diagnostic tests that detect any of the standard parasite biomarkers have all been developed for *P. falciparum* and/or *P. vivax*; all have poor sensitivity to *P. knowlesi*. Molecular confirmation is increasingly recommended and while there are a number of approaches, the most accurate appear to require initial amplification of DNA and subsequent sequencing, which may have logistical limitations for epidemiological use. In this context, measurement of *P. knowlesi*-specific antibodies to assess exposure to infection may prove a useful adjunct diagnostic test in highlighting demographic and spatial risk factors including defining areas with no apparent exposure (Fornace et al., 2019).

The review of vector bionomics has some intriguing observations where data on mosquito feeding times are presented alongside that from older studies examining the periodicity of infection to mosquitoes of controlled *P. knowlesi* infections. As in other nonhuman malaria systems, the peak biting time of mosquitoes appears to coincide with the highest densities of gametocytes in peripheral blood with the success of subsequent transmission to mosquitoes related to gametocyte density (Gautret and Motard, 1999). Understanding how this influences the overall transmission dynamics from infected non-human primates and humans has important implications particularly for the human-to-human transmission. If parasite densities, particularly those of gametocytes, are low and humans are unavailable or encouraged to use protection from mosquito bites at times of peak biting, then chances of onward transmission will be very limited. Chronic, untreated infections in nonhuman primates would seem to be the most likely source of mosquito infections. The molecular epidemiological analysis confirms this with the distribution of parasites largely dictated by the distribution of the nonhuman primate hosts (long and pig-tailed macaques). However, Divis et al. note that there is a real need for a prospective sampling of vector and primate hosts that allows a more thorough assessment of the extent and drivers of transmission.

One could argue that a concerted effort to establish prospective sampling is needed now more than ever. The unprecedented level of land-use and land-cover change has already been associated with changes in transmission dynamics of malaria and *P. knowlesi* in particular (Fornace et al., 2021). This alongside short- and long-term climate changes (Nissan et al., 2021) as well sociodemographic shifts including urbanisation will likely affect the risk profiles of those who get infected and where infections occur. The recent observations of infections with *P. cynomolgi, P. inui,* and other types of 'non-human primate' malaria in Malaysia (Yap et al., 2021) show that zoonosis can occur and probably does so more frequently than previously envisaged. There are numerous examples of spillover events from animal pathogens, including from nonhuman primates, some of which establish robust human-to-human transmission (Wolfe et al., 2007). It may be that in the case of malaria, biological limitations (restricted red cell invasion pathways, heterologous immunity), human protective behaviour, ecological niche restriction of vectors, and variable number of nonhuman primate hosts mean increases in infection prevalence are unlikely. However, as this volume shows, *P. knowlesi* is the only zoonotic malaria known to cause severe disease and fatalities, and there are numerous aspects of its biology and transmission that remain poorly defined to the extent that we cannot rule its spread, particularly in such changing times.

References

Ciuca, M., Chelarescu, M., Sofletea, A., Constaninesco, P., Teriteanu, E., Cortez, P., Balanovschi, G., Ilies, M., 1955. Contribution experimentale a l'etude de l'immunite dans le paludisme. Editions Acad. Rep. Pop. Roumaine, 1–108.

Fornace, K.M., Brock, P.M., Abidin, T.R., Grignard, L., Herman, L.S., Chua, T.H., Daim, S., William, T., Patterson, C., Hall, T., Grigg, M.J., Anstey, N.M., Tetteh, K.K.A., Cox, J., Drakeley, C.J., 2019. Environmental risk factors and exposure to the zoonotic malaria parasite *Plasmodium knowlesi* across northern Sabah, Malaysia: a population-based cross-sectional survey. Lancet Planet Health 3, e179–e186.

Fornace, K.M., Diaz, A.V., Lines, J., Drakeley, C.J., 2021. Achieving global malaria eradication in changing landscapes. Malar. J. 20, 69.

Gautret, P., Motard, A., 1999. Periodic infectivity of Plasmodium gametocytes to the vector. A review. Parasite 6, 103–111.

Mohring, F., Rawlinson, T.A., Draper, S.J., Moon, R.W., 2020. Multiplication and growth inhibition activity assays for the zoonotic malaria parasite, plasmodium knowlesi. Bio-Protoc. 10, e3743.

Ndegwa, D.N., Kundu, P., Hostetler, J.B., Marin-Menendez, A., Sanderson, T., Mwikali, K., Verzier, L.H., Coyle, R., Adjalley, S., Rayner, J.C., 2021. Using Plasmodium knowlesi as a model for screening Plasmodium vivax blood-stage malaria vaccine targets reveals new candidates. PLoS Pathog. 17, e1008864.

Nicol, W.D., 1935. Monkey malaria in GPI. Br. Med. J. 2, 760.

Nissan, H., Ukawuba, I., Thomson, M., 2021. Climate-proofing a malaria eradication strategy. Malar. J. 20, 190.

Singh, B., Kim Sung, L., Matusop, A., Radhakrishnan, A., Shamsul, S.S., Cox-Singh, J., Thomas, A., Conway, D.J., 2004. A large focus of naturally acquired Plasmodium knowlesi infections in human beings. Lancet 363, 1017–1024.

Wolfe, N.D., Dunavan, C.P., Diamond, J., 2007. Origins of major human infectious diseases. Nature 447, 279–283.

Yap, N.J., Hossain, H., Nada-Raja, T., Ngui, R., Muslim, A., Hoh, B.P., Khaw, L.T., Kadir, K.A., Simon Divis, P.C., Vythilingam, I., Singh, B., Lim, Y.A., 2021. Natural human infections with Plasmodium cynomolgi, *P. inui*, and 4 other simian malaria parasites, Malaysia. Emerg. Infect. Dis. 27, 2187–2191.

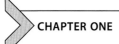

CHAPTER ONE

Knowlesi malaria: Human risk factors, clinical spectrum, and pathophysiology

Nicholas M. Anstey[a,*], Matthew J. Grigg[a], Giri S. Rajahram[b,c], Daniel J. Cooper[a,d], Timothy William[b,e], Steven Kho[a], and Bridget E. Barber[a,f]

[a]Menzies School of Health Research, Charles Darwin University, Darwin, NT, Australia
[b]Clinical Research Centre, Queen Elizabeth Hospital 1, Kota Kinabalu, Malaysia
[c]Queen Elizabeth Hospital 2, Kota Kinabalu, Malaysia
[d]Department of Medicine, University of Cambridge School of Medicine, Cambridge, United Kingdom
[e]Gleneagles Medical Centre, Kota Kinabalu, Malaysia
[f]QIMR Berghofer Medical Research Institute, Brisbane, QLD, Australia
*Corresponding author: e-mail address: nicholas.anstey@menzies.edu.au

Contents

1.	Introduction	2
2.	Transmission in humans	3
3.	Life cycle in humans	4
4.	Human risk factors for symptomatic infection	5
5.	Prepatent and incubation periods	6
6.	Clinical spectrum in malariotherapy and experimental human infection	7
7.	Clinical spectrum in natural infection	8
	7.1 Asymptomatic infections	9
	7.2 Symptoms in adults	9
	7.3 Clinical signs in adults	12
	7.4 Laboratory investigations in adults	13
	7.5 Severe knowlesi malaria	17
	7.6 Clinical and parasitological risk factors for severe disease	19
	7.7 Deaths from knowlesi malaria	20
	7.8 Knowlesi malaria in children	21
	7.9 Knowlesi malaria in pregnancy	22
	7.10 Congenital malaria	22
8.	Genetic risk factors	23
	8.1 Parasite genetics	23
	8.2 Host genetics	24
9.	Pathophysiology	24
	9.1 Microvascular accumulation of parasites	25
	9.2 Endothelial activation, dysfunction and glycocalyx breakdown	28
	9.3 Systemic inflammatory response	29

9.4	Intravascular haemolysis	29
9.5	Thrombocytopenia	30
9.6	Anaemia	31
10.	Conclusion	32
	Acknowledgements	32
	References	33

Abstract

Plasmodium knowlesi is endemic across Southeast Asia, and is the commonest cause of zoonotic malaria. The spectrum of clinical disease from *P. knowlesi* infection ranges from asymptomatic infection, through to severe malaria and death. Over 90% of clinical disease occurs in adults, mostly living in forest edge areas undergoing intensive land use change. With a 24-h asexual life cycle in humans, high parasite counts are possible, but most clinical cases of knowlesi malaria are uncomplicated with low parasitaemia. In co-endemic areas, median parasitaemia in knowlesi malaria is lower than that seen in vivax and falciparum malaria, suggesting a lower fever threshold. Severe malaria occurs in 6–9% of symptomatic adults. Manifestations of severe malaria from *P. knowlesi* are similar to those seen with falciparum malaria, with the notable absence of coma. Age, parasitaemia, cardiovascular comorbidities and delayed diagnosis are risk factors for severe disease and death, which are only seen in adults. Thrombocytopenia is near-universal in adults, likely related to platelet-red cell binding and clearance. Mechanisms underlying the microvascular sludging seen in fatal disease in non-natural primate hosts and the microvascular accumulation of parasites in fatal human disease are not clear. Marked reductions in deformability of both infected and uninfected red blood cells are associated with disease severity in both humans and other non-natural primate hosts, likely contributing to impaired microvascular perfusion and organ dysfunction. Endothelial activation, endothelial dysfunction, glycocalyx degradation and haemolysis are also associated with, and likely contribute to, severe disease and organ dysfunction, particularly acute kidney injury.

1. Introduction

Plasmodium knowlesi is the commonest cause of zoonotic malaria in humans. A simian malaria parasite, with the natural hosts being the long-tailed macaque and pig-tailed macaque, *Plasmodium knowlesi* was discovered in 1931 by Campbell and Napier in Calcutta, India, in a long-tailed macaque imported from Singapore (Napier and Campbell, 1932). The ability of *P. knowlesi* to infect humans was demonstrated around the same time by Knowles and Das Gutpa, through the inoculation of three volunteer patients (Knowles and Das Gupta, 1932). The first case of naturally acquired human infection with *P. knowlesi* was reported in 1965 in a US national working in Malaysia (Chin et al., 1965), and several years later the experimental mosquito transmission of *P. knowlesi* from man to monkey and man to man was reported (Chin et al., 1968). In 2004, Singh et al. reported a large focus of naturally acquired knowlesi malaria in humans in the eastern Malaysian state of Sarawak (Singh et al., 2004). Human cases of knowlesi malaria have now been reported throughout Southeast Asia, with the greatest number of cases reported from Malaysia, particularly the eastern Malaysian states of Sabah and Sarawak (Cooper et al., 2020; Hussin et al., 2020; Shearer et al., 2016). Knowlesi malaria is unique among the human zoonotic malarias in being able to cause severe and fatal disease (Cox-Singh et al., 2008; Rajahram et al., 2019), with a frequency similar to that occurring following infection with *P. falciparum* (Barber et al., 2013; Grigg et al., 2018a; Rajahram et al., 2016). *Plasmodium knowlesi* is now the commonest cause of death from malaria in Malaysia (Cooper et al., 2020; Rajahram et al., 2019). This chapter reviews the clinical spectrum, human risk factors, and pathophysiology of malaria from *Plasmodium knowlesi*.

2. Transmission in humans

P. knowlesi is predominantly a zoonotic infection, with humans presumed to be incidentally infected when bitten by a mosquito vector which has fed from an infected long-tail or pig-tail macaque reservoir host. While human-mosquito-human transmission has been demonstrated in a laboratory setting (Chin et al., 1968), it has not yet been proven to occur in the natural environment. The predominance of *P. knowlesi* as a zoonosis is further supported by: sequence data of the circumsporozoite protein (*csp*) gene and mtDNA demonstrating shared polymorphisms between human and macaques in Sarawak, and with no haplotypes unique to either species (Lee et al., 2011); mathematical modelling (Imai et al., 2014); and a lack of drug-resistant mutations detected in human isolates (Grigg et al., 2016a). Nonetheless, human cases of *P. knowlesi* have been reported to occur in domestic clusters, with individuals of all ages affected (Barber et al., 2012), and it remains possible that in endemic areas, human-mosquito-human transmission may be occurring to at least some degree. This is reviewed in more detail in the companion chapter by Cuenca et al. (2021).

Human to human transmission of *P. knowlesi* malaria through blood transfusion has also been reported in Thailand and Malaysia (Bird et al., 2016; Traipattanakul et al., 2014). The Thai case was considered probably transfusion-related, and resulted in uncomplicated knowlesi malaria

(Traipattanakul et al., 2014). The Malaysian case, confirmed as transfusion-related from a pre-symptomatic donor, occurred in a splenectomized thalassaemic patient who developed severe malaria with lactic acidosis and multi-organ failure (Bird et al., 2016).

3. Life cycle in humans

The life cycle of asexual stages of *P. knowlesi* infection in humans is similar to that of *P. falciparum*, with the exception of its 24-h erythrocytic cycle (Coatney et al., 1971). Transmission occurs when a female anopheline mosquito injects saliva containing sporozoites, which travel through the host's blood stream to the liver where they invade hepatocytes, undergo asexual replication and develop into schizonts. Hepatic schizonts rupture and release thousands of daughter merozoites into the blood stream. Merozoites then invade erythrocytes where they develop into young ring parasites and then trophozoites, which undergo further asexual multiplication to form schizonts, containing numerous merozoites. The infected erythrocyte then ruptures, causing fever and an inflammatory response in the host, with released merozoites reinvading uninfected erythrocytes, completing the first erythrocytic replication cycle. The 24-h erythrocytic cycle of *P. knowlesi* is the shortest of any of the *Plasmodium* species causing human malaria (Coatney et al., 1971). Thus, patients with *P. knowlesi* typically experience daily fever spikes. While high parasitaemia may develop rapidly in a minority of patients, most humans have relatively low circulating parasitaemia (Grigg et al., 2018a).

Plasmodium knowlesi does not have the latent hepatic hypnozoite stage seen in *P. vivax, P. ovale* and *P. cynomolgi*, and therefore relapses do not occur (Coatney et al., 1971). Within the erythrocyte some of the merozoites develop into male and female gametocytes. In contrast to their later appearance in *P. falciparum* infection, gametocytes appear early in human infection with *P. knowlesi*. In a recent clinical trial, 85% (82/97) of patients with knowlesi malaria had gametocyte mRNA transcripts detected by PCR on enrolment (Grigg et al., 2016b). Following a blood meal from a macaque host, gametocytes are taken up by a female mosquito and undergo sexual replication within the midgut of the mosquito, to complete the *Plasmodium* life cycle (Coatney et al., 1971). However, while onward mosquito-borne transmission of gametocytes circulating in humans to other humans has been demonstrated experimentally (Chin et al., 1968), the extent to which gametocytes from humans contribute to the transmission of knowlesi malaria in endemic areas is unknown.

4. Human risk factors for symptomatic infection

As *P. knowlesi* is predominantly a zoonotic parasite, infection is generally acquired in forest or forest-fringe areas. Hence, those at risk include farmers, plantation workers, or individuals undertaking other activities in forested areas (Barber et al., 2013; Grigg et al., 2017). Population-level epidemiological risk factors for infection are discussed in detail elsewhere (Cuenca et al., 2021). Symptomatic infection occurs more commonly in males, accounting for 75–85% of cases (Cooper et al., 2020; William et al., 2013, 2014). Clinical disease occurs far more commonly in adults than in children (Cooper et al., 2020; Daneshvar et al., 2009; Grigg et al., 2017, 2018a; William et al., 2013, 2014), with children <15 years accounting for only 9% of all *P. knowlesi* notifications in Sabah, Malaysia, during 2010–14 (Rajahram et al., 2016). More recent Sabah statewide reporting of *P. knowlesi* cases (2015–17) showed a continued adult predominance, with children less than 5 years old accounting for only 0.8% (25/3262) of PCR-confirmed infections and children aged 5–13 years accounting for only 5% (170/3262) of PCR-confirmed infections. Nonetheless, with the decline in the human-only *Plasmodium* species, *P. knowlesi* was the most common cause of malaria in children younger than 14 years, accounting for 195 of 253 (77%) cases (Cooper et al., 2020).

Human risk factors for acquiring symptomatic knowlesi malaria have been evaluated in a case–control study conducted in Sabah, Malaysia, involving 229 cases of *P. knowlesi* malaria, 91 cases of other *Plasmodium spp.*, and 953 controls (683 matched to *P. knowlesi* cases, 270 matched to non-*P. knowlesi* cases) (Grigg et al., 2017). Independent risk factors for symptomatic *P. knowlesi* infection included age ≥ 15 years, male gender, plantation work, sleeping outside, travel, being aware of the presence of monkeys in the past 4 weeks, and having open eaves or gaps in walls. Age ≥ 15 years, farming occupation, clearing vegetation, and having long grass around the house increased the risk for *P. knowlesi* infection but not for other *Plasmodium* spp. infection. G6PD deficiency protected against *P. knowlesi*, as did residual insecticide spraying of household walls, and the presence of sparse forest or rice paddies around the house. While adult men working in agricultural areas were at greatest risk of symptomatic knowlesi malaria, peridomestic transmission also occurred (Grigg et al., 2017). Notably, the use of bed nets was not found to be protective, highlighting the differences in control strategies that will likely be required for control of *P. knowlesi* malaria compared to falciparum and vivax malaria.

Travellers from non-endemic countries have acquired *P. knowlesi* infection in Malaysia, Thailand, Indonesia, Myanmar and the Philippines (Barber et al., 2017b; Froeschl et al., 2018; Ozbilgin et al., 2016). The large majority of these cases have been reported in adult males, who have mostly spent time in forested regions.

The extent to which past infection with human-only *Plasmodium* species protects against infection and disease from *P. knowlesi* is not known. Heterologous immunity was first suggested by data from early 20th century malariotherapy studies. Infection was particularly difficult to reproduce in three individuals who had been previously exposed to *P. vivax* (van Rooyen and Pile, 1935). This relative resistance to clinical disease among those previously exposed to malaria was also reported the same year by Nicol (Nicol, 1935), who found that among a total of 76 patients, only 1 of 16 with a previous history of malaria (with *P. vivax* being most commonly used at the time) developed fever following inoculation of *P. knowlesi* compared to 44% of non-immune patients. Heterologous immunity is supported by more recent studies demonstrating inhibition of *P. knowlesi* red cell invasion by *P. vivax* antibodies (Muh et al., 2018, 2020). The possibility that declining cross-protective immunity to *P. vivax* may contribute to rising incidence of knowlesi malaria has important implications for other Southeast Asian countries approaching malaria elimination (Anstey and Grigg, 2019).

5. Prepatent and incubation periods

Data from experimental human infection and neurosyphilis studies indicate that following intravenous inoculation of *P. knowlesi* the incubation period is usually around 8–12 days, although with a reported range of between 3 and 27 days (Milam and Kusch, 1938; van Rooyen and Pile, 1935). In the first three patients reported by Knowles and Das Gupta, fever and symptoms developed 10, 20 and 23 days after inoculation with parasites appearing in the blood up to 5 days after the first fever was recorded (Knowles and Das Gupta, 1932). The patient with the most severe disease had the shortest incubation time. Later studies confirmed that parasites normally appear in the blood several days after the initial temperature rise. In an early malariotherapy report, Van Rooyen and Pile detailed incubation periods of 3–14 days in 12 neurosyphilis patients inoculated with *P. knowlesi*, with fever recorded for most after 8 days, and patent parasitaemia developing around 10 days (van Rooyen and Pile, 1935). The first experimental transmission of *P. knowlesi* via infected mosquitoes to 7 humans not previously exposed to malaria described a pre-patent period of 9–12 days (Chin et al., 1968).

6. Clinical spectrum in malariotherapy and experimental human infection

In the first human experimental infection by Knowles and Das Gupta, three volunteer patients were infected, the first with "paretic symptoms" of uncertain aetiology, the second with a foot ulcer following a rat bite, and the third with lepromatous leprosy (Knowles and Das Gupta, 1932). Infection was associated with daily fever spikes and two patients experienced mild to moderate disease. However, the patient with the foot ulcer, who received blood passaged through the first patient, became "very seriously ill." Although reportedly comatose, clinical details were limited, and the patient made a spontaneous recovery (Knowles and Das Gupta, 1932).

Plasmodium knowlesi became widely used as a pyretic agent to treat neurosyphilis, with the first description provided in 1935 (van Rooyen and Pile, 1935). In their report of 12 patients inoculated with *P. knowlesi*, the authors noted the infection to be mild and "eminently suitable for the treatment of elderly debilitated patients." In the USA, Milam and Kusch noted that the clinical course in European Americans was mostly moderate, with daily fevers lasting about 10 days and with only half experiencing chills. Recovery was generally spontaneous, although 38% later experienced recrudescent infection, half of which were associated with mild clinical illness (Milam and Kusch, 1938). This report also described relative resistance to *P. knowlesi* infection and disease in all six African Americans enrolled (Milam and Kusch, 1938), confirmed by another report the same year of decreased susceptibility to infection and clinical disease in 12 African Americans compared to 30 European Americans (Milam and Coggleshall, 1938). In both these reports several African American patients were described as having subclinical infection, with no parasites seen on blood film and no fever experienced, but with infection produced in monkeys inoculated with their blood. Marked variability in susceptibility to infection and clinical illness was also reported in the UK, with Nicol questioning the utility of *P. knowlesi* for malariotherapy, because even in successfully infected patients, a quarter had low parasitaemias and spontaneously recovered within a week (Nicol, 1935).

In 1937 Ciuca et al. reported on their use of *P. knowlesi* to treat over 300 patients in Romania (Ciuca et al., 1937a,b). Among these patients, 46% and 80% of immune and non-immune patients respectively developed fever following exposure to *P. knowlesi* (Ciuca et al., 1937a,b). In contrast to Nicol who reported loss of pathogenicity of *P. knowlesi* with repeated passage from person-person (Nicol, 1935), Ciuca et al. later reported increased virulence of infection among patients infected by a single strain of *P. knowlesi* serially passaged 170 times through humans, with high parasite counts of up to 500,000/μL and severe disease necessitating antimalarial treatment (Ciuca et al., 1955). This led to the eventual discontinuation of malariotherapy, which in the meantime had been superseded by penicillin as treatment for neurosyphilis. Increased virulence with successive human transfers was also reported by Milam and Kusch, who noted high parasite counts (>10% infected RBCs) with "disease of serious proportions" in three of 15 (30%) patients infected after up to 22 serial human passages, in contrast to the low parasitaemia (<1%) and "moderate" clinical severity noted in patients treated with low-passage infections (Milam and Kusch, 1938). These authors speculated that the parasite may become better adapted to the human host with successive transfers (Milam and Kusch, 1938).

Chin et al. reported the clinical features of the first experimental sporozoite infections of humans in penitentiary volunteers (Chin et al., 1968). In the two European-American volunteers infected by mosquitoes fed on knowlesi-infected monkeys, the clinical course was reported to be mild, with maximum parasite counts of 1600 and 850/μL, and spontaneous resolution of patent infection after 11–12 days. In contrast, in a second group of volunteers infected with sporozoites from mosquitoes fed on experimentally-infected humans, maximum parasitaemias were higher (3450–6950/μL) and in three of the five infections, including in one African-American, the clinical illness was deemed severe enough to warrant chloroquine rescue therapy (Chin et al., 1968).

7. Clinical spectrum in natural infection

The spectrum of clinical disease from *Plasmodium knowlesi* infection ranges from asymptomatic infection, through to severe malaria and death. All prospective clinical and pathophysiology studies of knowlesi malaria have been performed in Malaysia where the incidence of clinical disease is highest, co-infections are less common than described elsewhere, and where host and parasite factors likely differ from other areas in the region.

Accordingly, the clinical spectrum may differ across knowlesi-endemic regions. In studies of symptomatic malaria reported from Malaysia and in reports of returned travellers from all regions, the majority have uncomplicated disease. However, severe and fatal cases can occur, particularly if commencement of antimalarial treatment is delayed (Barber et al., 2021a).

7.1 Asymptomatic infections

Similar to 20th century reports of asymptomatic infection in malariotherapy studies, asymptomatic infection has been reported in natural infection in a number of knowlesi-endemic areas (Jongwutiwes et al., 2011), Vietnam (Marchand et al., 2011), East Malaysia (Fornace et al., 2016; Grignard et al., 2019; Siner et al., 2017), West Malaysia (Noordin et al., 2020), Indonesia (Lubis et al., 2017), Myanmar (Ghinai et al., 2017) and Cambodia (Imwong et al., 2019). In the series reported from north of Malaysia, co-infections are common, which may contribute to the high proportion of asymptomatic infections described. With the limited number of community prevalence studies performed and the use of molecular methods with different sensitivities, the true prevalence across knowlesi-endemic regions is not well characterized. In one study of asymptomatic household contacts of symptomatic cases in northeastern Sabah, Malaysia prevalence of asymptomatic infection was 6.9% (Fornace et al., 2016). Interestingly, children aged <15 years and women accounted for a higher proportion of asymptomatic infections compared to symptomatic infections (Fornace et al., 2016). Subsequent larger cross-sectional studies in Sabah found a lower proportion of asymptomatic infections (Fornace et al., 2019; Grignard et al., 2019). Unanswered questions include how long these asymptomatic infections persist, the frequency with which these low-parasitaemia infections spontaneously resolve, their contribution to anaemia in knowlesi-endemic regions and the proportion subsequently progressing to symptomatic disease.

7.2 Symptoms in adults

Common presenting symptoms in knowlesi malaria in the three largest prospective series to date include fever (100%), chills, headache (89–94%), myalgia (47–88%), nausea, vomiting (24–34%), cough (35–56%) and abdominal pain (23–52%) (Barber et al., 2013; Daneshvar et al., 2009; Grigg et al., 2018a) (Table 1). The median duration of fever is 5 days (Barber et al., 2013; Daneshvar et al., 2009; Grigg et al., 2018a), comparable with malaria due to

Table 1 Demographic and clinical features in adults with knowlesi malaria enrolled in prospective studies.

Patient characteristic	District hospital studies		Tertiary referral hospital study
	Grigg et al. (2018a) Sabah, Malaysia $n = 481$ (437 adults)	Daneshvar et al. (2009) Sarawak, Malaysia $n = 121$ (113 adults)	Barber et al. (2013) Sabah, Malaysia $n = 130$
Adults (age $>$ 12 yrs), (%)	91	93	100
Age, years			
Median (IQR)	35 (25–50)	45 (14.9)[b]	46 (29–58)
Range	13–85	16–79	14–83
Male gender, (%)	79	56	74
Previous malaria (self-reported), (%)	21	26	28
History of chronic disease, (%)	8.0	NR	24
Days of fever, median (IQR)	4 (3–7)	5 (3–7)	5 (3–7)
Symptoms on enrolment, n (%)			
Rigors	82.3	89.7	84
Headache	89.0	94.4	91
Vomiting	24.0	33.6	30
Abdominal pain	23.3	52.3	31
Diarrhoea	8.2	29.0	18
Cough	35.0	56.1	48

Shortness of breath	16.0	NR	17
Myalgia	61.6	87.9	47
Arthralgia	66.1	NR	58
Examination findings on enrolment			
Temperature, °C, median (IQR)	37.4 (37.0–38.1)	37.6 (37–38.5)	37.5 (36.8–38.4)
Fever, temp $\geq$ 37.5 °C, (%)	49.3	NR	NR
Systolic blood pressure, mmHg, mean (SD)	120 (110–130)[a]	NR	118 (19.7)
Heart rate, beats/min, mean (SD)	88 (77–100)[a]	95 (16)	90 (15.1)
Respiratory rate, breaths/min, mean (SD)	20 (20–24)[a]	26 (22 – 31)[a]	27 (6.0)
Oxygen saturation, %, median (IQR)	98 (97–99)	NR	97.5 (96–99)
Palpable liver, n (%)	24.0	24.3	40
Palpable spleen, n (%)	5.9	15	33
Rash, n (%)	4.3	NR	NR

[a]Median (IQR)
[b]mean (SD)
NR: not reported

falciparum and vivax malaria (Grigg et al., 2018a). The symptoms of knowlesi malaria are non-specific and occur with similar frequency in falciparum and vivax malaria (Grigg et al., 2018a). The non-specific symptoms can also be attributed to other infections in knowlesi-endemic regions such as dengue, leptospirosis, COVID-19, typhoid and typhus. A high index of suspicion of knowlesi malaria is required in endemic areas, as presentations with abdominal pain, diarrhoea or cough can be misdiagnosed as organ-specific infections. Abdominal pain has led to a misdiagnosis of knowlesi malaria as acute gastroenteritis, with consequent delayed commencement of anti-malarial treatment, sometimes with fatal outcomes (Cox-Singh et al., 2008; Rajahram et al., 2013).

7.3 Clinical signs in adults

The common signs of knowlesi malaria include fever, tachycardia and tachypnoea (Table 1). In prospective series, splenomegaly and hepatomegaly are present in 6–33% and 24–40% of patients respectively (Barber et al., 2013; Daneshvar et al., 2009; Grigg et al., 2018a).

Patients can also present with hypotension, jaundice, or respiratory distress (Barber et al., 2013; Daneshvar et al., 2009; Grigg et al., 2018a), or develop these after commencement of therapy—see "severe knowlesi malaria" below.

In contrast to falciparum malaria (Dondorp et al., 2008; World Health Organization, 2014; Yeo et al., 2007), neurological signs are notably rare in knowlesi malaria. While altered mental state has been rarely reported (Barber et al., 2013), in the three largest prospective series of knowlesi malaria, none of 674 adults had unarousable coma or seizures, including the 76 patients who had severe disease (Barber et al., 2013; Daneshvar et al., 2009; Grigg et al., 2018a). In a retrospective case report of a single parasitemic patient presenting with coma (Rajahram et al., 2016), the absence of neuroimaging, lumbar puncture and other diagnostic workup meant alternative diagnoses could not be excluded. Similar diagnostic limitations were present for a knowlesi malaria case presenting with hemi-paresis, who had a history of uncontrolled hypertension (Daneshvar et al., 2009).

Retinal haemorrhages were observed on fundal photographs in 3/17 (18%) and 2/12 (17%) of patients hospitalized with uncomplicated and severe knowlesi malaria, respectively. These were associated with thrombo-cytopenia, but otherwise the retinopathy seen in knowlesi malaria is non-specific and the characteristic retinal whitening seen in severe falciparum malaria has not been reported to date (Govindasamy et al., 2016).

7.4 Laboratory investigations in adults

7.4.1 Haematology

Thrombocytopenia is near-universal in adult knowlesi malaria (Table 2). In the three largest prospective series, thrombocytopenia (platelets $<150 \times 10^3/\mu L$) occurred on presentation in 634/674 (94%) of adults hospitalized with knowlesi malaria (Barber et al., 2013; Daneshvar et al., 2009; Grigg et al., 2018a) (Table 2), with 29% and 60% of patients at district (Daneshvar et al., 2009) and tertiary referral hospitals (Barber et al., 2013), respectively, having a platelet count of $<50 \times 10^3/\mu L$. Platelet counts recover quickly, and bleeding is uncommon, occurring in only 5% of those with severe malaria (Barber et al., 2013; Daneshvar et al., 2009; Grigg et al., 2018a). An absence of thrombocytopenia has been reported in 3 of 7 splenectomized patients (Barber et al., 2013, 2016; Bird et al., 2016; Boo et al., 2016; Cheo et al., 2020).

Anaemia (based on WHO criteria (WHO, 2011)) is found on presentation in 36% of adults with knowlesi malaria (Grigg et al., 2018a), and can develop after treatment. In two randomized controlled trials, 63% (95% CI 55–71%) of artemisinin combination therapy-treated patients with uncomplicated malaria had anaemia at some point throughout 28 days of followup (Grigg et al., 2016b, 2018b). Severe anaemia ($<7\,g/dL$) is uncommon in adult knowlesi malaria, reported in only 1.7% and 1.5% overall in district and referral hospital series (Barber et al., 2013; Grigg et al., 2018a), though can occur in up to 28% of those with severe malaria (Grigg et al., 2018a).

The total white cell counts are usually normal although neutrophilia is often seen in severe and fatal disease (Barber et al., 2013, 2017a; Cox-Singh et al., 2011; Willmann et al., 2012) (Table 2). Coagulation studies can also be abnormal. In one series of severe knowlesi malaria, 32% of patients had significant elevations of the prothrombin and partial thromboplastin times, although none were reported to have clinically important bleeding (William et al., 2011).

7.4.2 Parasitaemia

Although *P. knowlesi* can cause high parasitaemia, parasite counts in most cases of knowlesi malaria are low. In the largest series of knowlesi malaria, median parasitaemia in adults presenting to a district hospital with knowlesi

Table 2 Clinical laboratory features in adults with knowlesi malaria enrolled in prospective studies.

Patient characteristic	District hospital studies		Tertiary referral hospital study	
	Grigg et al. (2018a) Sabah, Malaysia n = 481 (437 adults)	Daneshvar et al. (2009) Sarawak, Malaysia n = 121 (113 adults)	Barber et al. (2013) Sabah, Malaysia n = 130	
			Non-severe	Severe
Parasite count, parasites/µL, median (IQR)	2541 (478–8585)	1387 (6–222,570)	4837 (1576–14,641)	80,359 (25874–168,279)
Trophozoite proportion, mean % (SD)	NR	NR	49	42
Schizont proportion, mean % (SD)	2 (5.4)	NR	0 (0–1.25)[a]	0.79 (0–11.1)[a]
Parasite count >20,000/µL, (%)	15	NR	16	79
Haemoglobin, g/dL, mean (SD)	13.2 (12.1–14.3)[a]	13.3 (12–14.3)[a]	12.8 (1.6)[b]	12.1 (1.8)[b]
White blood cell count, ×103/µL, median (IQR)	6.1 (5.1–7.6)	5.6 (4.7–7.0)	6.1 (5.0–7.2)	6.6 (5.6–9.8)
Neutrophil count, ×103/µL, median (IQR)	3.5 (2.6–4.5)	3.7 (1.8)[b]	3.4 (2.5–4.4)	4.7 (3.5–7.6)
Lymphocyte count, ×103/µL, median (IQR)	1.4 (1.0–1.9)	1.5 (1.1–2.0)	1.6 (1.0–2.0)	1.4 (1.0–1.9)
Monocyte count, ×103/µL, median (IQR)	1.0 (0.7–1.4)	NR	0.9 (0.6–1.2)	1.0 (0.7–1.3)
Platelet count, ×103/µL, median (IQR)	70 (50–103)	71 (35)[b]	51 (35–81)	29 (20–49)
Platelet nadir, ×103/µL, median (IQR)	60 (42–83)	NR	42 (25–62)	27 (18–46)
Platelet nadir, median days (IQR)	1 (1–1)	NR	0 (0–1)	0 (0–1)

Thrombocytopenia (platelets <150 × 103/μL), (%)	92	98	99 (nadir)	100 (nadir)
Creatinine, μmol/L, median (IQR)	88 (75–103)	86 (73–100)	92 (78–110)	141 (101−213)
Sodium, mmol/L, median (IQR)	136 (134–139)	137 (135–140)	134 (3.2)[b]	131 (4.6)[b]
Bilirubin, μmol/L, median (IQR)	17.1 (11.8–24.6)	13 (9–18)	16.6 (12.9–24.8)	42.1 (26–66.8)
Glucose, mmol/L, median (IQR)	6.4 (5.6–7.4)	6.2 (5.3–6.7)	6.7 (5.8–7.8)	7.7 (6.4–9.5)
Albumin, g/dL, median (IQR)	36 (30–40)	36 (33–39)	30.5 (4.7)[b]	26.6 (5.3)[b]
AST, IU/L, median (IQR)	34 (23–47)	NR	39 (26–49)	58 (44–79)
ALT, IU/L, median (IQR)	37 (24–56)	36 (25–54)	35 (21–56)	36 (19–51)
Bicarbonate, mmol/L, median (IQR)	24 (21–27)	NR	24.8 (3.8)[b]	21.6 (4.9)[b]
Acute kidney injury, KDIGO criteria (%)	83 (19)	NR	NR	NR

[a]Median (IQR).
[b]mean (SD).
NR: not reported.

malaria (2541 parasites/μL [IQR 478–8585]) was lower than that seen in vivax (3765 [1755–8122]) and falciparum (9924 [2522–22,860]) malaria (Grigg et al., 2018a), suggesting a lower fever threshold in knowlesi malaria. Parasitaemia is strongly correlated with age (Barber et al., 2013, 2017a). Parasitaemia is independently associated with severe disease in *P. knowlesi* infections, with median parasitaemia in severe malaria of 42,224 parasites/μL compared with 2044 in non-severe knowlesi malaria (Grigg et al., 2018a). In tertiary hospital studies, the parasitaemias seen severe knowlesi malaria are comparable to those seen in severe falciparum malaria (Barber et al., 2013). Parasitaemia in severe malaria is discussed further below.

7.4.3 Liver function

Mild elevations of liver transaminases are common (Barber et al., 2013; Daneshvar et al., 2009) (Table 2). Hyperbilirubinemia (>42 μmol/L) was observed in 3% of district hospital presentations and in 53% of patients with severe knowlesi malaria (Daneshvar et al., 2009; Barber et al., 2013). Hypoalbuminemia occurs more frequently in severe disease compared to uncomplicated disease (Barber et al., 2013) and is universal in fatal cases (Rajahram et al., 2019). Transaminases may also increase after treatment, as has been observed in falciparum and vivax malaria (Odedra et al., 2020; Woodford et al., 2018).

7.4.4 Renal function

Acute kidney injury (AKI) is common in knowlesi malaria. In the largest prospective study to date, AKI of any severity, defined by KDIGO criteria, occurred in 83/437 (19%) adults with knowlesi malaria presenting to a district hospital (Grigg et al., 2018a). In a tertiary referral hospital study, AKI of any severity, by KDIGO criteria (with baseline creatinine estimated by the MDRD equation), was present on admission in 44/154 (29%) non-severe cases, and 40/48 (83%) severe cases (Barber et al., 2018a). A systematic review of fatal cases, showed that 100% of fatal cases had elevated creatinine on presentation (Rajahram et al., 2019). Higher creatinine is positively associated with parasitaemia and neutrophilia (Daneshvar et al., 2018). Hyponatremia is also common in severe malaria, and is universal in fatal cases (Rajahram et al., 2019).

7.5 Severe knowlesi malaria

Severe knowlesi malaria, defined by WHO criteria (WHO, 2014) (Table 3), has been reported in 6–9% of adults presenting to district hospitals (Daneshvar et al., 2009; Grigg et al., 2018a) and in 29% of adults treated at a tertiary referral hospital (Barber et al., 2013). The WHO epidemiological and research definition for severe knowlesi malaria (WHO, 2014) (Table 3) is a modification of that for severe falciparum malaria, with a lower parasite count of 100,000 parasites/μL used as the cut-off to define hyperparasitaemia and a parasitaemia threshold of 20,000/μL in the presence of jaundice (WHO, 2014). In adults, the most common manifestations of severe knowlesi malaria include acute kidney injury, hyperparasitaemia, jaundice, shock, respiratory distress and metabolic acidosis (Barber et al., 2013; Daneshvar et al., 2009; Grigg et al., 2018a; Singh and Daneshvar, 2013) (Table 3). In contrast to falciparum malaria, coma is not a feature of severe knowlesi malaria, with no case of coma, with exclusion of other causes, yet reported in PCR-confirmed knowlesi malaria. Also in contrast to falciparum malaria, severe disease from *P. knowlesi* has not been reported in children, and no paediatric deaths have been reported (Rajahram et al., 2016, 2019).

Severe acute kidney injury defining severe malaria (creatinine >265/μL) occurs in 24–36% of cases in prospective series of severe knowlesi malaria (Barber et al., 2013; Daneshvar et al., 2009; Grigg et al., 2018a) and in up to 94% in retrospective series (William et al., 2011; Willmann et al., 2012). Severe AKI is reported in 70% of fatal cases (Rajahram et al., 2019). Blackwater fever with acute kidney injury has been reported (Barber et al., 2013; William et al., 2011), including in a splenectomized patient with marked intravascular haemolysis (Barber et al., 2016).

Respiratory distress is a common feature in severe malaria, occurring in 7–70% of severe cases (Barber et al., 2013; Daneshvar et al., 2009; Grigg et al., 2018a; William et al., 2011; Willmann et al., 2012). Acute respiratory distress syndrome (ARDS) has been shown to occur with similar frequency to that seen in severe falciparum malaria (Barber et al., 2013) and is common in fatal cases (Rajahram et al., 2019). Respiratory distress is associated with both parasitaemia (Barber et al., 2013; Daneshvar et al., 2009) and neutrophilia (Barber et al., 2013). Development of respiratory distress has been reported to occur after commencement of antimalarial treatment, with either quinine (Daneshvar et al., 2009; William et al., 2011) or intravenous artesunate (Barber et al., 2013).

Table 3 Severe disease[d] in prospective studies of knowlesi malaria in adults.

	Daneshvar et al. (2009) Sarawak, Malaysia (n = 10)	Grigg et al. (2018a) Sabah, Malaysia (n = 28)	Barber et al. (2013) Sabah, Malaysia Tertiary referral hospital (n = 38)
Severe malaria[d] as % of all adult cases	9.3 (3.8–14.8)	6.4 (3.9–8.3)	29.2 (21.4–37)
Age (years) Median (IQR)[c]	63.5	53 (43–64)	55 (47–62)
Range	36–73	13–78	20–74
Male sex (%)	30	68	79
Severe criteria developed after treatment %	20	32	5
WHO severity Criteria[d], (%)			
Hyperparasitaemia (>100,000 parasites/μL)	30	29	47
Respiratory distress	70	7	37
Hypotension	20	18	34
Jaundice	40	29[a]	53[a]
Severe acute kidney injury	30	36	24
Metabolic acidosis	NR	11	11
Severe anaemia	0	29	5
Abnormal bleeding	NR	4	5
Multiple convulsions	NR	0	0
Hypoglycaemia	10	4	0
Coma	0	0	0
Death			
% of severe	20[b]	7.1[c]	0[c]
% of all cases	1.9	0.4	0

[a]With parasite count >20,000 parasites/μL for *P. knowlesi* and/or creatinine >132 μmol/L.
[b]Treated with intravenous quinine.
[c]Treated with intravenous artesunate.
[d]Severe malaria defined using WHO research and epidemiological definition of severe malaria (WHO, 2014).

Metabolic acidosis, including lactic acidosis, is common in severe malaria, occurring in 11–32% of cases (Barber et al., 2013; Grigg et al., 2018a; William et al., 2011), and 71% of fatal cases (Rajahram et al., 2019). Hematemesis has been reported in patients with severe and fatal disease (Barber et al., 2013; Boo et al., 2016; Cox-Singh et al., 2008). Other severe complications reported in knowlesi malaria include rhabdomyolysis (Takaya et al., 2018) and spontaneous splenic rupture (Chang et al., 2018). As in complicated falciparum malaria (Aung et al., 2018; Nyein et al., 2016), concurrent gram-negative bacteremia can occur in severe knowlesi malaria. Two cases of concurrent *Enterobacter* bacteraemia in severe and fatal disease have been reported (Rajahram et al., 2012; William et al., 2011), and another case of *Neisseria meningitidis* bacteraemia has been reported in uncomplicated knowlesi malaria (Grigg et al., 2018a).

7.6 Clinical and parasitological risk factors for severe disease

Parasitaemia is consistently higher in severe malaria than in uncomplicated knowlesi malaria (Barber et al., 2013, 2017a; Daneshvar et al., 2009; Grigg et al., 2018a; William et al., 2011; Willmann et al., 2012). In a tertiary-referral hospital study, severe disease occurred in 53% of patients with parasite counts of >20,000 and 83% of patients with parasite counts of >100,000/µL (Barber et al., 2013). Parasitaemia is strongly correlated with age (Barber et al., 2013, 2017a). In addition, although older adults have significantly higher parasitaemias and thus are at greater risk of severe disease, age has also been shown to be an independent risk factor for severe disease in a large tertiary hospital series (Barber et al., 2017a). In the largest prospective study of knowlesi malaria, parasitaemia, age, schizont proportion, abdominal pain and dyspnoea were independent predictors of severe disease (Grigg et al., 2018a). In this study a parasitaemia threshold of 15,000/µL had the best combined sensitivity (74%) and specificity (87%) for predicting severe knowlesi malaria, with an area under the curve of 0.80 and a negative predictive value of 98.5%. Thus, while a parasitaemia >100,000/µL has been defined as a WHO research criterion for severe disease in the absence of other severity criteria, in routine clinical practice, intravenous artesunate has been recommended for all patients with parasite counts >20,000/µL (WHO, 2014), and more recently >15,000/µL (Anstey et al., 2020; WHO, 2017).

Parasite counts have been found to be higher in farmers and plantation workers compared to other occupations, even when controlling for age and fever duration (Barber et al., 2017a). This may be due to a higher infective inoculum in these occupations. High parasitaemias and severe disease have also been observed in splenectomized patients (Barber et al., 2013, 2016; Bird et al., 2016; Boo et al., 2016; Cheo et al., 2020). HIV infection has been shown to be a risk factor for higher parasitaemia and severe disease in falciparum malaria (Berkley et al., 2009) but it is not known whether HIV infection increases risk of severe disease in *P. knowlesi* infections.

7.7 Deaths from knowlesi malaria

Deaths from knowlesi malaria are well documented (Cox-Singh et al., 2008; William et al., 2011), and *P. knowlesi* is now the most common cause of malaria deaths in Malaysia (WHO, 2020). In an analysis of malaria incidence and fatality data from the Sabah Department of Health from 2010 to 2017, the overall case fatality rate of knowlesi malaria was 2.5/1000 cases. For women, this was 6.0/000 compared to 1.7/1000 for men ($p = 0.01$). Age ≥ 45 years was associated with a fivefold increased risk of death, with a case fatality of 5.8/1000 in this age group, compared to 1.1/1000 for those aged <45 years (p > 0.001). On multivariate analysis, age >45 years and female sex were both independent risk factors for fatal disease (Rajahram et al., 2019).

Consistent with these data from Sabah, in a recent systematic review of all reported cases of fatal knowlesi malaria up to August 2018, median age of the 32 cases was 56 years (range 23–84) (Rajahram et al., 2019), and, in contrast to the predominance of males in studies of non-fatal knowlesi malaria (Barber et al., 2013; Grigg et al., 2018a), nearly half of all reported fatal cases were women. There was no difference in parasitaemia or fever duration between males and females, suggesting that the over-representation of females in this series of fatal cases was not due to delay in health-seeking behaviour (Rajahram et al., 2019).

Over a third (34%) of the fatal cases in this series had cardiovascular-metabolic chronic disease, including hypertension, diabetes, morbid obesity, ischemic heart disease and rheumatic heart disease (Rajahram et al., 2019). Abdominal pain was reported in over half of the cases, and elevated serum creatinine, hyponatremia and thrombocytopenia were seen in all. Of severe manifestations, severe acute kidney injury, jaundice and metabolic acidosis were found in >70% of the fatal cases (Rajahram et al., 2019).

Although 30/32 (94%) of the patients in this series met WHO criteria for severe disease at presentation, only 19 (63%) were recognized as having severe malaria by the treating clinician, leading to inappropriate oral therapy and delay in initiation of intravenous artesunate (Rajahram et al., 2019). In addition, species diagnosis on admission microscopy was incorrect in 90% of cases, with 69% diagnosed as *P. malariae*, 14% as *P. falciparum*, and 7% as *P. vivax* (Rajahram et al., 2019). Consistent with earlier reports, the misidentification of *P. knowlesi* by microscopy, particularly as the more benign *P. malariae* (Barber et al., 2013; Lee et al., 2009; Rajahram et al., 2012), likely contributed to inappropriate oral therapy and delayed initiation of parenteral therapy (Rajahram et al., 2019). Inadequate access to healthcare in endemic settings was also associated with fatal outcomes, including unavailability of intravenous artesunate despite prompt recognition and diagnosis (Rajahram et al., 2019). In Sabah, Malaysia, a fall in case-fatality rate of PCR-confirmed knowlesi malaria in adults coincided with greater recognition of disease, earlier diagnosis and rollout of artesunate therapy (Rajahram et al., 2016).

7.8 Knowlesi malaria in children

As outlined earlier, knowlesi malaria is predominantly a disease of adults, with prospective clinical series reporting <10% of cases in children (Daneshvar et al., 2009; Grigg et al., 2018a) Clinical presentations in children are usually non-specific, most commonly with a history of fever (Barber et al., 2011). In the first prospective study of clinical presentations in children ($n = 44$), presenting symptoms were similar to those of falciparum and vivax malaria, including fever (100%), rigors (66%), headache (77%), vomiting (32%) and cough (34%) (Grigg et al., 2018a). In this series, abdominal pain was notably more common in knowlesi malaria (43%) than falciparum or vivax malaria. Hepatomegaly (32%) and splenomegaly (21%) occurred with similar frequency as in falciparum and vivax malaria (Grigg et al., 2018a). As in adults, children with knowlesi malaria have lower parasitaemias than malaria from other species. Median parasitaemia in 44 children presenting to a district hospital with knowlesi malaria (1722 parasites/µL [IQR 386-4830]) was lower than that seen in vivax (5967 [1829-13,901]) and falciparum (7392[1462-36,546]) malaria (Grigg et al., 2018a).

In children, thrombocytopenia (platelet count <150,000/µL) occurs frequently (Barber et al., 2011), but is less common in paediatric knowlesi malaria (68%) than in adults (92%) (Grigg et al., 2018a). In Sabah, 84% of children with knowlesi malaria had nonsevere anaemia, with the lowest haemoglobin concentration of 5.1 g/dL occurring in a 4-year old child. In a retrospective series, post-treatment haemoglobin nadir occurred later than that seen in falciparum malaria (Barber et al., 2011). Severe anaemia (haemoglobin of 4.9 g/dL) has been reported in child with microscopy-diagnosed knowlesi malaria, although this was not confirmed with PCR (Barber et al., 2011). While overall clinical illness in the prospective series was milder than in adults, and no cases of severe malaria were reported, children had a 11-fold higher risk of anaemia at presentation and a similar risk of mild-moderate acute kidney injury (by KDIGO criteria) than adults (Grigg et al., 2018a).

It is notable that there have been no cases reported to date of severe PCR-confirmed knowlesi malaria in children (Barber et al., 2011; Grigg et al., 2018a). In contrast to the risk of death in knowlesi malaria in adults, and in contrast to the significant mortality associated with falciparum and vivax malaria in children (Douglas et al., 2014; Marsh et al., 1995), no deaths from knowlesi malaria have been reported among children to date (Rajahram et al., 2016, 2019).

7.9 Knowlesi malaria in pregnancy

In co-endemic areas, the risk of *P. knowlesi* infection in pregnancy appears to be lower than that of *P. falciparum* and *P. vivax* infection (Barber et al., 2015a). This has been hypothesized to be due to behavioural changes in pregnancy resulting in less occupational and forest exposure, and differences among species in peridomestic exposure (Barber et al., 2015a). Only seven cases of *P. knowlesi* infection in pregnancy have been reported (Barber et al., 2015a; Rajahram et al., 2019; William et al., 2011). This makes assessment of the risk of adverse maternal and foetal outcomes uncertain. Nevertheless, two of the seven cases presented with severe malaria in the third trimester, with both having acute kidney injury and hypotension, and one with acute respiratory distress syndrome and fatal outcome (Rajahram et al., 2019; William et al., 2011). This suggests that there is an increased risk of severe disease resulting from *P. knowlesi* infection in pregnancy, as also seen in falciparum malaria (WHO, 2014). Adverse foetal outcomes have also been reported, including intrauterine death, preterm delivery and low birth weight (Barber et al., 2015a; Rajahram et al., 2019; William et al., 2011).

7.10 Congenital malaria

Congenital malaria due to *P. falciparum* and *P. vivax* is well-described (Poespoprodjo et al., 2011). The extent to which congenital malaria occurs with *P. knowlesi* is not known. In a baboon model of *P. knowlesi* infection, placental infiltration of parasitized erythrocytes and inflammatory cells was seen but parasitized erythrocytes in cord blood and the foetal-placental region were absent, suggesting that the risk of congenital malaria may be low (Onditi et al., 2015). A possible case of congenital malaria has been reported in Sabah in an anaemic 6 week-old (haemoglobin 7.4 g/dL) with no epidemiological risk factors for post-natal infection (Grigg et al., 2018a).

8. Genetic risk factors
8.1 Parasite genetics

P. knowlesi parasites show greater genetic diversity than the two major human malaria species, *P. falciparum* and *P. vivax* (Benavente et al., 2018). Multilocus microsatellite genotyping and whole genome sequencing studies have confirmed the presence of three major subpopulations of *P. knowlesi* in human clinical isolates from Malaysia (Assefa et al., 2015; Divis et al., 2015, 2017). Two highly divergent clusters have been identified in humans from Malaysian Borneo, associated with long-tailed and pig-tailed macaque reservoir hosts respectively, and with significant geographical differentiation occurring between the two subpopulations (Assefa et al., 2015; Divis et al., 2015). A third highly divergent cluster has been identified in clinical isolates from humans and most macaques in Peninsular Malaysia (Divis et al., 2017). Whether these subpopulations are associated with different clinical phenotypes has not yet been reported.

Because disease severity in knowlesi malaria is closely linked with parasitaemia (Barber et al., 2013, 2017a; Grigg et al., 2018a) there has been significant interest in whether parasite genes encoding more efficient erythrocyte invasion are linked to malaria disease severity. Mathematical modelling predicts that parasite adaptation for invasion of older human red cells may be a major factor allowing the high parasitaemias associated with disease severity (Lim et al., 2013). Sequence diversity has been demonstrated in the *P. knowlesi* normocyte binding proteins (*Pknbpxa* and *Pknpbxb*) (Ahmed et al., 2016) that are required for human erythrocyte invasion (Moon et al., 2016). Certain alleles of *Pknbpxa* and *Pknpbxb* have been associated with high parasitaemias and other features of disease severity, suggesting a link between invasion gene variants and parasite virulence (Ahmed et al., 2014). Sequence diversity has also been demonstrated in merozoite surface protein-1 (*Pkmsp1*) (Yap et al., 2017), *Pkmsp3* (De Silva et al., 2017) and Duffy binding protein (*PkDBP*) (Putaporntip et al., 2016) and differences in PkDBPαII binding activity with human erythrocytes have been identified (Lim et al., 2017). To date no links with disease severity have been reported for these latter genes.

8.2 Host genetics

Human genetic polymorphisms influencing risk of *P. falciparum* infection and severe disease are well-described (Mackinnon et al., 2005). Much less is known about host genetic factors influencing risk of *P. knowlesi* infection and its disease severity. Glucose-6-phosphate dehydrogenase (G6PD) deficiency linked to mutations in the X chromosome is known to be associated with protection from malaria due to the human-only species *P. falciparum* and *P. vivax* (Leslie et al., 2010; Manjurano et al., 2015). In a large case-control study in Sabah, Malaysia, G6PD deficiency was also found to be associated with protection against acquisition of symptomatic *P. knowlesi* infection in multivariate models, conferring a fivefold lower risk of knowlesi malaria (Grigg et al., 2017).

Southeast Asian ovalocytosis (SAO) is widely distributed in knowlesi-endemic Malaysia and Indonesia (Paquette et al., 2015). *In vitro* studies have shown that human SAO ovalocytes are highly resistant to invasion by *P. knowlesi* merozoites, making it likely that SAO protects against knowlesi malaria (Hadley et al., 1983). This has not yet been shown in case-control studies. It may be anticipated that other genetic erythrocyte abnormalities and haemoglobinopathies prevalent in knowlesi-endemic regions may also confer protection from knowlesi malaria but this remains to be shown.

9. Pathophysiology

The pathophysiology of severe knowlesi malaria in humans is not as well understood as that of severe falciparum malaria. Disease severity in malaria from the human-only species, *P. falciparum* and *P. vivax*, is associated with parasite biomass (Barber et al., 2015b; Dondorp et al., 2005), and this is clearly also the case in knowlesi malaria (Barber et al., 2013; Daneshvar et al., 2009; Grigg et al., 2018a; William et al., 2011; Willmann et al., 2012). The relative distribution of parasite biomass between the circulating compartment and deep tissue microvasculature in human knowlesi malaria is less well defined. In the following sections, we review pathophysiological mechanisms associated with disease severity in knowlesi malaria.

9.1 Microvascular accumulation of parasites

In rhesus macaques, another non-natural primate host for *P. knowlesi* susceptible to severe disease, infection with *P. knowlesi* is characterized by widespread microvascular accumulation of infected red blood cells, with malarial pigment seen in multiple organs including the small intestine, liver, brain, spleen, heart, lung, kidney, adipose tissue and skeletal muscle, and associated with widespread cellular necrosis (Chen et al., 2001; Miller et al., 1971a; Miller and Chien, 1971; Spangler et al., 1978). The occurrence of deep vascular schizogony (the cyclic disappearance of infected red blood cells from the peripheral circulation as the parasite matures), with infected red blood cells accumulating in multiple organs at higher parasitaemia, has also been described in rhesus macaques (Miller et al., 1971a). To-date only a single autopsy in human severe knowlesi malaria has been reported (Cox-Singh et al., 2010). In this report, a lack of peripheral parasitaemia precluded calculation of a sequestration index, but there was widespread marked accumulation of pigmented infected red blood cells in the microvasculature of vital organs including the brain, heart and kidney as well as in the liver sinusoids and the splenic red pulp, without evidence of chronic inflammatory response in the brain or other organs (Cox-Singh et al., 2010). Further investigation with electron microscopy was not able to be conducted.

In macaques, microvascular accumulation of *P. knowlesi*-infected red blood cells appears to occur first in the small intestine (Miller et al., 1971a; Miller and Chien, 1971). Of note, abdominal pain is more common in human knowlesi malaria than malaria from other species, at least in children (Grigg et al., 2018a). Parasitaemia is associated with abdominal pain in adults (Barber et al., 2013; Daneshvar et al., 2009, 2018), and the majority of fatal cases have had abdominal pain, hypothesized to be from microvascular accumulation of parasites in the gut and/or stress ulceration (Rajahram et al., 2019).

The mechanisms underlying the microvascular accumulation of *P. knowlesi*-infected red blood cells are not clear. In *P. falciparum* infection, infected red blood cells express surface knob-like protrusions expressing variant parasite derived proteins of the PfEMP1 *var* family, which cytoadhere to multiple microvascular endothelial cell receptors, including CD36, ICAM-1, and EPCR (Su et al., 1995; Turner et al., 1994), with clear evidence for cytoadherence to activated endothelial cells mediating microvascular sequestration and obstruction (MacPherson et al., 1985; Marchiafava and Bignami, 1894; Taylor et al., 2004; White et al., 2013). In *P. knowlesi*, schizont-infected cell agglutination ligands (SICA) are red blood cell surface proteins encoded by the SICA*var* gene family, and while phylogenetically distinct, share some binding protein motifs with PfEMP1 proteins (Korir and Galinski, 2006), with antigenic variant expression hypothesized to be related to parasite virulence (Barnwell et al., 1983; Howard et al., 1983; Korir and Galinski, 2006). However, evidence for endothelial cytoadherence of *P. knowlesi*-infected red blood cells is limited. Electron microscopy of microvascular *P. knowlesi*-infected red blood cells in severe disease in rhesus macaques does not show the knobs that mediate cytoadherence in *P. falciparum* or *P. coatneyi*, and, while closely associated with the endothelium, *P. knowlesi*-infected red cells "were not held by extensions of the endothelial cells" (Miller et al., 1971a). Lack of surface knobs has been confirmed on atomic force microscopy of circulating *P. knowlesi*-infected red cells from humans with both uncomplicated and severe knowlesi malaria (Barber et al., 2018b). Instead, caveolae pits were observed (Barber et al., 2018b).

In the single human autopsy case, while there was intense accumulation of parasitized red cells within the microvasculature, clear evidence of cytoadherence to endothelial cells was not apparent, with interspersion of infected red blood cells with uninfected red blood cells, and a lack of clear marginalization of parasitized cells (Cox-Singh et al., 2010). Furthermore, ICAM-1, which mediates cytoadherence to brain endothelial cells in falciparum malaria (Berendt et al., 1989; Turner et al., 1994), was not detected on brain endothelium (Cox-Singh et al., 2010). A subsequent small study showed that *P. knowlesi*-infected red blood cells could, variably, bind *in vitro* to ICAM-1 and VCAM-1 but not CD36 (Fatih et al., 2012). A paucity of falciparum-like cytoadherence of infected red blood cells in knowlesi malaria is also suggested by the notable lack of coma in reported cases of severe knowlesi malaria to-date (Barber et al., 2013; Cox-Singh et al., 2008; Daneshvar et al., 2009; Grigg et al., 2018a; Rajahram et al., 2012, 2016, 2019; William et al., 2011) and the lack of the specific malarial retinopathy and characteristic retinal whitening seen in severe falciparum malaria (Govindasamy et al., 2016). Thus, important differences likely exist between the pathophysiology of severe knowlesi and severe falciparum malaria, particularly the mechanisms by which infected red blood cells accumulate in the microvasculature.

If not sequestration through falciparum-like endothelial cytoadherence, what other mechanisms might account for the marked accumulation of *P. knowlesi*-infected red cells in the microvasculature? Early 1940s "motion picture" microscopy studies in rhesus macaques demonstrated marked microcirculatory changes in *P. knowlesi*-infected monkeys, with impairment of microvascular flow reported to be a critical factor in fatal outcomes (Knisely and Stratman-Thomas, 1945, 1948). These studies reported coating of parasitized red cells with a "precipitate," progressing at higher parasitaemias to a further coating of both infected and uninfected red blood cells, binding infected and uninfected red cells together, and changing blood to a "thick, muck-like sludge," leading to microvascular obstruction and widespread tissue hypoxia (Knisely and Stratman-Thomas, 1945, 1948). Whether such agglutination and sludging contributes to microvascular obstruction and severe disease in human knowlesi malaria is not clear.

Autogglutination and clumping of infected red blood cells is associated with disease severity in falciparum malaria (Pain et al., 2001). Agglutinates of infected red blood cells have been recently observed in blood from a knowlesi malaria patient, in association with platelets (Kho et al., 2018). In falciparum malaria, agglutination of infected red blood cells is mediated by platelet-expressed CD36 (Pain et al., 2001), however, the inability of *P. knowlesi*-infected red blood cells to bind CD36 *in vitro* (Fatih et al., 2012) suggests a distinct mechanism may mediate such agglutination in knowlesi malaria in humans.

Increased viscosity and resistance to flow of red blood cells from *P. knowlesi*- infected macaques has also been demonstrated, suggestive of reduced deformability of RBCs (Miller et al., 1971b). Reduced deformability of red blood cells is a key feature of severe falciparum malaria (Dondorp et al., 1997) (Dondorp et al., 1999) and has recently been reported in human knowlesi malaria (Barber et al., 2018b). In this study, ektacytometry demonstrated overall red blood cell deformability was reduced in Malaysian adults with knowlesi malaria, in proportion to disease severity, and comparable to that seen in severe falciparum malaria (Barber et al., 2018b). Red blood cell deformability was reduced in proportion to parasite biomass and lactate (as a measure of tissue perfusion). Micropipette aspiration confirmed that in humans, *P. knowlesi* infection causes increased stiffness of both infected and uninfected red blood cells, with the latter mostly as a result of echinocytosis (Barber et al., 2018b). Single-event flow cytometry and atomic force microscopy each showed sphericity was increased in infected red blood cells *vs* uninfected red blood cells. These findings were in contrast to parallel studies done in the natural host *Macaca fascicularis*, in which the deformability of uninfected red blood cells was not impaired and echinocyte formation was not seen (Barber et al., 2018b). *In vitro* studies using the human red blood cell-adapted *P. knowlesi* A1 strain have shown *P. knowlesi* infection results in a 20% increase in volume of the human red blood cell and an 11% decrease in the surface area to volume ratio, which combine to cause a markedly decreased deformability (Liu et al., 2019). Taken together, findings suggest that in humans, and other non-natural primate hosts of *P. knowlesi*, reduced deformability of both infected and uninfected red blood cells may be a major mechanism contributing to microvascular accumulation of parasites and impaired organ perfusion in severe knowlesi malaria.

In falciparum malaria, additional processes contributing to microvascular sequestration of infected red blood cells and reduced microvascular flow include adherence of infected red blood cells to uninfected red blood cells to form rosettes (David et al., 1988; Kaul et al., 1991; Udomsangpetch et al., 1989), however, rosetting has not been investigated to date in knowlesi malaria.

9.2 Endothelial activation, dysfunction and glycocalyx breakdown

Endothelial activation, impaired nitric oxide (NO) bioavailability and microvascular dysfunction are key features of severe falciparum malaria (Yeo et al., 2007, 2008, 2010, 2013, 2014), with endothelial activation and parasite biomass independent predictors of impaired organ perfusion, severe malaria and malaria mortality (Hanson et al., 2015). Endothelial activation, impaired NO bioavailability and microvascular dysfunction are also associated with severe disease in knowlesi malaria (Barber et al., 2017a, 2018a). In Malaysian adults with knowlesi malaria, parasitaemia and endothelial activation (measured by plasma angiopoietin-2) were independent predictors of severe disease, including acute kidney injury (Barber et al., 2017a). In this study, Barber et al. also found that endothelial activation and microvascular dysfunction were both associated with age, independent of parasitaemia; thus these mechanisms may also contribute to the more severe presentation of knowlesi malaria observed in older adults (Barber et al., 2017a). Because knowlesi malaria affects a wide age range from children through to the elderly, and because the pathogen biomass can be readily quantitated, human knowlesi malaria is an ideal model to evaluate the effects of aging on pathogenic mechanisms in all the human malarias.

The glycocalyx is a gel-like layer lining endothelial cells, essential in maintaining NO-dependent vascular homeostasis (Yeo et al., 2019b). Breakdown of the endothelial glycocalyx is associated with malaria severity, acute kidney injury and mortality in severe falciparum malaria (Yeo et al., 2019a,b). Recent studies show that endothelial glycocalyx degradation is also increased in knowlesi malaria in proportion to disease severity, and associated with impaired NO-dependent microvascular reactivity and acute kidney injury (Barber et al., 2021b). Glycocalyx breakdown is likely an additional mechanism of microvascular dysfunction and acute kidney injury in knowlesi malaria.

Cardiovascular disease and metabolic syndrome are known to be associated with increased endothelial activation, systemic inflammation, albuminuria, glycocalyx degradation and microvascular dysfunction (Rabelink and de Zeeuw, 2015). This may contribute to the increased risk of severe and fatal disease from *P. knowlesi* in those with cardiovascular-metabolic disease (Rajahram et al., 2019), as has also been reported in falciparum malaria (Wyss et al., 2017).

9.3 Systemic inflammatory response

As with falciparum malaria, the host inflammatory response has been associated with disease severity in knowlesi malaria, with both inflammatory and anti-inflammatory cytokines increased in severe disease, and with IL-6, IL-10 and IL-ra associated with parasitaemia (Barber et al., 2017a; Cox-Singh et al., 2011). Systemic inflammation (IL-6, and the IL-6/IL-10 ratio) in knowlesi malaria is also associated with age, independent of parasitaemia (Barber et al., 2017a). The causal role of systemic inflammation in pathogenesis is not clear. *Plasmodium knowlesi* infection also impairs protective human immune responses. Recent studies show that *P. knowlesi* infection of adults causes a decline in all subsets of circulating dendritic cells, key activators of the adaptive immune response to infection (Loughland et al., 2021).

9.4 Intravascular haemolysis

In severe falciparum malaria intravascular haemolysis is a key pathogenic mechanism in heme-induced acute kidney injury (Plewes et al., 2017, 2018) and endothelial dysfunction (Yeo et al., 2009). Haemolysis is associated with release of cell-free haemoglobin in proportion to disease severity leading to quenching of NO and endothelial dysfunction (Yeo et al., 2009). The scavenging capacity of haptoglobin and haemopexin are exceeded (Yeo et al., 2009), leading to circulation of free haemoglobin and free heme, which upon filtration through the kidney glomeruli, appear in the urine.

Heme is rapidly oxidized from its ferrous (Fe^{2+}) form to ferric (Fe^{3+}) heme. Further oxidation of ferric to ferryl (Fe^{4+}) heme generates lipid radical species, leading to oxidative stress and oxidative injury to glomeruli and renal tubular cells (Reeder and Wilson, 2005). Acute kidney injury in falciparum malaria is associated with both cell-free haemoglobin and measures of lipid peroxidation, supporting the hypothesis that heme-induced lipid peroxidation contributes to acute kidney injury in falciparum malaria (Plewes et al., 2017).

Intravascular haemolysis has been shown to be increased in severe knowlesi malaria, to a greater degree than that seen in falciparum malaria, and is thought to be a key mechanism of acute kidney injury in knowlesi malaria (Barber et al., 2018a). In Malaysian adults with knowlesi malaria, intravascular haemolysis (measured by cell free haemoglobin) is independently associated with clinical measures of disease severity including lactate and acute kidney injury, and with microvascular dysfunction and the endothelial activation markers osteoprotegerin and angiopoietin-2 (Barber et al., 2018a). Given the magnitude of haemolysis in knowlesi malaria, it is likely a significant contributor to impaired tissue perfusion, organ dysfunction and acute kidney injury in severe disease (Barber et al., 2018a).

9.5 Thrombocytopenia

Thrombocytopenia is near-universal in knowlesi malaria (Barber et al., 2013; Daneshvar et al., 2009; Grigg et al., 2018a) but the underlying cause is not certain. The reported absence of thrombocytopenia in three of seven splenectomized patients with knowlesi malaria (Barber et al., 2013, 2016; Bird et al., 2016; Boo et al., 2016; Cheo et al., 2020) suggests a role of the spleen in platelet destruction or accumulation. Recent studies in patients with knowlesi malaria have shown that platelets bind to both *P. knowlesi*-infected red blood cells and uninfected red blood cells in the circulation, with platelets killing parasites through a platelet factor 4-mediated mechanism (Kho et al., 2018). Platelet-red blood cell complexes comprised a median of 12.5%, and up to 47.7% of the total circulating platelet pool in knowlesi malaria and are likely to contribute considerably to malaria thrombocytopenia (Kho et al., 2018). Platelets complexed with red blood cells are not recognized in platelet counts generated by automated haematology analyzers and therefore complex formation leads to apparent platelet loss. If there is an accelerated splenic clearance of these complexes this would further add to the contribution of complexes to platelet loss (Kho et al., 2018).

It was notable in this study that the proportion of infected red blood cells bound to platelets was significantly higher in *P. knowlesi* infection than infection with *P. falciparum* or *P. vivax*, and that platelet-RBC complexes therefore formed the greatest proportion of the circulating platelet pool in knowlesi malaria (Kho et al., 2018). This is consistent with knowlesi malaria having the highest frequency of thrombocytopenia of all the *Plasmodium* species (Barber et al., 2013; Grigg et al., 2018a).

9.6 Anaemia

Intravascular and extravascular haemolysis of infected red blood cells contributes to anaemia in knowlesi malaria (Barber et al., 2018a). Unlike falciparum and vivax malaria (Jakeman et al., 1999), the relative contribution to anaemia of loss of infected *vs* uninfected red blood cells has not been modelled. Mechanisms underlying the loss of uninfected red blood cells in knowlesi malaria are not clear. Knisely's early "motion picture" microscopy studies in rhesus macaques demonstrated increased phagocytosis by the spleen and liver of "coated" *P. knowlesi*-infected and uninfected red blood cells contributing to anaemia (Knisely and Stratman-Thomas, 1945, 1948). Reduced deformability of red blood cells is associated with severe anaemia in falciparum malaria (Dondorp et al., 1999). The reduced deformability of both infected and uninfected red blood cells seen in both uncomplicated and severe knowlesi malaria (Barber et al., 2018b) likely enhances splenic clearance of both infected and uninfected red blood cells. Reduced red blood cell deformability was associated with haemoglobin nadir, independent of parasitaemia, suggesting a significant contribution to the anaemia of knowlesi malaria (Barber et al., 2018b). In chronic falciparum and vivax malaria, a hidden endosplenic lifecycle of asexual-stage parasites and the splenic accumulation of uninfected red blood cells are both significant contributors to anaemia (Kho et al., 2021a,b). The extent to which this occurs in knowlesi malaria is uncertain, but splenic congestion of both infected and uninfected red blood cells was seen in the single human autopsy case of fatal knowlesi malaria (Cox-Singh et al., 2010). In falciparum and vivax malaria, neutrophil extracellular traps mediate loss of bystander uninfected red blood cells and may be a mechanism contributing to anaemia (Kho et al., 2019). The role of neutrophil extracellular traps in the pathogenesis of anaemia or organ dysfunction in knowlesi malaria is unknown. Barber et al. have shown that concentrations of anti-phosphatidylserine IgM and IgG antibodies are elevated in knowlesi malaria, but unlike *P. falciparum* and

P. vivax, these are not associated with anaemia (Barber et al., 2019). Loss of red blood cell complement regulatory proteins is an age-independent mechanism of loss of uninfected red blood cells in both falciparum and vivax malaria (Oyong et al., 2018), but its contribution to uninfected red blood cell loss and anaemia in knowlesi malaria is not yet known. While platelet-red blood cell complexes contribute significantly to thrombocytopenia in knowlesi malaria, they comprise only a small minority of the total circulating red blood cell pool in knowlesi malaria (up to 1%) and are therefore unlikely to be a significant contributor to anaemia (Kho et al., 2018).

10. Conclusion

Plasmodium knowlesi is the commonest cause of zoonotic malaria, and the only zoonotic malaria to cause severe and fatal disease. The clinical spectrum and risk factors for severe disease and death have been well described in high-incidence settings in Malaysia. While known to be endemic across Southeast Asia, the true burden and spectrum of clinical disease outside Malaysia is not well characterized. As the human-only *Plasmodium* species decline in these regions, the burden of clinical disease from knowlesi malaria will likely increase. Enhanced molecular surveillance of *Plasmodium* species from both symptomatic and asymptomatic infections is required across Southeast Asia. The neonatal and maternal impacts of knowlesi malaria in pregnancy are poorly understood and require further study.

Parasite and host factors associated with the risk of infection, high parasite counts and severe disease need further characterization. While significant advances in our understanding of pathogenesis of human disease have been made over the last decade, further work is needed, particularly in understanding mechanisms of microvascular accumulation of parasitized red blood cells, impaired organ perfusion and organ dysfunction. Such understanding will guide the development of appropriate adjunctive therapies to complement existing strategies to improve clinical outcomes, including rapid and accurate diagnosis and prompt initiation of artemisinin-based antimalarial therapy.

Acknowledgements

This work was supported by the Australian National Health and Medical Research Council (grant numbers 1037304 and 1045156; fellowships to NMA [1042072], BEB [1088738]; MJG [1138860] and "Improving Health Outcomes in the Tropical North: A multidisciplinary collaboration (HOT NORTH)," [grant 1131932]), and the ZOOMAL project ("Evaluating zoonotic malaria and agricultural land use in Indonesia"; #LS-2019-116), Australian Centre for International Agricultural Research and Department of Foreign Affairs, Australian Government. The Sabah Malaria Research Program is supported by the US NIH.

References

Ahmed, A.M., Pinheiro, M.M., Divis, P.C., Siner, A., Zainudin, R., Wong, I.T., Lu, C.W., Singh-Khaira, S.K., Millar, S.B., Lynch, S., Willmann, M., Singh, B., Krishna, S., Cox-Singh, J., 2014. Disease progression in Plasmodium knowlesi malaria is linked to variation in invasion gene family members. PLoS Negl. Trop. Dis. 8 (8), e3086.

Ahmed, M.A., Fong, M.Y., Lau, Y.L., Yusof, R., 2016. Clustering and genetic differentiation of the normocyte binding protein (nbpxa) of Plasmodium knowlesi clinical isolates from Peninsular Malaysia and Malaysia Borneo. Malar. J. 15, 241.

Anstey, N.M., Grigg, M.J., 2019. Zoonotic malaria: the better you look, the more you find. J Infect Dis 219 (5), 679–681.

Anstey, N.M., William, T., Barber, B.E., 2020. In: Baron, E. (Ed.), Non-Falciparum Malaria: Plasmodium Knowlesi. Wolters Kluwer. UpToDate.

Assefa, S., Lim, C., Preston, M.D., Duffy, C.W., Nair, M.B., Adroub, S.A., Kadir, K.A., Goldberg, J.M., Neafsey, D.E., Divis, P., Clark, T.G., Duraisingh, M.T., Conway, D.J., Pain, A., Singh, B., 2015. Population genomic structure and adaptation in the zoonotic malaria parasite Plasmodium knowlesi. Proc. Natl. Acad. Sci. U. S. A. 112 (42), 13027–13032.

Aung, N.M., Nyein, P.P., Htut, T.Y., Htet, Z.W., Kyi, T.T., Anstey, N.M., Kyi, M.M., Hanson, J., 2018. Antibiotic therapy in adults with malaria (ANTHEM): high rate of clinically significant bacteremia in hospitalized adults diagnosed with falciparum malaria. Am. J. Trop. Med. Hyg. 99 (3), 688–696.

Barber, B.E., William, T., Jikal, M., Jilip, J., Dhararaj, P., Menon, J., Yeo, T.W., Anstey, N.M., 2011. Plasmodium knowlesi malaria in children. Emerg. Infect. Dis. 17 (5), 814–820.

Barber, B.E., William, T., Dhararaj, P., Anderios, F., Grigg, M.J., Yeo, T.W., Anstey, N.M., 2012. Epidemiology of Plasmodium knowlesi malaria in North-East Sabah, Malaysia: family clusters and wide age distribution. Malar. J. 11, 401.

Barber, B.E., William, T., Grigg, M.J., Menon, J., Auburn, S., Marfurt, J., Anstey, N.M., Yeo, T.W., 2013. A prospective comparative study of knowlesi, falciparum, and vivax malaria in Sabah, Malaysia: high proportion with severe disease from Plasmodium knowlesi and Plasmodium vivax but no mortality with early referral and artesunate therapy. Clin. Infect. Dis. 56 (3), 383–397.

Barber, B.E., Bird, E., Wilkes, C.S., William, T., Grigg, M.J., Paramaswaran, U., Menon, J., Jelip, J., Yeo, T.W., Anstey, N.M., 2015a. Plasmodium knowlesi malaria during pregnancy. J Infect Dis 211 (7), 1104–1110.

Barber, B.E., William, T., Grigg, M.J., Parameswaran, U., Piera, K.A., Price, R.N., Yeo, T.W., Anstey, N.M., 2015b. Parasite biomass-related inflammation, endothelial activation, microvascular dysfunction and disease severity in vivax malaria. PLoS Pathog. 11 (1), e1004558.

Barber, B.E., Grigg, M.J., William, T., Yeo, T.W., Anstey, N.M., 2016. Intravascular haemolysis with haemoglobinuria in a splenectomized patient with severe Plasmodium knowlesi malaria. Malar. J. 15, 462.

Barber, B.E., Grigg, M.J., William, T., Piera, K.A., Boyle, M.J., Yeo, T.W., Anstey, N.M., 2017a. Effects of aging on parasite biomass, inflammation, endothelial activation, microvascular dysfunction and disease severity in Plasmodium knowlesi and Plasmodium falciparum Malaria. J Infect Dis 215 (12), 1908–1917.

Barber, B.E., Grigg, M.J., William, T., Yeo, T.W., Anstey, N.M., 2017b. The treatment of Plasmodium knowlesi malaria. Trends Parasitol. 33 (3), 242–253.

Barber, B.E., Grigg, M.J., Piera, K.A., William, T., Cooper, D.J., Plewes, K., Dondorp, A.M., Yeo, T.W., Anstey, N.M., 2018a. Intravascular haemolysis in severe Plasmodium knowlesi malaria: association with endothelial activation, microvascular dysfunction, and acute kidney injury. Emerg. Microb. Infect. 7 (1), 106.

Barber, B.E., Russell, B., Grigg, M.J., Zhang, R., William, T., Amir, A., Lau, Y.L., Chatfield, M.D., Dondorp, A.M., Anstey, N.M., Yeo, T.W., 2018b. Reduced red blood cell deformability in Plasmodium knowlesi malaria. Blood Adv. 2 (4), 433–443.

Barber, B.E., Grigg, M.J., Piera, K., Amante, F.H., William, T., Boyle, M.J., Minigo, G., Dondorp, A.M., McCarthy, J.S., Anstey, N.M., 2019. Antiphosphatidylserine immunoglobulin M and immunoglobulin G antibodies are higher in vivax than falciparum malaria, and associated with early anemia in both species. J Infect Dis 220 (9), 1435–1443.

Barber, B.E., Grigg, M.J., Cooper, D.J., van Schalkwyk, D.A., William, T., Rajahram, G.S., Anstey, N.M., 2021a. Clinical management of *Plasmodium knowlesi* malaria. Adv. Parasitol. 113, 45–76.

Barber, B.E., Grigg, M.J., Piera, K.A., Chen, Y., William, T., Weinberg, J.B., Yeo, T.W., Anstey, N.M., 2021b. Endothelial glycocalyx degradation and disease severity in Plasmodium vivax and Plasmodium knowlesi malaria. Sci. Rep. 11 (1), 9741.

Barnwell, J.W., Howard, R.J., Coon, H.G., Miller, L.H., 1983. Splenic requirement for antigenic variation and expression of the variant antigen on the erythrocyte membrane in cloned Plasmodium knowlesi malaria. Infect. Immun. 40 (3), 985–994.

Benavente, E.D., de Sessions, P.F., Moon, R.W., Grainger, M., Holder, A.A., Blackman, M.J., Roper, C., Drakeley, C.J., Pain, A., Sutherland, C.J., Hibberd, M.L., Campino, S., Clark, T.G., 2018. A reference genome and methylome for the Plasmodium knowlesi A1-H.1 line. Int. J. Parasitol. 48 (3–4), 191–196.

Berendt, A.R., Simmons, D.L., Tansey, J., Newbold, C.I., Marsh, K., 1989. Intercellular adhesion molecule is an endothelial cell adhesion receptor for *Plasmodium falciparum*. Nature 341, 57–59.

Berkley, J.A., Bejon, P., Mwangi, T., Gwer, S., Maitland, K., Williams, T.N., Mohammed, S., Osier, F., Kinyanjui, S., Fegan, G., Lowe, B.S., English, M., Peshu, N., Marsh, K., Newton, C.R., 2009. HIV infection, malnutrition, and invasive bacterial infection among children with severe malaria. Clin. Infect. Dis. 49 (3), 336–343.

Bird, E.M., Parameswaran, U., William, T., Khoo, T.M., Grigg, M.J., Aziz, A., Marfurt, J., Yeo, T.W., Auburn, S., Anstey, N.M., Barber, B.E., 2016. Transfusion-transmitted severe Plasmodium knowlesi malaria in a splenectomized patient with beta-thalassaemia major in Sabah, Malaysia: a case report. Malar. J. 15 (1), 357.

Boo, Y.L., Lim, H.T., Chin, P.W., Lim, S.Y., Hoo, F.K., 2016. A case of severe Plasmodium knowlesi in a splenectomized patient. Parasitol. Int. 65 (1), 55–57.

Chang, C.Y., Pui, W.C., Kadir, K.A., Singh, B., 2018. Spontaneous splenic rupture in Plasmodium knowlesi malaria. Malar. J. 17 (1), 448.

Chen, L., Li, G., Lu, Y., Luo, Z., 2001. Histopathological changes of *Macaca mulatta* infected with Plasmodium knowlesi. Chin Med J (Engl) 114 (10), 1073–1077.

Cheo, S.W., Khoo, T.T., Tan, Y.A., Yeoh, W.C., Low, Q.J., 2020. A case of severe Plasmodium knowlesi malaria in a post-splenectomy patient. Med. J. Malaysia 75 (4), 447–449.

Chin, W., Contacos, P.G., Coatney, G.R., Kimball, H.R., 1965. A naturally acquired quotidian-type malaria in man transferable to monkeys. Science 149, 865.

Chin, W., Contacos, P.G., Collins, W.E., Jeter, M.H., Alpert, E., 1968. Experimental mosquito-transmission of Plasmodium knowlesi to man and monkey. Am. J. Trop. Med. Hyg. 17 (3), 355–358.

Ciuca, M., Ballif, L., Chelarescu, M., Lavrinenko, M., Zotta, E., 1937a. Contributions a l'étude de l'action pathogene de Pl. knowlesi pour l'homme (considerations sur l'immunite naturelle et l'immunité acquise contre cette espece de parasite). Bull. Soc. Pathol. Exot. 30, 305–315.

Ciuca, M., Tomescu, P., Badenski, G., Badenski, A., Terintianu, P.I.M., 1937b. Contribution à l'étude de la virulence du Pl. knowlesi chez l'homme. Caractères de la maladie et biologie du parasitie. Arch. Roum. Pathol. Exp. Microbiol. 10, 5–28.

Ciuca, M., Chelarescu, M., Sofletes, A., Constantinescu, P., Teritaenu, E., Cortez, P., Balanovschi, G., Ilies, M. (Eds.), 1955. Contribution experimentale a l'etude de l'immunite dans le paludisme. Editions Acad. Rep. Pop. Roumaine. L'Academie, Bucharest, Romania.

Coatney, G., Collins, W., Warren, M., Contacos, P., 1971. The Primate Malarias. US Departmnet of Health Eduation and Welfare, Bethesda, USA.

Cooper, D.J., Rajahram, G.S., William, T., Jelip, J., Mohammad, R., Benedict, J., Alaza, D.A., Malacova, E., Yeo, T.W., Grigg, M.J., Anstey, N.M., Barber, B.E., 2020. Plasmodium knowlesi malaria in Sabah, Malaysia, 2015–2017: ongoing increase in incidence despite near-elimination of the human-only plasmodium species. Clin. Infect. Dis. 70 (3), 361–367.

Cox-Singh, J., Davis, T.M., Lee, K.S., Shamsul, S.S., Matusop, A., Ratnam, S., Rahman, H.A., Conway, D.J., Singh, B., 2008. Plasmodium knowlesi malaria in humans is widely distributed and potentially life threatening. Clin. Infect. Dis. 46 (2), 165–171.

Cox-Singh, J., Hiu, J., Lucas, S.B., Divis, P.C., Zulkarnaen, M., Chandran, P., Wong, K.T., Adem, P., Zaki, S.R., Singh, B., Krishna, S., 2010. Severe malaria—a case of fatal Plasmodium knowlesi infection with post-mortem findings: a case report. Malar. J. 9 (1), 10.

Cox-Singh, J., Singh, B., Daneshvar, C., Planche, T., Parker-Williams, J., Krishna, S., 2011. Anti-inflammatory cytokines predominate in acute human Plasmodium knowlesi infections. PLoS One 6 (6), e20541.

Cuenca, P.R., Key, S., Jumail, A., Surendra, H., Ferguson, H.M., Drakeley, C.J., Fornace, K., 2021. Epidemiology of the zoonotic malaria Plasmodium knowlesi in changing landscapes. Adv. Parasitol. 113, 225–286.

Daneshvar, C., Davis, T.M., Cox-Singh, J., Rafa'ee, M.Z., Zakaria, S.K., Divis, P.C., Singh, B., 2009. Clinical and laboratory features of human Plasmodium knowlesi infection. Clin. Infect. Dis. 49 (6), 852–860.

Daneshvar, C., William, T., Davis, T.M.E., 2018. Clinical features and management of Plasmodium knowlesi infections in humans. Parasitology 145 (1), 18–31.

David, P., Handunnetti, S., Leech, J., 1988. Rosetting: a new cytoadherence property of malaria-infected erythrocytes. Am. J. Trop. Med. Hyg. 38, 289–297.

De Silva, J.R., Lau, Y.L., Fong, M.Y., 2017. Genetic clustering and polymorphism of the merozoite surface protein-3 of Plasmodium knowlesi clinical isolates from Peninsular Malaysia. Parasit. Vectors 10 (1), 2.

Divis, P.C., Singh, B., Anderios, F., Hisam, S., Matusop, A., Kocken, C.H., Assefa, S.A., Duffy, C.W., Conway, D.J., 2015. Admixture in humans of two divergent Plasmodium knowlesi populations associated with different macaque host species. PLoS Pathog. 11 (5), e1004888.

Divis, P.C., Lin, L.C., Rovie-Ryan, J.J., Kadir, K.A., Anderios, F., Hisam, S., Sharma, R.S., Singh, B., Conway, D.J., 2017. Three divergent subpopulations of the malaria parasite Plasmodium knowlesi. Emerg. Infect. Dis. 23 (4), 616–624.

Dondorp, A.M., Angus, B.J., Hardeman, M.R., Chotivanich, K.T., Silamut, K., Ruangveerayuth, R., Kager, P.A., White, N.J., Vreeken, J., 1997. Prognostic significance of reduced red blood cell deformability in severe falciparum malaria. Am. J. Trop. Med. Hyg. 57 (5), 507–511.

Dondorp, A.M., Angus, B.J., Chotivanich, K., Silamut, K., Ruangveerayuth, R., Hardeman, M.R., Kager, P.A., Vreeken, J., White, N.J., 1999. Red blood cell deformability as a predictor of anemia in severe falciparum malaria. Am. J. Trop. Med. Hyg. 60 (5), 733–737.

Dondorp, A.M., Desakorn, V., Pongtavornpinyo, W., Sahassananda, D., Silamut, K., Chotivanich, K., Newton, P.N., Pitisuttithum, P., Smithyman, A.M., White, N.J., Day, N.P., 2005. Estimation of the total parasite biomass in acute falciparum malaria from plasma PfHRP2. PLoS Med. 2, e204.

Dondorp, A.M., Lee, S.J., Faiz, M.A., Mishra, S., Price, R., Tjitra, E., Than, M., Htut, Y., Mohanty, S., Yunus, E.B., Rahman, R., Nosten, F., Anstey, N.M., Day, N.P., White, N.J., 2008. The relationship between age and the manifestations of and mortality associated with severe malaria. Clin. Infect. Dis. 47 (2), 151–157.

Douglas, N.M., Pontororing, G.J., Lampah, D.A., Yeo, T.W., Kenangalem, E., Poespoprodjo, J.R., Ralph, A.P., Bangs, M.J., Sugiarto, P., Anstey, N.M., Price, R.N., 2014. Mortality attributable to Plasmodium vivax malaria: a clinical audit from Papua, Indonesia. BMC Med. 12, 217.

Fatih, F.A., Siner, A., Ahmed, A., Woon, L.C., Craig, A.G., Singh, B., Krishna, S., Cox-Singh, J., 2012. Cytoadherence and virulence—the case of Plasmodium knowlesi malaria. Malar. J. 11, 33.

Fornace, K.M., Nuin, N.A., Betson, M., Grigg, M.J., William, T., Anstey, N.M., Yeo, T.W., Cox, J., Ying, L.T., Drakeley, C.J., 2016. Asymptomatic and submicroscopic carriage of Plasmodium knowlesi malaria in household and community members of clinical cases in Sabah, Malaysia. J Infect Dis 213 (5), 784–787.

Fornace, K.M., Brock, P.M., Abidin, T.R., Grignard, L., Herman, L.S., Chua, T.H., Daim, S., William, T., Patterson, C., Hall, T., Grigg, M.J., Anstey, N.M., Tetteh, K.K.A., Cox, J., Drakeley, C.J., 2019. Environmental risk factors and exposure to the zoonotic malaria parasite Plasmodium knowlesi across northern Sabah, Malaysia: a population-based cross-sectional survey. Lancet Planet. Health 3 (4), e179–e186.

Froeschl, G., Nothdurft, H.D., von Sonnenburg, F., Bretzel, G., Polanetz, R., Kroidl, I., Seilmaier, M., Orth, H.M., Jordan, S., Kremsner, P., Vygen-Bonnet, S., Pritsch, M., Hoelscher, M., Rothe, C., 2018. Retrospective clinical case series study in 2017 identifies Plasmodium knowlesi as most frequent Plasmodium species in returning travellers from Thailand to Germany. Euro Surveill. 23 (29), 1700619.

Ghinai, I., Cook, J., Hla, T.T., Htet, H.M., Hall, T., Lubis, I.N., Ghinai, R., Hesketh, T., Naung, Y., Lwin, M.M., Latt, T.S., Heymann, D.L., Sutherland, C.J., Drakeley, C., Field, N., 2017. Malaria epidemiology in Central Myanmar: identification of a multi-species asymptomatic reservoir of infection. Malar. J. 16 (1), 16.

Govindasamy, G., Barber, B.E., Ghani, S.A., William, T., Grigg, M.J., Borooah, S., Dhillon, B., Dondorp, A.M., Yeo, T.W., Anstey, N.M., Maude, R.J., 2016. Retinal changes in uncomplicated and severe Plasmodium knowlesi malaria. J Infect Dis 213 (9), 1476–1482.

Grigg, M.J., Barber, B.E., Marfurt, J., Imwong, M., William, T., Bird, E., Piera, K.A., Aziz, A., Boonyuen, U., Drakeley, C.J., Cox, J., White, N.J., Cheng, Q., Yeo, T.W., Auburn, S., Anstey, N.M., 2016a. Dihydrofolate-reductase mutations in Plasmodium knowlesi appear unrelated to selective drug pressure from putative human-to-human transmission in Sabah, Malaysia. PLoS One 11 (3), e0149519.

Grigg, M.J., William, T., Menon, J., Dhanaraj, P., Barber, B.E., Wilkes, C.S., von Seidlein, L., Rajahram, G.S., Pasay, C., McCarthy, J.S., Price, R.N., Anstey, N.M., Yeo, T.W., 2016b. Artesunate-mefloquine versus chloroquine for treatment of uncomplicated Plasmodium knowlesi malaria in Malaysia (ACT KNOW): an open-label, randomised controlled trial. Lancet Infect. Dis. 16 (2), 180–188.

Grigg, M.J., Cox, J., William, T., Jelip, J., Fornace, K.M., Brock, P.M., von Seidlein, L., Barber, B.E., Anstey, N.M., Yeo, T.W., Drakeley, C.J., 2017. Individual-level factors associated with the risk of acquiring human Plasmodium knowlesi malaria in Malaysia: a case-control study. Lancet Planet. Health 1 (3), e97–e104.

Grigg, M.J., William, T., Barber, B.E., Rajahram, G.S., Menon, J., Schimann, E., Piera, K., Wilkes, C.S., Patel, K., Chandna, A., Drakeley, C.J., Yeo, T.W., Anstey, N.M., 2018a. Age-related clinical spectrum of Plasmodium knowlesi malaria and predictors of severity. Clin. Infect. Dis. 67 (3), 350–359.

Grigg, M.J., William, T., Barber, B.E., Rajahram, G.S., Menon, J., Schimann, E., Wilkes, C.S., Patel, K., Chandna, A., Price, R.N., Yeo, T.W., Anstey, N.M., 2018b. Artemether-Lumefantrine versus chloroquine for the treatment of uncomplicated Plasmodium knowlesi malaria: an open-label randomized controlled trial CAN KNOW. Clin. Infect. Dis. 66 (2), 229–236.

Grignard, L., Shah, S., Chua, T.H., William, T., Drakeley, C.J., Fornace, K.M., 2019. Natural human infections with Plasmodium cynomolgi and other malaria species in an elimination setting in Sabah, Malaysia. J Infect Dis 220 (12), 1946–1949.

Hadley, T., Saul, A., Lamont, G., Hudson, D.E., Miller, L.H., Kidson, C., 1983. Resistance of Melanesian elliptocytes (ovalocytes) to invasion by Plasmodium knowlesi and Plasmodium falciparum malaria parasites in vitro. J. Clin. Invest. 71 (3), 780–782.

Hanson, J., Lee, S.J., Hossain, M.A., Anstey, N.M., Charunwatthana, P., Maude, R.J., Kingston, H.W., Mishra, S.K., Mohanty, S., Plewes, K., Piera, K., Hassan, M.U., Ghose, A., Faiz, M.A., White, N.J., Day, N.P., Dondorp, A.M., 2015. Microvascular obstruction and endothelial activation are independently associated with the clinical manifestations of severe falciparum malaria in adults: an observational study. BMC Med. 13, 122.

Howard, R.J., Barnwell, J.W., Kao, V., 1983. Antigenic variation of Plasmodium knowlesi malaria: identification of the variant antigen on infected erythrocytes. Proc. Natl. Acad. Sci. U. S. A. 80 (13), 4129–4133.

Hussin, N., Lim, Y.A., Goh, P.P., William, T., Jelip, J., Mudin, R.N., 2020. Updates on malaria incidence and profile in Malaysia from 2013 to 2017. Malar. J. 19 (1), 55.

Imai, N., White, M.T., Ghani, A.C., Drakeley, C.J., 2014. Transmission and control of Plasmodium knowlesi: a mathematical modelling study. PLoS Negl. Trop. Dis. 8 (7), e2978.

Imwong, M., Madmanee, W., Suwannasin, K., Kunasol, C., Peto, T.J., Tripura, R., von Seidlein, L., Nguon, C., Davoeung, C., Day, N.P.J., Dondorp, A.M., White, N.J., 2019. Asymptomatic natural human infections with the simian malaria parasites Plasmodium cynomolgi and Plasmodium knowlesi. J Infect Dis 219 (5), 695–702.

Jakeman, G.N., Saul, A., Hogarth, W.L., Collins, W.E., 1999. Anaemia of acute malaria infections in non-immune patients primarily results from destruction of uninfected erythrocytes. Parasitology 119 (Pt 2), 127–133.

Jongwutiwes, S., Buppan, P., Kosuvin, R., Seethamchai, S., Pattanawong, U., Sirichaisinthop, J., Putaporntip, C., 2011. Plasmodium knowlesi malaria in humans and macaques, Thailand. Emerg. Infect. Dis. 17 (10), 1799–1806.

Kaul, D., Roth, E., Nagel, R., 1991. Rosetting of *Plasmodium falciparum* infected red blood cells with uninfected red blood cells enhances microvascular obstruction under flow conditions. Blood 78, 812–819.

Kho, S., Barber, B.E., Johar, E., Andries, B., Poespoprodjo, J.R., Kenangalem, E., Piera, K.A., Ehmann, A., Price, R.N., William, T., Woodberry, T., Foote, S., Minigo, G., Yeo, T.W., Grigg, M.J., Anstey, N.M., McMorran, B.J., 2018. Platelets kill circulating parasites of all major Plasmodium species in human malaria. Blood 132 (12), 1332–1344.

Kho, S., Minigo, G., Andries, B., Leonardo, L., Prayoga, P., Poespoprodjo, J.R., Kenangalem, E., Price, R.N., Woodberry, T., Anstey, N.M., Yeo, T.W., 2019. Circulating neutrophil extracellular traps and neutrophil activation are increased in proportion to disease severity in human malaria. J Infect Dis 219 (12), 1994–2004.

Kho, S., Qotrunnada, L., Leonardo, L., Andries, B., Wardani, P.A.I., Fricot, A., Henry, B., Hardy, D., Margyaningsih, N.I., Apriyanti, D., Puspitasari, A.M., Prayoga, P., Trianty, L., Kenangalem, E., Chretien, F., Brousse, V., Safeukui, I., Del Portillo, H.A., Fernandez-Becerra, C., Meibalan, E., Marti, M., Price, R.N., Woodberry, T., Ndour, P.A., Russell, B.M., Yeo, T.W., Minigo, G., Noviyanti, R., Poespoprodjo, J.R., Siregar, N.C., Buffet, P.A., Anstey, N.M., 2021a. Evaluation of splenic accumulation and colocalization of immature reticulocytes and Plasmodium vivax in asymptomatic malaria: a prospective human splenectomy study. PLoS Med. 18 (5), e1003632.

Kho, S., Qotrunnada, L., Leonardo, L., Andries, B., Wardani, P.A.I., Fricot, A., Henry, B., Hardy, D., Margyaningsih, N.I., Apriyanti, D., Puspitasari, A.M., Prayoga, P., Trianty, L., Kenangalem, E., Chretien, F., Safeukui, I., Del Portillo, H.A., Fernandez-Becerra, C., Meibalan, E., Marti, M., Price, R.N., Woodberry, T., Ndour, P.A., Russell, B.M., Yeo, T.W., Minigo, G., Noviyanti, R., Poespoprodjo, J.R., Siregar, N.C., Buffet, P.A., Anstey, N.M., 2021b. Hidden biomass of intact malaria parasites in the human spleen. N. Engl. J. Med. 384 (21), 2067–2069.

Knisely, M., Stratman-Thomas, W., 1945. Knowlesi malaria in monkeys: microscopic pathological circulatory physiology of rhesus monkeys during acute Plasmodium knowlesi malaria. J. Natl. Malar. Soc. 4, 285–300.

Knisely, M., Stratman-Thomas, W.K., 1948. Microscopic observations of intravascular agglutination of red cells and consequent sludging of blood in rhesus monkeys infected with knowlesi malaria. Anat. Rec. 101, 701.

Knowles, R., Das Gupta, B., 1932. A study of monkey-malaria and its experimental transmission to man. Ind. Med. Gaz. 67, 301–321.

Korir, C.C., Galinski, M.R., 2006. Proteomic studies of Plasmodium knowlesi SICA variant antigens demonstrate their relationship with P. falciparum EMP1. Infect. Genet. Evol. 6 (1), 75–79.

Lee, K.S., Cox-Singh, J., Singh, B., 2009. Morphological features and differential counts of Plasmodium knowlesi parasites in naturally acquired human infections. Malar. J. 8, 73.

Lee, K.S., Divis, P.C., Zakaria, S.K., Matusop, A., Julin, R.A., Conway, D.J., Cox-Singh, J., Singh, B., 2011. Plasmodium knowlesi: reservoir hosts and tracking the emergence in humans and macaques. PLoS Pathog. 7 (4), e1002015.

Leslie, T., Briceno, M., Mayan, I., Mohammed, N., Klinkenberg, E., Sibley, C.H., Whitty, C.J., Rowland, M., 2010. The impact of phenotypic and genotypic G6PD deficiency on risk of plasmodium vivax infection: a case-control study amongst Afghan refugees in Pakistan. PLoS Med. 7 (5), e1000283.

Lim, C., Hansen, E., DeSimone, T.M., Moreno, Y., Junker, K., Bei, A., Brugnara, C., Buckee, C.O., Duraisingh, M.T., 2013. Expansion of host cellular niche can drive adaptation of a zoonotic malaria parasite to humans. Nat. Commun. 4, 1638.

Lim, K.L., Amir, A., Lau, Y.L., Fong, M.Y., 2017. The Duffy binding protein (PkDBPalphaII) of Plasmodium knowlesi from Peninsular Malaysia and Malaysian Borneo show different binding activity level to human erythrocytes. Malar. J. 16 (1), 331.

Liu, B., Blanch, A.J., Namvar, A., Carmo, O., Tiash, S., Andrew, D., Hanssen, E., Rajagopal, V., Dixon, M.W.A., Tilley, L., 2019. Multimodal analysis of Plasmodium knowlesi-infected erythrocytes reveals large invaginations, swelling of the host cell, and rheological defects. Cell. Microbiol. 21 (5), e13005.

Loughland, J.R., Woodberry, T., Oyong, D., Piera, K.A., Amante, F.H., Barber, B.E., Grigg, M.J., William, T., Engwerda, C.R., Anstey, N.M., McCarthy, J.S.,

Boyle, M.J., Minigo, G., 2021. Reduced circulating dendritic cells in acute Plasmodium knowlesi and Plasmodium falciparum malaria despite elevated plasma Flt3 ligand levels. Malar. J. 20 (1), 97.

Lubis, I.N.D., Wijaya, H., Lubis, M., Lubis, C.P., Divis, P.C.S., Beshir, K.B., Sutherland, C.J., 2017. Contribution of Plasmodium knowlesi to multispecies human malaria infections in North Sumatera, Indonesia. J Infect Dis 215 (7), 1148–1155.

Mackinnon, M.J., Mwangi, T.W., Snow, R.W., Marsh, K., Williams, T.N., 2005. Heritability of malaria in Africa. PLoS Med. 2 (12), e340.

MacPherson, G.G., Warrell, M.J., White, N.J., Looareesuwan, S., Warrell, D.A., 1985. Human cerebral malaria. A quantitative ultrastructural analysis of parasitized erythrocyte sequestration. Am. J. Pathol. 119 (3), 385–401.

Manjurano, A., Sepulveda, N., Nadjm, B., Mtove, G., Wangai, H., Maxwell, C., Olomi, R., Reyburn, H., Riley, E.M., Drakeley, C.J., Clark, T.G., Malaria, G.E.N.C., 2015. African glucose-6-phosphate dehydrogenase alleles associated with protection from severe malaria in heterozygous females in Tanzania. PLoS Genet. 11 (2), e1004960.

Marchand, R.P., Culleton, R., Maeno, Y., Quang, N.T., Nakazawa, S., 2011. Co-infections of Plasmodium knowlesi, P. falciparum, and P. vivax among humans and Anopheles dirus mosquitoes, Southern Vietnam. Emerg. Infect. Dis. 17 (7), 1232–1239.

Marchiafava, E., Bignami, A., 1894. On Summer-Autumnal Malaria Fevers. The New Sydenham Society, London.

Marsh, K., Forster, D., Waruiru, C., Mwangi, I., Winstanley, M., Marsh, V., Newton, C., Winstanley, P., Warn, P., Peshu, N., et al., 1995. Indicators of life-threatening malaria in African children. N. Engl. J. Med. 332 (21), 1399–1404.

Milam, D.F., Coggleshall, L.T., 1938. Duration of *Plasmodium knowlesi* infections in man. Am. J. Trop. Med. Hyg. 18, 331–338.

Milam, D.F., Kusch, E., 1938. Observations on *Plasmodium knowlesi* malaria in general paresis. South. Med. J. 31, 947–949.

Miller, L.H., Chien, S., 1971. Density distribution of red cells infected by Plasmodium knowlesi and Plasmodium coatneyi. Exp. Parasitol. 29 (3), 451–456.

Miller, L.H., Fremount, H.N., Luse, S.A., 1971a. Deep vascular schizogony of Plasmodium knowlesi in *Macaca mulatta*. Distribution in organs and ultrastructure of parasitized red cells. Am. J. Trop. Med. Hyg. 20 (6), 816–824.

Miller, L.H., Usami, S., Chien, S., 1971b. Alteration in the rheologic properties of Plasmodium knowlesi—infected red cells. A possible mechanism for capillary obstruction. J. Clin. Invest. 50 (7), 1451–1455.

Moon, R.W., Sharaf, H., Hastings, C.H., Ho, Y.S., Nair, M.B., Rchiad, Z., Knuepfer, E., Ramaprasad, A., Mohring, F., Amir, A., Yusuf, N.A., Hall, J., Almond, N., Lau, Y.L., Pain, A., Blackman, M.J., Holder, A.A., 2016. Normocyte-binding protein required for human erythrocyte invasion by the zoonotic malaria parasite Plasmodium knowlesi. Proc. Natl. Acad. Sci. U. S. A. 113 (26), 7231–7236.

Muh, F., Ahmed, M.A., Han, J.H., Nyunt, M.H., Lee, S.K., Lau, Y.L., Kaneko, O., Han, E.T., 2018. Cross-species analysis of apical asparagine-rich protein of Plasmodium vivax and Plasmodium knowlesi. Sci. Rep. 8 (1), 5781.

Muh, F., Kim, N., Nyunt, M.H., Firdaus, E.R., Han, J.H., Hoque, M.R., Lee, S.K., Park, J.H., Moon, R.W., Lau, Y.L., Kaneko, O., Han, E.T., 2020. Cross-species reactivity of antibodies against Plasmodium vivax blood-stage antigens to Plasmodium knowlesi. PLoS Negl. Trop. Dis. 14 (6), e0008323.

Napier, L.E., Campbell, H.G.M., 1932. Observations on a plasmodium infection which causes haemoglobinuria in certain species of monkey. Ind. Med. Gaz. 67 (5), 246–249.

Nicol, W.D., 1935. Monkey malaria in GPI. Br. Med. J. 2 (3902), 760.

Noordin, N.R., Lee, P.Y., Mohd Bukhari, F.D., Fong, M.Y., Abdul Hamid, M.H., Jelip, J., Mudin, R.N., Lau, Y.L., 2020. Prevalence of asymptomatic and/or low-density malaria infection among high-risk groups in peninsular Malaysia. Am. J. Trop. Med. Hyg. 103 (3), 1107–1110.

Nyein, P.P., Aung, N.M., Kyi, T.T., Htet, Z.W., Anstey, N.M., Kyi, M.M., Hanson, J., 2016. High frequency of clinically significant bacteremia in adults hospitalized with falciparum malaria. Open Forum Infect. Dis. 3 (1), ofw028.

Odedra, A., Webb, L., Marquart, L., Britton, L.J., Chalon, S., Moehrle, J.J., Anstey, N.M., William, T., Grigg, M.J., Lalloo, D.G., Barber, B.E., McCarthy, J.S., 2020. Liver function test abnormalities in experimental and clinical Plasmodium vivax infection. Am. J. Trop. Med. Hyg. 103 (5), 1910–1917.

Onditi, F.I., Nyamongo, O.W., Omwandho, C.O., Maina, N.W., Maloba, F., Farah, I.O., King, C.L., Moore, J.M., Ozwara, H.S., 2015. Parasite accumulation in placenta of non-immune baboons during Plasmodium knowlesi infection. Malar. J. 14, 118.

Oyong, D.A., Kenangalem, E., Poespoprodjo, J.R., Beeson, J.G., Anstey, N.M., Price, R.N., Boyle, M.J., 2018. Loss of complement regulatory proteins on uninfected erythrocytes in vivax and falciparum malaria anemia. JCI Insight 3 (22), e124854.

Ozbilgin, A., Cavus, I., Yildirim, A., Gunduz, C., 2016. The first monkey malaria in Turkey: a case of Plasmodium knowlesi. Mikrobiyol. Bul. 50 (3), 484–490.

Pain, A., Ferguson, D.J., Kai, O., Urban, B.C., Lowe, B., Marsh, K., Roberts, D.J., 2001. Platelet-mediated clumping of Plasmodium falciparum-infected erythrocytes is a common adhesive phenotype and is associated with severe malaria. Proc. Natl. Acad. Sci. U. S. A. 98, 1805–1810.

Paquette, A.M., Harahap, A., Laosombat, V., Patnode, J.M., Satyagraha, A., Sudoyo, H., Thompson, M.K., Yusoff, N.M., Wilder, J.A., 2015. The evolutionary origins of Southeast Asian Ovalocytosis. Infect. Genet. Evol. 34, 153–159.

Plewes, K., Kingston, H.W.F., Ghose, A., Maude, R.J., Herdman, M.T., Leopold, S.J., Ishioka, H., Hasan, M.M.U., Haider, M.S., Alam, S., Piera, K.A., Charunwatthana, P., Silamut, K., Yeo, T.W., Faiz, M.A., Lee, S.J., Mukaka, M., Turner, G.D.H., Anstey, N.M., Jackson Roberts 2nd, L., White, N.J., Day, N.P.J., Hossain, M.A., Dondorp, A.M., 2017. Cell-free hemoglobin mediated oxidative stress is associated with acute kidney injury and renal replacement therapy in severe falciparum malaria: an observational study. BMC Infect. Dis. 17 (1), 313.

Plewes, K., Kingston, H.W.F., Ghose, A., Wattanakul, T., Hassan, M.M.U., Haider, M.S., Dutta, P.K., Islam, M.A., Alam, S., Jahangir, S.M., Zahed, A.S.M., Sattar, M.A., Chowdhury, M.A.H., Herdman, M.T., Leopold, S.J., Ishioka, H., Piera, K.A., Charunwatthana, P., Silamut, K., Yeo, T.W., Lee, S.J., Mukaka, M., Maude, R.J., Turner, G.D.H., Faiz, M.A., Tarning, J., Oates, J.A., Anstey, N.M., White, N.J., Day, N.P.J., Hossain, M.A., Roberts Ii, L.J., Dondorp, A.M., 2018. Acetaminophen as a renoprotective adjunctive treatment in patients with severe and moderately severe falciparum malaria: a randomized, controlled, open-label trial. Clin. Infect. Dis. 67 (7), 991–999.

Poespoprodjo, J.R., Fobia, W., Kenangalem, E., Hasanuddin, A., Sugiarto, P., Tjitra, E., Anstey, N.M., Price, R.N., 2011. Highly effective therapy for maternal malaria associated with a lower risk of vertical transmission. J Infect Dis 204, 1613–1619.

Putaporntip, C., Kuamsab, N., Jongwutiwes, S., 2016. Sequence diversity and positive selection at the Duffy-binding protein genes of Plasmodium knowlesi and P. cynomolgi: analysis of the complete coding sequences of Thai isolates. Infect. Genet. Evol. 44, 367–375.

Rabelink, T.J., de Zeeuw, D., 2015. The glycocalyx—linking albuminuria with renal and cardiovascular disease. Nat. Rev. Nephrol. 11 (11), 667–676.

Rajahram, G.S., Barber, B.E., William, T., Menon, J., Anstey, N.M., Yeo, T.W., 2012. Deaths due to Plasmodium knowlesi malaria in Sabah, Malaysia: association with reporting as Plasmodium malariae and delayed parenteral artesunate. Malar. J. 11 (1), 284.

Rajahram, G.S., Barber, B.E., Yeo, T.W., Tan, W.W., William, T., 2013. Case report: fatal Plasmodium knowlesi malaria following an atypical clinical presentation and delayed diagnosis. Med. J. Malaysia 68 (1), 71–72.

Rajahram, G.S., Barber, B.E., William, T., Grigg, M.J., Menon, J., Yeo, T.W., Anstey, N.M., 2016. Falling Plasmodium knowlesi malaria death rate among adults despite rising incidence, Sabah, Malaysia, 2010–2014. Emerg. Infect. Dis. 22 (1), 41–48.

Rajahram, G.S., Cooper, D.J., William, T., Grigg, M.J., Anstey, N.M., Barber, B.E., 2019. Deaths from Plasmodium knowlesi malaria: case series and systematic review. Clin. Infect. Dis. 69 (10), 1703–1711.

Reeder, B.J., Wilson, M.T., 2005. Hemoglobin and myoglobin associated oxidative stress: from molecular mechanisms to disease states. Curr. Med. Chem. 12 (23), 2741–2751.

Shearer, F.M., Huang, Z., Weiss, D.J., Wiebe, A., Gibson, H.S., Battle, K.E., Pigott, D.M., Brady, O.J., Putaporntip, C., Jongwutiwes, S., Lau, Y.L., Manske, M., Amato, R., Elyazar, I.R., Vythilingam, I., Bhatt, S., Gething, P.W., Singh, B., Golding, N., Hay, S.I., Moyes, C.L., 2016. Estimating geographical variation in the risk of zoonotic Plasmodium knowlesi infection in countries eliminating malaria. PLoS Negl. Trop. Dis. 10 (8), e0004915.

Siner, A., Liew, S.T., Kadir, K.A., Mohamad, D.S.A., Thomas, F.K., Zulkarnaen, M., Singh, B., 2017. Absence of Plasmodium inui and Plasmodium cynomolgi, but detection of Plasmodium knowlesi and Plasmodium vivax infections in asymptomatic humans in the Betong division of Sarawak, Malaysian Borneo. Malar. J. 16 (1), 417.

Singh, B., Daneshvar, C., 2013. Human infections and detection of Plasmodium knowlesi. Clin. Microbiol. Rev. 26 (2), 165–184.

Singh, B., Lee, K., Matusop, A., Radhakrishnan, A., Shamsul, S., Cox-Singh, J., Conway, T., 2004. A large focus of naturally acquired *Plasmodium knowlesi* infections in human beings. Lancet 363, 1017–1024.

Spangler, W.L., Gribble, D., Abildgaard, C., Harrison, J., 1978. Plasmodium knowlesi malaria in the Rhesus monkey. Vet. Pathol. 15 (1), 83–91.

Su, X., Heatwole, V., Wertheimer, S., 1995. The large diverse gene family var encodes proteins involved in cytoadherence and antigenic variation of *Plasmodium falciparum*-infected erythrocytes. Cell 82, 89–100.

Takaya, S., Kutsuna, S., Suzuki, T., Komaki-Yasuda, K., Kano, S., Ohmagari, N., 2018. Case report: Plasmodium knowlesi infection with rhabdomyolysis in a Japanese traveler to Palawan, the Philippines. Am. J. Trop. Med. Hyg. 99 (4), 967–969.

Taylor, T.E., Fu, W.J., Carr, R.A., Whitten, R.O., Mueller, J.S., Fosiko, N.G., Lewallen, S., Liomba, N.G., Molyneux, M.E., 2004. Differentiating the pathologies of cerebral malaria by postmortem parasite counts. Nat. Med. 10, 143–145.

Traipattanakul, J., Changpradub, D., Trakulhun, K., Phiboonbanakit, D., Mungthin, M., 2014. A frst case of Plasmodium knowlesi malaria in Phramongkutklao hospital. J. Infect. Dis. Antimicrob. Agents 31, 91–100.

Turner, G.D., Morrison, H., Jones, M., Davis, T.M., Looareesuwan, S., Buley, I.D., Gatter, K.C., Newbold, C.I., Pukritayakamee, S., Nagachinta, B., et al., 1994. An immunohistochemical study of the pathology of fatal malaria. Evidence for widespread endothelial activation and a potential role for intercellular adhesion molecule-1 in cerebral sequestration. Am. J. Pathol. 145, 1057–1069.

Udomsangpetch, R., Wahlin, B., Carlson, J., 1989. *Plasmodium falciparum*-infected erythrocytes form spontaneous erythrocyte rosettes. J. Exp. Med. 169, 1835–1840.

van Rooyen, C.E., Pile, G.R., 1935. Observations on infection by Plasmodium knowlesi (ape malaria) in the treatment of general paralysis of the insane. Br. Med. J. 2 (3901), 662–666.

White, N.J., Turner, G.D., Day, N.P., Dondorp, A.M., 2013. Lethal malaria: Marchiafava and Bignami were right. J Infect Dis 208 (2), 192–198.

WHO, 2011. Haemoglobin Concentrations for the Diagnosis of Anaemia and Assessment of Severity 2011. World Health Organization, Geneva. http://www.who.int/vmnis/indicators/haemoglobin.pdf.

WHO, 2014. Severe and complicated malaria. Trop. Med. Int. Health 19, 7–131.

WHO, 2017. Expert consultation on Plasmodium knowlesi Malaria to guide malaria elimination strategies, Kota Kinabalu, Malaysia,1–2 March 2017: meeting report. Manila. https://apps.who.int/iris/handle/10665/259130.

WHO, 2020. World malaria report. World Health Organization, Geneva.

William, T., Menon, J., Rajahram, G., Chan, L., Ma, G., Donaldson, S., Khoo, S., Frederick, C., Jelip, J., Anstey, N.M., Yeo, T.W., 2011. Severe Plasmodium knowlesi malaria in a tertiary care hospital, Sabah, Malaysia. Emerg. Infect. Dis. 17 (7), 1248–1255.

William, T., Rahman, H.A., Jelip, J., Ibrahim, M.Y., Menon, J., Grigg, M.J., Yeo, T.W., Anstey, N.M., Barber, B.E., 2013. Increasing incidence of Plasmodium knowlesi malaria following control of P. falciparum and P. vivax Malaria in Sabah, Malaysia. PLoS Negl. Trop. Dis. 7 (1), e2026.

William, T., Jelip, J., Menon, J., Anderios, F., Mohammad, R., Awang Mohammad, T.A., Grigg, M.J., Yeo, T.W., Anstey, N.M., Barber, B.E., 2014. Changing epidemiology of malaria in Sabah, Malaysia: increasing incidence of Plasmodium knowlesi. Malar. J. 13, 390.

Willmann, M., Ahmed, A., Siner, A., Wong, I.T., Woon, L.C., Singh, B., Krishna, S., Cox-Singh, J., 2012. Laboratory markers of disease severity in Plasmodium knowlesi infection: a case control study. Malar. J. 11, 363.

Woodford, J., Shanks, G.D., Griffin, P., Chalon, S., McCarthy, J.S., 2018. The dynamics of liver function test abnormalities after malaria infection: a retrospective observational study. Am. J. Trop. Med. Hyg. 98 (4), 1113–1119.

Wyss, K., Wangdahl, A., Vesterlund, M., Hammar, U., Dashti, S., Naucler, P., Farnert, A., 2017. Obesity and diabetes as risk factors for severe Plasmodium falciparum malaria: results from a Swedish Nationwide Study. Clin. Infect. Dis. 65 (6), 949–958.

Yap, N.J., Goh, X.T., Koehler, A.V., William, T., Yeo, T.W., Vythilingam, I., Gasser, R.B., Lim, Y.A.L., 2017. Genetic diversity in the C-terminus of merozoite surface protein 1 among Plasmodium knowlesi isolates from Selangor and Sabah Borneo, Malaysia. Infect. Genet. Evol. 54, 39–46.

Yeo, T.W., Lampah, D.A., Gitawati, R., Tjitra, E., Kenangalem, E., McNeil, Y.R., Darcy, C.J., Granger, D.L., Weinberg, J.B., Lopansri, B.K., Price, R.N., Duffull, S.B., Celermajer, D.S., Anstey, N.M., 2007. Impaired nitric oxide bioavailability and L-arginine reversible endothelial dysfunction in adults with falciparum malaria. J. Exp. Med. 204 (11), 2693–2704.

Yeo, T.W., Lampah, D.A., Gitawati, R., Tjitra, E., Kenangalem, E., Piera, K., Price, R., Duffull, S.B., Celermajer, D.S., Anstey, N., 2008. Angiopoietin-2 is associated with decreased endothelial nitric oxide and poor clinical outcome in severe falciparum malaria. Proc. Natl. Acad. Sci. U. S. A. 105, 17097–17102.

Yeo, T.W., Lampah, D.A., Tjitra, E., Gitawati, R., Kenangalem, E., Piera, K., Granger, D.L., Lopansri, B.K., Weinberg, J.B., Price, R.N., Duffull, S.B., Celermajer, D.S., Anstey, N.M., 2009. Relationship of cell-free hemoglobin to impaired endothelial nitric oxide bioavailability and perfusion in severe falciparum malaria. J Infect Dis 200 (10), 1522–1529.

Yeo, T.W., Lampah, D.A., Tjitra, E., Gitawati, R., Darcy, C.J., Jones, C., Kenangalem, E., McNeil, Y.R., Granger, D.L., Lopansri, B.K., Weinberg, J.B., Price, R.N., Duffull, S.B., Celermajer, D.S., Anstey, N.M., 2010. Increased asymmetric dimethylarginine in severe falciparum malaria: association with impaired nitric oxide bioavailability and fatal outcome. PLoS Pathog. 6 (4), e1000868.

Yeo, T.W., Lampah, D.A., Kenangalem, E., Tjitra, E., Price, R.N., Anstey, N.M., 2013. Impaired skeletal muscle microvascular function and increased skeletal muscle oxygen consumption in severe falciparum malaria. J Infect Dis 207 (3), 528–536.

Yeo, T.W., Lampah, D.A., Kenangalem, E., Tjitra, E., Weinberg, J.B., Granger, D.L., Price, R.N., Anstey, N.M., 2014. Decreased endothelial nitric oxide bioavailability, impaired microvascular function, and increased tissue oxygen consumption in children with falciparum malaria. J Infect Dis 210 (10), 1627–1632.

Yeo, T.W., Bush, P.A., Chen, Y., Young, S.P., Zhang, H., Millington, D.S., Granger, D.L., Mwaikambo, E.D., Anstey, N.M., Weinberg, J.B., 2019a. Glycocalyx breakdown is increased in African children with cerebral and uncomplicated falciparum malaria. FASEB J. 33 (12), 14185–14193.

Yeo, T.W., Weinberg, J.B., Lampah, D.A., Kenangalem, E., Bush, P., Chen, Y., Price, R.N., Young, S., Zhang, H.Y., Millington, D., Granger, D.L., Anstey, N.M., 2019b. Glycocalyx breakdown is associated with severe disease and fatal outcome in Plasmodium falciparum malaria. Clin. Infect. Dis. 69 (10), 1712–1720.

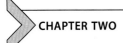

CHAPTER TWO

Clinical management of *Plasmodium knowlesi* malaria

Bridget E. Barber[a,b,*], Matthew J. Grigg[b], Daniel J. Cooper[b,c], Donelly A. van Schalkwyk[d], Timothy William[e,f], Giri S. Rajahram[f,g], and Nicholas M. Anstey[b]

[a]QIMR Berghofer Medical Research Institute, Brisbane, QLD, Australia
[b]Menzies School of Health Research, Charles Darwin University, Darwin, NT, Australia
[c]Department of Medicine, University of Cambridge School of Medicine, Cambridge, United Kingdom
[d]London School of Hygiene and Tropical Medicine, London, United Kingdom
[e]Gleneagles Medical Centre, Kota Kinabalu, Malaysia
[f]Clinical Research Centre, Queen Elizabeth Hospital 1, Kota Kinabalu, Malaysia
[g]Queen Elizabeth Hospital 2, Kota Kinabalu, Malaysia
*Corresponding author: e-mail address: bridget.barber@qimrberghofer.edu.au

Contents

1. Introduction	46
2. Diagnosis of *Plasmodium knowlesi*	46
3. *In vitro* susceptibility of *P. knowlesi* to antimalarial agents	47
4. Drug resistance mutations	55
5. Treatment of uncomplicated knowlesi malaria	56
5.1 Artemisinin combination treatment (ACT)	56
5.2 Chloroquine	61
5.3 Other agents	62
5.4 Primaquine	62
6. Clinical management of severe knowlesi malaria	63
6.1 Intravenous artesunate	63
6.2 Paracetamol as a renoprotective agent	65
6.3 Other adjunctive and supportive treatment	67
7. Treatment of knowlesi malaria in children	67
8. Treatment of knowlesi malaria in pregnancy	68
9. Conclusions	69
Acknowledgements	70
References	70

Abstract

The zoonotic parasite *Plasmodium knowlesi* has emerged as an important cause of human malaria in parts of Southeast Asia. The parasite is indistinguishable by microscopy from the more benign *P. malariae*, but can result in high parasitaemias with multiorgan failure, and deaths have been reported. Recognition of severe knowlesi malaria, and prompt initiation of effective therapy is therefore essential to prevent adverse outcomes. Here we review all studies reporting treatment of uncomplicated and severe knowlesi malaria. We report that although chloroquine is effective for the treatment of uncomplicated knowlesi malaria, artemisinin combination treatment is associated with faster parasite clearance times and lower rates of anaemia during follow-up, and should be considered the treatment of choice, particularly given the risk of administering chloroquine to drug-resistant *P. vivax* or *P. falciparum* misdiagnosed as *P. knowlesi* malaria in co-endemic areas. For severe knowlesi malaria, intravenous artesunate has been shown to be highly effective and associated with reduced case-fatality rates, and should be commenced without delay. Regular paracetamol may also be considered for patients with severe knowlesi malaria or for those with acute kidney injury, to attenuate the renal damage resulting from haemolysis-induced lipid peroxidation.

1. Introduction

The zoonotic parasite *Plasmodium knowlesi* is endemic throughout Southeast Asia, with human cases reported in all countries where both the *Anopheles leucosphyrus* mosquito vector and the simian hosts reside. In Malaysia *P. knowlesi* accounts for nearly all cases of human malaria, with over 3000 cases reported in 2019 (World Health Organization, 2020). The 24 h asexual replication cycle of *P. knowlesi* is the shortest of any human malaria, and high parasitaemias can develop rapidly. In adults the rate of severe disease from *P. knowlesi* is at least as high as that of falciparum malaria (Barber et al., 2013a), and fatal cases have been reported (Rajahram et al., 2019). Prompt initiation of effective treatment is therefore essential to avoid poor outcomes. This review discusses the treatment of uncomplicated and severe knowlesi malaria, highlighting the benefits of artemisinin–combination therapy (ACT) for uncomplicated knowlesi malaria, and the importance of prompt initiation of intravenous artesunate for all severe malaria regardless of species. The role of adjunctive paracetamol in severe knowlesi malaria is also discussed.

2. Diagnosis of *Plasmodium knowlesi*

The diagnosis of *P. knowlesi* is limited by the difficulties with distinguishing the parasite from other *Plasmodium* species by microscopy. Ring forms of *P. knowlesi* may resemble those of *P. falciparum*, while *P. knowlesi* trophozoites and schizonts are nearly indistinguishable from *P. malariae* (Lee et al., 2009). Misidentification of *P. knowlesi* as *P. vivax*, and vice-versa, is also common in co-endemic areas (Barber et al., 2013c; Coutrier et al., 2018). Misdiagnosis of *P. knowlesi* as the more benign *P. malariae* has been associated with failure to recognise severe disease, with subsequent delay in administering parenteral therapy (Rajahram et al., 2012). For this reason, in areas where *P. knowlesi* is prevalent, parasites resembling *P. malariae* should be reported as *P. knowlesi*. Rapid diagnostic tests evaluated to date are insensitive for *P. knowlesi*, particularly at low parasitaemias, and are not able to distinguish *P. knowlesi* from other non-falciparum species (Barber et al., 2013b; Grigg et al., 2014). Given these limitations of microscopy and rapid diagnostic tests, species confirmation using molecular methods such as PCR should be performed where possible (Grigg et al., 2021). In addition to facilitating accurate reporting and surveillance, PCR confirmation of species enables any patient with *P. vivax* misdiagnosed with *P. knowlesi* to receive appropriate anti-hypnozoital treatment with primaquine for prevention of relapses.

3. *In vitro* susceptibility of *P. knowlesi* to antimalarial agents

The recent adaption of *P. knowlesi* to long-term *in vitro* culture (Grüring et al., 2014; Lim et al., 2013; Moon et al., 2013) has enabled the detailed evaluation of the susceptibility of this species to both approved and investigational antimalarial agents. Importantly, *P. knowlesi* is closely related phylogenetically to *P. vivax* and other non-falciparum species (Loy et al., 2017), and thus susceptibility of *P. knowlesi* to antimalarial agents may be indicative of the drug susceptibility of other non-falciparum *Plasmodium* species. This is particularly important given that the development of novel antimalarial agents generally involves extensive testing only on *P. falciparum*. Demonstrating susceptibility of *P. knowlesi* to antimalarial agents will support the further development of these agents and their use in areas endemic for non-falciparum species.

The susceptibilities of culture-adapted A1–H1 *P. knowlesi* (isolated in the 1960s) to a range of approved and investigational antimalarial agents have been recently evaluated in a series of studies by van Schalkwyk et al., with the authors comparing drug susceptibilities to those of *P. falciparum* 3D7 using identical assay conditions (van Schalkwyk et al., 2017, 2019, 2020). The EC_{50} values reported in these and other studies (Arnold et al., 2016; Burns et al., 2020; Fatih et al., 2012) are listed in Table 1. The large majority of antimalarial agents evaluated by van Schalkwyk et al. were highly potent

Table 1 *In vitro* susceptibility of *P. knowlesi* and *P. falciparum* to approved and investigational antimalarial agents.

Compound	EC$_{50}$ values (nM)		Fold difference (Pk/Pf)	*P* value	Refs.
	P. knowlesi	*P. falciparum* 3D7			
Artemisinins and synthetic endoperoxides					
Dihydroartemisinin	2.35±0.23	5.16±0.62	0.46	0.0017	van Schalkwyk et al. (2019)
	2.0±0.3	4.2±0.5	0.48	0.0098	van Schalkwyk et al. (2017)
	2.1 (0.4)[a]				van Schalkwyk et al. (2019)
	1.6±0.92[b]				Fatih et al. (2012)
	0.79 (0.62–1.0)[c]				Fatih et al. (2012)
	1.52±0.07	3.64±0.42	0.42	0.0112	Van Schalkwyk et al. (2020)
	2.4±1[d]	0.8±0.1[d]	3.0	ND	Burns et al. (2020)
Artemisinin	7.39±1.87	11.00±1.32	0.67	0.1667	van Schalkwyk et al. (2019)
	2.1±0.99[b]				Fatih et al. (2012)
	0.80 (0.35–1.9)[c]				Fatih et al. (2012)
Artemisone	0.47±0.14	0.72±0.15	0.65	0.2701	van Schalkwyk et al. (2019)
Artesunate	10.30±1.9	8.28±1.05	1.24	0.3552	van Schalkwyk et al. (2019)
	10.9±1.7	9.0±1.5	1.20	0.4280	van Schalkwyk et al. (2017)
	13.8 (3.6)[a]				van Schalkwyk et al. (2019)
	0.90±0.12[b]				Fatih et al. (2012)
	2.0 (0.93–4.2)[c]				Fatih et al. (2012)

Artemether	4.56±0.55	6.93±0.73	0.66	0.0413	van Schalkwyk et al. (2019)
	0.90±0.19[b]				Fatih et al. (2012)
	0.84 (0.34–2.1)[c]				Fatih et al. (2012)
Arterolane (OZ277)	2.27±0.42	4.03±0.59	0.56	0.0407	van Schalkwyk et al. (2019)
Artefenomel (OZ439)	4.76±0.40	4.82±0.62	0.99	0.9350	van Schalkwyk et al. (2019)
	6.6±1.4	7.4±1.2	0.89	0.6750	van Schalkwyk et al. (2017)
	4.4 (1.6)[a]				van Schalkwyk et al. (2019)
Deoxyartemisinin	>10,000	>10,000	ND	ND	van Schalkwyk et al. (2019)
Aminoquinolines and amino-alcohols					
Chloroquine	29.3±4.7	15.9±3.0	1.85	0.0303	van Schalkwyk et al. (2017)
	23±4.8[b]				Fatih et al. (2012)
	3.2 (2.2–4.7)[c]				Fatih et al. (2012)
	10.9±3.1[e]				Arnold et al. (2016)
	33.1±2.0	17.7±1.3	1.87	<0.0001	Van Schalkwyk et al. (2020)
	21.5 (4.9)[a]				van Schalkwyk et al. (2019)
	17±5[d]	52±6[d]	0.34	ND	Burns et al. (2020)
	38±8[f]	53±7[f]			Gilson et al. (2019)
Amodiaquine	9.3±1.7	5.9±0.6	1.59	0.0662	van Schalkwyk et al. (2017)
Desethylamodiaquine	12.4±1.4	12.4±3.1	1.00	0.9973	van Schalkwyk et al. (2017)
Quinine	54.8±3.0	57.9±6.9	0.94	0.7177	van Schalkwyk et al. (2017)
	40.3 0.4)[a]				van Schalkwyk et al. (2019)

Continued

Table 1 *In vitro* susceptibility of *P. knowlesi* and *P. falciparum* to approved and investigational antimalarial agents.—cont'd

| Compound | EC$_{50}$ values (nM) | | Fold difference (Pk/Pf) | P value | Refs. |
	P. knowlesi	P. falciparum 3D7			
Quinidine	38.4 ± 10.5	52.9 ± 10.7	0.73	0.3704	van Schalkwyk et al. (2019)
AQ 13	11.4 ± 2.82	5.1 ± 1.15	2.23	0.1091	van Schalkwyk et al. (2019)
Mefloquine	10.9 ± 1.1	26.2 ± 4.2	0.42	0.0090	van Schalkwyk et al. (2017)
	26 ± 3.1[b]				Fatih et al. (2012)
	25 (7.4–81)[c]				Fatih et al. (2012)
	13.1 2.5)[a]				van Schalkwyk et al. (2019)
	3 ± 1[f]	18 ± 4[f]			Gilson et al. (2019)
Primaquine	3871 ± 887	5627 ± 1195	0.69	0.2847	van Schalkwyk et al. (2017)
Bisquinoline	2.2 ± 1.4	2.3 ± 0.94	0.97	0.9715	van Schalkwyk et al. (2019)
Lumefantrine	90.4 ± 13	152 ± 26	0.60	0.0424	van Schalkwyk et al. (2017)
Piperaquine	21.0 ± 3.1	39.8 ± 4.9	0.53	0.0115	van Schalkwyk et al. (2017)
Pyronaridine	10.7 ± 1.6	4.4 ± 1.6	2.44	0.0268	van Schalkwyk et al. (2017)
	4.9 (0.84)				van Schalkwyk et al. (2019)
Ferroquine	12.2 ± 1.6	4.7 ± 0.6	2.60	0.0068	van Schalkwyk et al. (2017)
	9.8 (2.32)[a]				van Schalkwyk et al. (2019)
Halofantrine	0.92 ± 0.25	3.60 ± 0.40	0.31	0.0174	van Schalkwyk et al. (2019)
Naphthoquine	117 ± 83	111 ± 23	1.05	0.5544	van Schalkwyk et al. (2019)
New Isoquine	15.9 ± 2.4	11.4 ± 2.38	1.39	0.2474	van Schalkwyk et al. (2019)

DHFR inhibitors					
Pyrimethamine	5.1±0.8	54.0±5.0	0.09	<0.0001	van Schalkwyk et al. (2017)
	3.2 (0.5)[a]				van Schalkwyk et al. (2019)
Cycloguanil	1.3±0.3	11.8±0.6	0.11	<0.0001	van Schalkwyk et al. (2017)
	3.9±0.7[e]				Arnold et al. (2016)
	0.7 (0.1)[a]				van Schalkwyk et al. (2019)
Trimethoprim	265±47	3098±229	0.09	<0.0001	van Schalkwyk et al. (2017)
	137 (54)[a]				van Schalkwyk et al. (2019)
P218	4.1±0.7	3.5±0.2	1.18	0.4884	van Schalkwyk et al. (2017)
	0.68 (0.04)[a]				van Schalkwyk et al. (2019)
Quinolones					
Atovaquone	2.6±0.4	2.3±0.5	1.13	0.6366	van Schalkwyk et al. (2017)
	0.71±0.02[g]	0.74±0.09	0.99	0.1211	Van Schalkwyk et al. (2020)
	4.1 (0.04)[a]				van Schalkwyk et al. (2019)
Endochin	18.9±1.2	18.1±0.5	1.04	0.6233	van Schalkwyk et al. (2020)
ELQ-300	15.4±0.9	23.1 ±1.2	0.67	0.0215	van Schalkwyk et al. (2020)
ATP4 inhibitors					
Cipargamin (KAE609)	6.1±0.5	0.89±0.08	6.83	<0.0001	van Schalkwyk et al. (2019)
	3.8 (1.6)[a]				van Schalkwyk et al. (2019)
SJ733	386±34	64.3±4.3	6.00	<0.0001	van Schalkwyk et al. (2019)

Continued

Table 1 *In vitro* susceptibility of *P. knowlesi* and *P. falciparum* to approved and investigational antimalarial agents.—cont'd

| Compound | EC$_{50}$ values (nM) | | Fold difference (Pk/Pf) | *P* value | Refs. |
	P. knowlesi	*P. falciparum* 3D7			
PA21A092	63.8±7.6	10.2±1.4	6.25	0.0002	van Schalkwyk et al. (2019)
	35.7 (2.8)[a]				van Schalkwyk et al. (2019)
Others					
Clindamycin	>10,000				Arnold et al. (2016)
	>10,000	>10,000	ND	ND	van Schalkwyk et al. (2017)
Doxycycline	>10,000	>10,000	ND	ND	van Schalkwyk et al. (2017)
Azithromycin[h]	5662±725	6003±323	0.94	ND	van Schalkwyk et al. (2017)
	16,000±1800	11,310±490	1.41	ND	Burns et al. (2020)
Proguanil	2461±236[g]	228±29	10.79	0.0007	Van Schalkwyk et al. (2020)
AN13762	2762±296	41.3±3.8	66.88	<0.0001	van Schalkwyk et al. (2019)
	3618 (110)[a]				van Schalkwyk et al. (2019)
Pentamidine	331±20	99±4	3.34	0.0003	van Schalkwyk et al. (2019)
Cladosporin	411±134	133±10	3.09	0.0831	van Schalkwyk et al. (2019)
Ganaplacide (KAF156)	1.7±0.16	7.9±0.12	0.22	<0.0001	van Schalkwyk et al. (2019)
Methylene Blue	5.38±1.8	3.31±0.7	1.63	0.3543	van Schalkwyk et al. (2019)
NMT MMV884705	46.2±16	206±44	0.22	0.0266	van Schalkwyk et al. (2019)
MMV253	13.0±1.9	7.4±1.5	1.76	0.0810	van Schalkwyk et al. (2019)
MMV048	17.2±0.9	29.5±2.5	0.58	0.0103	van Schalkwyk et al. (2019)
Cyclohexamide	117±40	188±35	0.62	0.2544	van Schalkwyk et al. (2019)

Benzylquine	31.53 ± 10.88	22.05 ± 2.02	1.43	0.3469	van Schalkwyk et al. (2019)
WR194965	282 ± 111	539 ± 236	0.52	0.3633	van Schalkwyk et al. (2019)
BIX-01294	22.6 ± 4.4	21.2 ± 4.1	1.07	0.8207	van Schalkwyk et al. (2019)
Sitamaquine	112 ± 25	72 ± 15	1.56	0.2350	van Schalkwyk et al. (2019)
Methotrexate	1991 ± 125	693 ± 48	2.87	0.0006	van Schalkwyk et al. (2019)
MK-4815	47.6 ± 6	127 ± 16	0.37	0.0100	van Schalkwyk et al. (2019)
MMV688558	17.5 ± 2.0	42.4 ± 1.6	0.41	0.0006	van Schalkwyk et al. (2019)
DSM1	509 ± 11	149 ± 5	3.4	≤ 0.0018	van Schalkwyk et al. (2017)
DSM265	303 ± 15	37 ± 3	8.2	≤ 0.0018	van Schalkwyk et al. (2017)
	170 (66)[a]				van Schalkwyk et al. (2019)
DSM421	194 ± 23	72 ± 5	2.7	≤ 0.0018	van Schalkwyk et al. (2017)
	142 (71)[a]				van Schalkwyk et al. (2019)
2-Anilinoquinazoline compounds WEB-484, 485, 486 and 487	59 ± 10 to 95 ± 8	87 ± 1 to 110 ± 37			Gilson et al. (2019)

[a]EC_{50} of UM01 clinical isolate. Data are the mean of 2 independent experiments, each performed in duplicate. Numbers in parenthesis are the range/2.
[b]Mean from 6 clinical isolates, schizont maturation assay.
[c]Mean (95% CI) from a single experiment repeated 5 times, laboratory H strain, pLDH assay.
[d]In-cycle assay using the *P. knowlesi* YH1 strain, and the *P. falciparum* PHG strain.
[e]Utilising a [^{3}H]hypoxanthine uptake assay.
[f]Evaluated by flow-cytometry after 48 h exposure for *P. knowlesi* YH1, or 72 h exposure for *P. falciparum* 3D7.
[g]Drug exposure over 2.5 life-cycles.
[h]The susceptibility of *P. knowlesi* YH1 to a number of azithromycin analogues has also been evaluated, with EC_{50} values of 12–360 nM (Burns et al., 2020).
Numbers are mean $\pm$ SEM unless otherwise specified. The *P. knowlesi* strain is A1-H1 unless otherwise specified. Drug exposure is over one life-cycle unless otherwise specified.

against *P. knowlesi*, with EC_{50} values similar to those of *P. falciparum* 3D7, including chloroquine ($EC_{50} < 30\,nM$), quinine ($EC_{50} < 55\,nM$), amodiaquine ($EC_{50} < 10\,nM$), the artemisinin derivatives (EC_{50} values $<11\,nM$), and the synthetic endoperoxides arterolane (OZ277) and artefenomel (OZ439) (EC_{50} values both $<5\,nM$) (van Schalkwyk et al., 2019). Compared to *P. falciparum*, *P. knowlesi* was significantly more susceptible to several artemisinin partner drugs, including mefloquine ($EC_{50} < 11\,nM$), lumefantrine ($EC_{50} < 91\,nM$), and piperaquine ($EC_{50} < 22\,nM$) (van Schalkwyk et al., 2017). This is in contrast to an earlier study which assessed *P. knowlesi* growth using a modified schizont maturation assay and reported reduced susceptibility of *P. knowlesi* to mefloquine (Fatih et al., 2013). However, this earlier study included only six clinical isolates, and did not assess stage specificity of the drugs, which is an important confounder of susceptibility of non-falciparum *Plasmodium* species (Kerlin et al., 2012; Russell et al., 2008).

Although the clinical significance is uncertain, van Schalkwyk et al. did find that compared to *P. falciparum*, *P. knowlesi* had reduced susceptibility to inhibitors of dihydroorotate dehydrogenase (DHODH), a target of several new antimalarials under development including DSM421 and DSM265 (van Schalkwyk et al., 2017). DSM265 in particular was 8-fold less potent against *P. knowlesi* than *P. falciparum*. Importantly, compared to *P. falciparum* this agent has also been demonstrated to be 5-fold less potent against *P. vivax* field isolates ex vivo (Phillips et al., 2016). Furthermore, in a phase 2a study in Peru, DSM265 rapidly cleared most *P. falciparum* infections in patients while none of the doses tested cleared *P. vivax* infections (Llanos–Cuentas et al., 2018). This highlights the utility of *P. knowlesi* as a model to test drug susceptibilities of non-falciparum species. *P. knowlesi* also had reduced susceptibility to ATP4 inhibitors cipargamin, SJ733 and PA21A092, with EC_{50} values ~ 6 fold higher than those of *P. falciparum* (van Schalkwyk et al., 2017). The greatest difference in susceptibility between *P. knowlesi* and *P. falciparum* was observed with the oxaborole AN13762 (van Schalkwyk et al., 2019). This agent was 67-fold less potent against *P. knowlesi* than against *P. falciparum,* suggesting either differences in the drug target or a species-specific resistance mechanism.

In a more recent study van Schalkwyk et al. also evaluated the susceptibility of *P. knowlesi* to quinolones, including atovaquone as well as the more recently developed endochin–like quinolones (ELQs) (Van Schalkwyk et al., 2020). The quinolones were found to be equally potent against *P. knowlesi* ($EC_{50} < 117\,nM$) as *P. falciparum*. However, *P. knowlesi* was 10-fold less susceptible to the quinolone partner drug proguanil, with an EC_{50} of

2461 nM compared to 228 nM for *P. falciparum*. Furthermore, in contrast to *P. falciparum*, no synergy against *P. knowlesi* was observed between the quinolones and proguanil. Importantly however, synergy between proguanil and the novel ELQ-300 was demonstrated against both species. In addition, ELQ-300 was synergistic with atovaquone against both *P. falciparum* and *P. knowlesi*.

Given the potential limitations of using a culture-adapted strain of *P. knowlesi* to evaluate drug susceptibilities, van Schalkwyk et al. also evaluated the drug susceptibilities of a new culture-adapted *P. knowlesi* line, UM01, isolated from a human host in Malaysia in 2013 (Amir et al., 2016; van Schalkwyk et al., 2019). Compared to the A1-H1 strain, EC_{50} values for the UM01 line were similar or lower to all antimalarial agents evaluated (Table 1), suggesting that the 1960s culture-adapted A1-H1 strain may continue to be suitable for evaluating drug susceptibilities of *P. knowlesi*. Van Schalkwyk et al. also evaluated several drug combinations against the *P. knowlesi* A1-H1, and showed similar drug interactions to those with *P. falciparum* (van Schalkwyk et al., 2019).

4. Drug resistance mutations

The emergence and spread of drug resistant mutations in *P. falciparum* and *P. vivax* presents a major threat to malaria control. However, given that transmission of *P. knowlesi* is largely, if not exclusively, zoonotic (Cuenca et al., 2021; Imai et al., 2014; Lee et al., 2011), drug resistant mutations are not expected to emerge. The lack of orthologous *P. knowlesi* drug resistant mutations has been confirmed by a number of studies. These include a study by Assefa et al., where 48 isolates from Sarawak, Malaysia, were analysed for mutations in the chloroquine resistance transporter (CRT) gene, the multidrug resistant protein 1 (MDR1) gene, the dihydrofolate reductase gene (DHFR), the dihydropteroate synthase (DHPS) gene, and the kelch 13 gene (Assefa et al., 2015). No drug resistant mutations were found, suggesting lack of drug pressure from chloroquine, mefloquine, pyrimethamine, sulphadoxine, and artemisinin derivatives, respectively. An additional 6 clinical isolates from Sarawak were analysed by Fatih et al., who also found no drug-resistance mutations in either the CRT or the MDR1 gene (Fatih et al., 2013). In over 400 samples from Sabah, Malaysia, Grigg et al. analysed the sequences of the DFHR gene, and although non-synonymous *pkdhfr* polymorphisms were frequently present, homology modelling demonstrated that these were not associated with pyrimethamine drug binding (Grigg et al., 2016a). Tyagi et al. also found no drug resistance mutations in either the DHFR gene or the CRT gene in 53 isolates from the Andaman and Nicobah Islands in India (Tyagi et al., 2013). Finally, although Pinheiro et al. reported dimorphism and polymorphism among *P. knowlesi* isolates in the multidrug resistance associated protein MRP1 and the multidrug resistance protein MDR2, both members of the ATP-binding cassette transporter family of genes associated with mefloquine resistance in *P. falciparum* (Pinheiro et al., 2015), the functional implications in *P. knowlesi* are not clear.

5. Treatment of uncomplicated knowlesi malaria

Uncomplicated knowlesi malaria is defined as detectable *P. knowlesi* parasitaemia without any of the clinical or laboratory criteria meeting the definition of severe knowlesi malaria (Table 2). For the purposes of treatment recommendations, this also incorporates asymptomatic parasitaemia. Treatment should be initiated as soon as a diagnosis is confirmed. The preferred treatment regimen consists of an oral artemisinin combination therapy (ACT). While chloroquine is also effective against *P. knowlesi*, ACT is associated with faster parasite clearance times (detailed below). Furthermore, administration of chloroquine to those with a diagnosis of knowlesi malaria is associated with a risk of inadvertently administering chloroquine to those with misdiagnosed vivax or falciparum malaria. Given the high prevalence of chloroquine-resistant vivax and falciparum malaria in knowlesi-endemic regions (Grigg et al., 2016b; Price et al., 2014), use of chloroquine as an antimalarial treatment is not recommended.

5.1 Artemisinin combination treatment (ACT)

Artemether-lumefantrine is the most widely used ACT for the treatment of knowlesi malaria, and is listed by the Malaysian Ministry of Health as the preferred treatment (Ministry of Health Malaysia, 2014). Artemether-lumefantrine has been evaluated in one of only two randomised controlled trials evaluating antimalarial treatment for uncomplicated knowlesi malaria (Table 3). In this study, 123 patients with PCR-confirmed uncomplicated knowlesi malaria in 3 district hospitals in Sabah, Malaysia, were randomised to receive either artemether-lumefantrine (total dose 12 mg/kg of artemether and 60 mg/kg of lumefantrine) or chloroquine (25 mg/kg) (Grigg et al., 2018b). To ensure applicability of results to a real-world

Table 2 Severe malaria definitions.

(1) Epidemiological and Research definition for severe knowlesi malaria.
One or more of the following criteria (World Health Organization, 2014, 2021):

Unrousable coma[a]	Glasgow coma scale <11
Respiratory distress	Oxygen saturation <92% with respiratory rate >30 breaths/min
Shock	Systolic blood pressure <80 mmHg with cool peripheries or impaired capillary refill
Jaundice	Bilirubin >50 μmol/L, with parasitaemia >20,000/μL and/or creatinine >132 μmol/L
Severe anaemia	Haemoglobin <7.0 g/dL (adults) Haemoglobin <5.0 g/dL (children)[a]
Significant abnormal bleeding	
Hypoglycaemia	Blood glucose <2.2 mmol/L
Metabolic acidosis	Bicarbonate <15 mmol/L or lactate >5 mmol/L
Acute kidney injury	Creatinine >265 μmol/L
Hyperparasitaemia	Parasite count >100,000/μL (or >2% or infected red blood cells)

(2) Clinical definition requiring treatment with intravenous artesunate:
One or more of the following criteria (World Health Organization, 2014) in settings where clinical or laboratory criteria of severity cannot be fully assessed.

- Inability to tolerate oral therapy
- Warning signs or clinical severity criteria as above
- Parasitaemia >20,000/μL, particularly in settings where clinical or laboratory criteria of severity cannot be fully assessed

[a]Not yet reported in PCR-confirmed knowlesi malaria.

setting, co-administration of artemether-lumefantrine with fatty food (a biscuit or milk) was encouraged but not mandated. Participants of all ages were included if they weighed >10 kg, had a parasite count of <20,000/μL, and had a negative rapid diagnostic test result for *P. falciparum*. The primary outcome was parasite clearance at 24 h, which was achieved in 76% (95% CI 63–86%) of patients administered artemether-lumefantrine, compared to 60% (95% CI 47–72%) of those administered chloroquine ($P = 0.06$).

Table 3 Studies reporting antimalarial chemotherapy used in the treatment of knowlesi malaria in adults and children in endemic areas.[a]

	Study design	Number of patients	Per cent male	Median age (range)	Median (range) parasitaemia (parasites/µL)	PCT50 (hours), median	PCT90 (hours), median	Parasite reduction ratio at 24h (%, 95% CI)	% negative at 24h (95% CI)	Time to parasite clearance (<5/µL), median (range)	Died	Refs.
Uncomplicated malaria												
Chloroquine and primaquine	Prospective observational	33	58	46	3724 (1845–7480)	3.1 (range 2.8–3.4)	10.3 (range 9.4–11.4)	99.4 (97.0–99.9)	33	36 (31–51) hours	0	Daneshvar et al. (2010)
Chloroquine	Randomised controlled trial	125	75	32 (7–85)	1329 (33–35,873)	6.3 (95% CI 5.1–7.5)	14.8 (95% CI 13.4–16.1)	97.5 (96.6–98.4)	55 (45–64)	24 (6–60) hours	0	Grigg et al. (2016c)
Chloroquine	Retrospective	16	50	9 (4–14)	2240 (200–14,400)	NR	NR	NR	6[b]	2 days (range 1–5)[b]		Barber et al. (2011)
Chloroquine	Randomised controlled trial	65	71	31 (4–75)	1485 (89–32,660)	8.2 (95% CI 6.4–10.1)	15.6 (95% CI 3.6–17.7)	98.1 (97.2–99.1)[c]	60 (47–72)	24 (12–48) hours		Grigg et al. (2018b)
Artesunate/ mefloquine	Randomised controlled trial	115	81	33 (3–82)	1457 (36–35,008)	3.4 (95% CI 2.9–4.0)	8.9 (95% CI 8.2–9.6)	99.8 (99.7–100)	84 (76–91)	18 (6–48) hours	0	Grigg et al. (2016c)
Artemether-lumefantrine	Prospective observational	27	70	31 (17–70)	4066 (232–60,840)	NR	NR	NR	33[b]	2 days (range 1–3)[b]	0	Barber et al. (2013a)[c]
Artemether-lumefantrine	Retrospective	6	100	30	NR	NR	NR	NR	66[b]	1 day (range 0–3)[b]	0	William et al. (2011)[c]

Treatment	Study type	N	Age	Parasitemia						Time to negative	Deaths	Reference
Artemether–lumefantrine	Randomised controlled trial	58	85	30 (7–79)	1437 (57–44,744)	7.2 (95% CI 5.6–8.9)	13.7 (95% CI 11.8–14.7)	99.6 (99.2–100)[c]	76 (63–86)	24 (12–42) hours		Grigg et al. (2018b)
Oral quinine	Retrospective	11	83	45	NR	NR	NR	NR	12[b]	2.5 days (range 1–3)[b]	0	William et al. (2011)[c]

Severe malaria

Intravenous artesunate	Prospective observational	36	75	55 (20–74)	100,995 (32–584,015)	NR	NR	NR	33[b]	NR[b,d]	0	Barber et al. (2013a)[c]
Intravenous artesunate	Retrospective	6	63	56	NR	NR	NR	NR	50%	2 days (range 1–3)[b]	1 (17%)	William et al. (2011)[c]
Intravenous quinine	Prospective observational	10	30	64 (36–73)	NR	NR	NR	NR	NR	NR	2 (20%)	Daneshvar et al. (2010)
Intravenous quinine	Retrospective	16	69	55	4+	NR	NR	NR	30%	4 days (range 2–7)[b]	5 (27%)	William et al. (2011)

[a]Does not include case reports.
[b]Based on daily routine hospital microscopy.
[c]Supplementary data.
[d]NR, not recorded.

Median parasite clearance was shorter after artemether-lumefantrine than chloroquine (18 vs. 24 h, $P = 0.02$), and all patients were aparasitaemic by 48 h. Patients were followed up to day 42, and there were no treatment failures with either artemether-lumefantrine or chloroquine. Adverse events were similar between the two groups, although dyspepsia occurred more commonly in those who received artemether-lumefantrine (7% vs. 0%, $P = 0.03$). There were no serious adverse events. When applying the Malaysian national hospital policy of 2 negative blood films on 2 consecutive days prior to discharge, the predicted bed occupancy was 2414 days per 1000 patients treated with artemether-lumefantrine compared to 2800 days per 1000 patients treated with chloroquine (incidence rate ratio 0.86, 95% CI 0.82–0.91, $P < 0.001$).

In the only other randomised controlled trial to have evaluated antimalarial treatment for uncomplicated knowlesi malaria, 252 patients older than 1 year presenting to the same district hospitals as the study above were randomised to receive either artesunate-mefloquine (12 mg/kg artesunate and 25 mg/kg mefloquine) or chloroquine (25 mg/kg) (Grigg et al., 2016c). The primary endpoint of parasite clearance at 24 h was achieved in 84% (95% CI 76–91) of patients in the artesunate-mefloquine group, compared to 55% (95% CI 45–64) in the chloroquine group ($P < 0.0001$). Median parasite clearance was faster with artesunate-mefloquine compared to chloroquine (18 vs 24 h, $P < 0.0001$). The risk of anaemia within 28 days was also lower in the artesunate-mefloquine group compared to the chloroquine group (62% vs 71%, $P = 0.035$). Two patients had serious adverse events. The first was in a 41 year old man in the artesunate-mefloquine group who developed an acute psychosis on day 3, with auditory hallucinations, nausea, dizziness, and subsequent minor attempts at self-harm. The symptoms resolved over a period of 2 weeks, and the patient remained well over the next 6 months of follow-up. The event was considered probably related to mefloquine. The second serious adverse event also occurred in the artesunate-mefloquine arm, in a 55 year old man with cardiovascular risk factors who died after being readmitted to hospital with severe pneumonia 24 days after his enrolment in the trial. The event was considered unrelated to the study drug. Adverse events were otherwise similar between the two groups.

A meta-analysis of the two studies above found that compared to chloroquine, both ACTs were associated with a similar increase in the proportion of patients who were parasite negative at 24 h, and there were no significant differences in treatment outcomes between artemether-lumefantrine and artesunate-mefloquine (Grigg et al., 2018b). The results of these randomised controlled trials are consistent with earlier non-randomised studies reporting efficacy of artemether-lumefantrine and artesunate-mefloquine for the treatment of uncomplicated malaria at a tertiary referral hospital in Sabah, Malaysia (Table 3; Barber et al., 2013a; William et al., 2011).

Several other ACTs have been used successfully for the treatment of uncomplicated knowlesi malaria, including dihydroartemisinin-piperaquine (Setiadi et al., 2016). Given the similar *in vitro* susceptibilities of *P. knowlesi* and *P. falciparum* to artemisinin derivatives (detailed above) and most partner drugs (Table 1), it is highly likely that most ACTs effective against artemisinin-sensitive strains of *P. falciparum* will be also highly effective against *P. knowlesi*.

5.2 Chloroquine

Prior to the increasing recognition of knowlesi malaria in Malaysia over the past decade, knowlesi malaria was commonly diagnosed as the micro-scopically near-identical *P. malariae*, and was thus treated with chloroquine, previously the first-line treatment for *P. malariae* in Malaysia. The large majority of patients included in early case series of knowlesi malaria there-fore received treatment with chloroquine. Consistent with the findings from the randomised controlled trials described above, these early studies demon-strated chloroquine to be effective for the treatment of uncomplicated knowlesi malaria. In the first report of a large focus of human infections with knowlesi malaria, Singh et al. reported 92 patients with knowlesi malaria treated with chloroquine at a district hospital in Sarawak, Malaysia, with primaquine given at 24 and 48 h (Singh et al., 2004). Median parasite clearance time was 2.4 days (range 1–5 days) and no deaths were reported. In a prospective observational study at the same hospital, chloroquine was administered to 96 adults with uncomplicated knowlesi malaria (Daneshvar et al., 2010). All patients had cleared their parasites by day 3, and all were negative by PCR on day 7, 14, 21 and 28.

Despite the efficacy of chloroquine for treating uncomplicated knowlesi malaria, administration of chloroquine to patients with unsuspected severe knowlesi malaria has resulted in adverse outcomes, including deaths (Rajahram et al., 2012). For this reason, in addition to the risk of administering chloroquine to patients with misdiagnosed vivax or falciparum malaria, ACT is the preferred option for treatment of uncomplicated knowlesi malaria.

5.3 Other agents

Atovaquone-proguanil has been used for the treatment of uncomplicated knowlesi malaria in returned travellers, with rapid recovery reported in all cases (Ehrhardt et al., 2013; Figtree et al., 2010; Hoosen and Shaw, 2011; Mackroth et al., 2016). However, although atovaquone is highly potent *in vitro* against *P. knowlesi* ($EC_{50} < 5$ nM) (van Schalkwyk et al., 2017, 2019), proguanil has been shown to be more than 10-fold less potent against the laboratory adapted *P. knowlesi* A1-H1 strain than *P. falciparum* (EC_{50} of 2461 nM compared to 228 nM for *P. falciparum*) (Van Schalkwyk et al., 2020). Furthermore, the synergy between proguanil and atovaquone that occurs with *P. falciparum* was not observed with *P. knowlesi* (Van Schalkwyk et al., 2020). Therefore, atovaquone-proguanil should be used for the treatment of knowlesi malaria only if ACTs are not readily available.

5.4 Primaquine

Primaquine is not generally indicated for the treatment of knowlesi malaria. *P. knowlesi* does not form hypnozoites, thus anti-relapse therapy is not required. The use of primaquine to reduce transmission is also not considered necessary, given that *P. knowlesi* exists primarily as a zoonosis without evidence of substantial human–human transmission. Furthermore, gametocytes have been shown to be cleared rapidly in knowlesi malaria without use of primaquine. In a clinical trial, gametocytes were detected by PCR at day 7 in only 2/48 (4%) and 3/49 (6%) patients treated with chloroquine and artesunate-mefloquine respectively, despite gametocytes having been present at baseline in 39/48 (81%) and 43/49 (88%) of these patients (Grigg et al., 2016c). In another clinical trial, although PCR was not done, gametocytes were present by microscopy at baseline in 15/58 (26%) and 17/65 (26%) of patients treated with artemether-lumefantrine and chloroquine, respectively, and negative by microscopy in all patients at all follow-up time points (including 6 hourly blood films until parasite clearance) (Grigg et al., 2018b). Primaquine should be used to prevent *P. vivax* relapses in cases of *P. knowlesi*/*P. vivax* mixed infections, and should also be used to prevent transmission in cases of *P. knowlesi*/*P. falciparum* mixed infections.

6. Clinical management of severe knowlesi malaria

Although the majority of patients with knowlesi malaria have uncomplicated disease, in Malaysia severe disease has been shown to occur in ~6–9% of patients at district hospitals (Daneshvar et al., 2009; Grigg et al., 2018a), and up to 29% of patients at a tertiary referral hospital (Barber et al., 2013a). In the tertiary hospital study, risk of severe disease was at least as high as that of *P. falciparum*. Age and parasitaemia have both been shown to be independent risk factors for severe disease (Barber et al., 2017; Grigg et al., 2018a). In a recent review of knowlesi malaria cases in Sabah, Malaysia, during 2010–2017, the overall case-fatality rate was 2.5/1000: 6.0/1000 for women, and 1.7/1000 for men (Rajahram et al., 2019). Independent risk factors for death included female sex (OR 2.6 [95% CI 1.0–6.7], $P = 0.04$) and age > 45 years (OR 4.7 [95% CI 1.8–12.5], $P < 0.01$). Parasitaemia as a risk factor for death was not able to be evaluated in this analysis, although this association could be assumed, given the strong association between parasitaemia and disease severity. Other factors contributing to fatal outcomes included cardiovascular comorbidities, microscopic misdiagnoses, and delays in administering intravenous therapy. Thus, early recognition and diagnosis of severe disease, and early initiation of appropriate treatment is essential to avoid fatal outcomes.

Severe knowlesi malaria has been defined according to modified criteria for severe falciparum malaria, with a lower parasite count of 100,000/μL used as a cut-off to define hyperparasitaemia. In adults, the most common severity criteria include hyperparasitaemia, jaundice, acute kidney injury, shock, and respiratory distress (Barber et al., 2013a; Daneshvar et al., 2009; Grigg et al., 2018a). Anaemia occurs less commonly. Metabolic acidosis is common in fatal cases (Rajahram et al., 2019).

6.1 Intravenous artesunate

The WHO recommends intravenous artesunate for all patients with severe malaria regardless of species (World Health Organization, 2021), based on 8 randomised controlled trials in African and Asian countries in adults ($n = 1664$) and children ($n = 5765$) demonstrating reduced mortality with intravenous artesunate compared to intravenous quinine for the treatment of severe falciparum malaria (Sinclair et al., 2012). Intravenous artesunate has also been shown to be highly effective for the treatment of severe knowlesi malaria, with no deaths occurring in a prospective tertiary hospital involving 38 patients with severe knowlesi malaria in Sabah, Malaysia (Barber et al., 2013a). In an earlier retrospective study conducted at the same hospital, 1/6 (17%) patients treated with intravenous artesunate died, compared to 5/16 (31%) treated with intravenous quinine (William et al., 2011). In another prospective observational study in Sarawak, Malaysia, 2/10 (20%) patients with severe knowlesi malaria treated with intravenous quinine died (Daneshvar et al., 2010). This lower case-fatality rate associated with the use of intravenous artesunate was also supported by a state-wide study conducted in Sabah, that demonstrated a fall in the *P. knowlesi* case-fatality rate from 9.2/1000 case notifications in 2010 (when local guidelines changed to recommend intravenous artesunate) to 1.6/1000 case notifications in 2014 (Rajahram et al., 2016). It is likely that this reduction was due at least in part to the increasing use of intravenous artesunate for severe knowlesi malaria.

While intravenous artesunate should clearly be administered to patients with clinical or laboratory evidence of severe knowlesi malaria (Table 1), and to those not tolerating oral medications, the optimal treatment for patients with moderately high parasite counts in the absence of other evidence of severe disease is less certain. In a tertiary hospital study, severe disease occurred in 24/45 (53%) patients with a parasite count of $>20,000/\mu L$, including in 9/27 (33%) of those who had parasite counts of between 20,000 and $100,000/\mu L$. The sensitivity and specificity of $20,000/\mu L$ as a cut-off for predicting severe disease was 75% and 79%, respectively (Barber et al., 2013a). Similar results were observed in a district hospital study, where severe disease occurred in 22/54 (41%) patients with parasite counts over 15,000 parasites/μL, with this cut-off having a sensitivity and specificity of 74% and 87%, respectively (Grigg et al., 2018a). In a third study, severe disease occurred in 11/25 (44%) in patients with a parasite count above 35,000 parasites/μL, including 3/9 (33%) with a parasitaemia between 35,000 and $100,000/\mu L$; the $35,000/\mu L$ parasitaemia cut-off had a sensitivity and specificity of 65% and 85%, respectively, for predicting severe disease (Willmann et al., 2012). In the two randomised controlled trials by Grigg et al. evaluating artemether-lumefantrine (Grigg et al., 2018b) or artesunate-mefloquine (Grigg et al., 2016c) versus chloroquine for the treatment of uncomplicated knowlesi malaria, patients with parasite counts $>20,000/\mu L$ on screening hospital microscopy were excluded due to uncertainty about the safety of administering oral treatment to these patients.

However, research cross check of enrolment slides and recalculation of parasite counts using individual patient WBC measurements indicated that 17 patients had parasite counts of between 20,000 and 45,000 parasites/μL and no other severity criteria and were safely treated with either chloroquine ($n = 7$), artesunate-mefloquine ($n = 9$), or artemether-lumefantrine ($n = 4$) (Grigg et al., 2016c, 2018b). Nonetheless, because of the higher risk of severe disease at these moderately high parasitaemias, WHO has recommended intravenous artesunate for patients with parasitaemias >20,000/μL, particularly if other laboratory criteria for severe disease cannot be evaluated (World Health Organization, 2014). More recently, based on the largest of the studies above (Grigg et al., 2018a), a lower parasitaemia cut-off of >15,000/μL has also been recommended (Anstey et al., 2021; World Health Organization & Regional Office for the Western Pacific, 2017).

For patients fulfilling criteria for severe knowlesi malaria, intravenous artesunate should be given for a minimum of 3 doses (2.4 mg/kg), 12 h apart (World Health Organization, 2021). This should be followed by a 3 day course of oral ACT such as artemether-lumefantrine once oral intake is tolerated, according to local guidelines and availability. For patients commenced on intravenous artesunate in the absence of criteria for severe malaria, oral ACT should be substituted as soon as oral intake is tolerated.

In severe falciparum malaria intravenous artesunate has in some cases been associated with post-treatment haemolysis, presenting as severe anaemia 7–14 days after treatment (Fanello et al., 2017; Gómez-Junyent et al., 2015; Jauréguiberry et al., 2014). While early haemolysis with haemoglobinuria has been reported following artesunate use in severe knowlesi malaria (Barber et al., 2016b), post-artesunate delayed haemolysis has not yet been reported in *P. knowlesi* infection. WHO recommends that all hyperparasitaemic patients who have received intravenous artesunate be monitored for delayed haemolytic anaemia (World Health Organization, 2021).

6.2 Paracetamol as a renoprotective agent

Acute kidney injury (AKI) is a common complication of knowlesi malaria. In a tertiary-hospital study, AKI by KDIGO criteria (with baseline creatinine estimated by the MDRD equation) was present on admission in 44/154 (29%) non-severe cases, and 40/48 (83%) severe cases (Barber et al., 2018). In another district hospital study where severe malaria was less common, AKI by the same criteria was present in 109/396 (30%) hospitalised patients with knowlesi malaria (Cooper et al., 2018a). As with falciparum malaria, haemolysis is increased in severe knowlesi malaria, and is thought to be a key contributing factor to AKI (Barber et al., 2018). Haemolysis is associated with release of cell-free haemoglobin (CFHb), leading to rapid oxidation of ferrous (Fe^{2+}) to ferric (Fe^{3+}) haemoglobin. Further oxidation of ferric to ferryl (Fe^{4+}) haemoglobin generates lipid radical species, leading to oxidative stress and oxidative injury.

In falciparum malaria, acute kidney injury has been shown to be associated with both CFHb and measures of lipid peroxidation, supporting the hypothesis that CFHb-induced lipid peroxidation contributes to AKI in falciparum malaria (Plewes et al., 2017). Paracetamol inhibits CFHb-mediated lipid peroxidation by reducing heme-ferryl radicals, and hence has been proposed as a renoprotective agent in severe malaria complicated by haemolysis. Building on this hypothesis, a Phase 2 RCT evaluating the ability of regularly dosed paracetamol (1 g 6 hourly) to improve renal function was conducted in 62 Bangladeshi adults with moderate to severe falciparum malaria (Plewes et al., 2018). After 72 h creatinine had reduced by 23% (IQR 37–18%) in patients randomised to paracetamol, compared to 14% (IQR 0–29%) in those randomised to no paracetamol ($P = 0.043$). The difference was more marked in those with CFHb > 45,000 ng/mL compared to those with a CFHb < 45,000 ng/mL (37% [IQR 22–48%] reduction vs 14% [IQR −71–30%), $P = 0.01$).

In a larger RCT in Malaysian adults with knowlesi malaria of any severity, 396 hospitalised patients were randomised to paracetamol (1 g 6 hourly for 72 h), or no paracetamol (Cooper et al., 2018a, b). While the primary endpoint of improved change in creatinine at 72 h was not met in the overall group, regularly-dosed paracetamol was associated with greater improvements in creatinine in certain pre-defined subgroups, including those with severe malaria, and in those with AKI and haemolysis (defined in this study as a CFHb ≥77,600 ng/mL). Regularly dosed paracetamol was shown to be safe and well-tolerated. While the median alanine transaminase (ALT) was higher following treatment in the paracetamol arm compared to the control arm, no patient met the criteria for Hy's law for hepatotoxicity (Temple, 2006). Based on these results, regularly-dosed paracetamol may be considered as a renoprotective agent for patients with severe knowlesi malaria, and is recommended in current guidelines (Antibiotic Expert Group, 2019). Regularly dosed paracetamol may also be considered for patients with knowlesi malaria complicated by AKI, even in the absence of other criteria for severe malaria.

6.3 Other adjunctive and supportive treatment

Like falciparum malaria, severe knowlesi malaria is frequently associated with multiorgan failure requiring intensive supportive management. However, with the exception of the paracetamol trial discussed above, there have been no other clinical trials of adjunctive therapy in severe knowlesi malaria, and no other adjunctive therapy that has proven effective in severe falciparum malaria (World Health Organization, 2021). Supportive treatment for severe knowlesi malaria is therefore limited to inotropic and ventilatory support (Barber et al., 2013a; William et al., 2011), haemodialysis for acute kidney injury (Barber et al., 2013a, William et al., 2011), and blood transfusions as required (World Health Organization, 2021). Thrombocytopenia is universal in severe knowlesi malaria; however, platelet counts recover rapidly after commencement of antimalarial treatment (Barber et al., 2013a), and significant abnormal bleeding is uncommon (Barber et al., 2013a; Cox-Singh et al., 2008; Daneshvar et al., 2009; Grigg et al., 2018a; Lee et al., 2010; Ninan et al., 2012). Thus, platelet transfusions are not generally required. There have been no clinical trials to guide intravenous fluid management in knowlesi malaria. In severe falciparum malaria liberal administration of intravenous fluids has been shown to be deleterious (Hanson et al., 2013, 2014), while conservative fluid regimens have been shown to be safe (Aung et al., 2015; Ishioka et al., 2020). Because the risk of acute respiratory distress syndrome and non-cardiogenic pulmonary oedema is at least as high in severe knowlesi malaria as in severe falciparum malaria (Barber et al., 2013a), a conservative intravenous fluid regimen is generally recommended (Barber et al., 2016a; Hanson et al., 2014; World Health Organization, 2021).

There are no clinical trials to guide the use of empirical antibiotics in severe knowlesi malaria. Concurrent bacteraemia, predominantly gram negative, occurs in up to 15% of adults hospitalised with falciparum malaria (Aung et al., 2015, 2018); in knowlesi malaria, *Enterobacter* bacteremia has been reported in two series of severe knowlesi malaria (Barber et al., 2013a, William et al., 2011), and *Neisseria meningitides* in another (Grigg et al., 2018a). Empirical intravenous broad-spectrum antibiotics are commonly administered in severe knowlesi malaria with multiorgan failure until blood cultures are negative (Barber et al., 2013a).

7. Treatment of knowlesi malaria in children

Plasmodium knowlesi occurs less commonly in children than in adults. In Sabah, Malaysia, children aged <5 years accounted for only 25/3262

(0.8%) of PCR confirmed *P. knowlesi* cases reported during 2015–2017, while children 5–13 years accounted for another 170 (5%) cases (Cooper et al., 2019). The disease is also of lower severity. Parasite counts are lower (Grigg et al., 2018a), and the multi-organ failure that characterises severe disease in adults does not appear to occur in children, nor the severe anaemia commonly seen with falciparum and vivax malaria in this age group (Douglas et al., 2013). Indeed, there have been no cases of severe paediatric PCR-confirmed knowlesi malaria reported to date (Barber et al., 2011; Grigg et al., 2018a; Singh and Daneshvar, 2013). Moderate severity disease is however not uncommon. In a recent district hospital in Sabah, children <13 years accounted for 44/481 (9%) of patients hospitalised with knowlesi malaria (Grigg et al., 2018a). Abdominal pain was more common in children than in adults (43% vs 23%), as was anaemia, occurring in 82% of children compared to 36% of adults. AKI was common in both children and adults (26% vs 19%).

The treatment recommendations for knowlesi malaria in children are the same as for adults. In the two RCTs conducted by Grigg et al., 12, 13 and 7 children ≤12 years old were treated with artesunate-mefloquine, chloroquine, and artemether-lumefantrine, respectively (Grigg et al., 2016c, 2018b). Median (range) parasite counts in these children were 377 (36–9998), 2455 (274–32,320), and 487 (183–9229) parasites/µL, respectively, and all were aparasitaemic by 48 h (Grigg et al., 2016c). The use of chloroquine in an additional 16 children with uncomplicated knowlesi malaria was reported in a retrospective study; median parasite clearance time was 2 days, although a parasite clearance time of 5 days was reported in an 8 year old boy with an admission parasitaemia of 14,400/µL (Barber et al., 2011). Successful use of oral and intravenous quinine for knowlesi malaria in children was also reported (Barber et al., 2011). In the absence of reported severe knowlesi malaria in children, the use of intravenous artesunate for this indication has not been described, but would be recommended based on its known efficacy in children with severe falciparum malaria (Dondorp et al., 2005, 2010), and in adults with severe knowlesi malaria (Barber et al., 2013a). If artesunate is required, children weighing <20 kg should receive a higher dose (3 mg/kg per dose) to ensure adequate drug exposure (World Health Organization, 2021).

8. Treatment of knowlesi malaria in pregnancy

In contrast to *P. falciparum* and *P. vivax*, *P. knowlesi* infection during pregnancy appears to be relatively rare, with only 6 cases reported to date

(Barber et al., 2014; Rajahram et al., 2019; William et al., 2011). However, despite its rarity, adverse maternal and infant outcomes have been reported, including severe maternal malaria, foetal loss and low birth weight (Barber et al., 2014; William et al., 2011), and a single maternal fatality, occurring in a 32 year old woman at 35 weeks gestation (Rajahram et al., 2019). Prompt and effective treatment is therefore essential, and any woman with severe malaria in pregnancy should be treated with immediate intravenous artesunate, regardless of species and including those in the first trimester (World Health Organization, 2021). Women with uncomplicated knowlesi malaria in the second or third trimester of pregnancy may be treated with oral ACT, as per the guidelines for treatment of uncomplicated falciparum malaria in pregnancy (World Health Organization, 2021). In the first trimester of pregnancy uncomplicated knowlesi malaria may be treated with chloroquine. If there is any doubt as to the microscopic diagnosis, alternative treatments include quinine and clindamycin, as per WHO guidelines for falciparum and vivax malaria (World Health Organization, 2021). These guidelines are based on published prospective data from 700 women exposed to ACT in the first trimester of pregnancy (Dellicour et al., 2015; McGready et al., 2012; Moore et al., 2016; Mosha et al., 2014), which indicate no adverse effects on the pregnancy or the health of the foetus or neonate, and are sufficient to exclude a $\geq$4.2-fold increase in risk of any major birth defect (background prevalence assumed to be 0.9%), if half the exposures occur during the embryo-sensitive period (4–9 weeks post conception) (World Health Organization, 2021). These data can be used to reassure women who are accidentally exposed to ACT during the first trimester of pregnancy.

9. Conclusions

The zoonotic parasite *P. knowlesi* has emerged as a major cause of human malaria in Southeast Asia, particularly in eastern Malaysia. Diagnosis by microscopy can be challenging, and for treatment purposes, in knowlesi endemic areas any patient with parasites resembling *P. malariae* should be considered to have *P. knowlesi*. Recognition of the ability of *P. knowlesi* to cause severe disease is paramount for ensuring prompt initiation of effective treatment to prevent adverse outcomes. Given the zoonotic nature of the parasite, drug resistance has not emerged as a concern, and the first line ACTs artesunate-mefloquine and artemether-lumefantrine have both been shown to be highly effective for treatment of uncomplicated disease. For severe disease, intravenous artesunate must be initiated without delay. Recent data also indicate a role for paracetamol as a renoprotective agent for those with severe disease.

Acknowledgements

This work was supported by the Australian National Health and Medical Research Council (grant numbers 1037304 and 1045156; fellowships to NMA [1042072], BEB [1088738]; MJG [1138860] and 'Improving Health Outcomes in the Tropical North: A multidisciplinary collaboration 'Hot North', [grant 1131932]). The Sabah Malaria Research Program is supported by the US NIH, and by the Australian Centre for International Agricultural Research and Department of Foreign Affairs, Australian Government (#LS-2019-116).

References

Amir, A., Russell, B., Liew, J.W.K., Moon, R.W., Fong, M.Y., Vythilingam, I., Subramaniam, V., Snounou, G., Lau, Y.L., 2016. Invasion characteristics of a *Plasmodium knowlesi* line newly isolated from a human. Sci. Rep. 6, 24623.

Anstey, N.M., Barber, B.E., William, T., 2021. Non-Falciparum Malaria: *Plasmodium knowlesi*. UpToDate, Waltham, MA. https://www.uptodate.com/contents/non-falciparum-malaria-plasmodium-knowlesi.

Antibiotic Expert Group, 2019. Treatment of severe malaria. In: eTG Complete [Digital]. Therapeutic Guidelines Limited.

Arnold, M.S., Engel, J.A., Chua, M.J., Fisher, G.M., Skinner-Adams, T.S., Andrews, K.T., 2016. Adaptation of the [3H] hypoxanthine uptake assay for in vitro-cultured *Plasmodium knowlesi* malaria parasites. Antimicrob. Agents Chemother. 60, 4361–4363.

Assefa, S., Lim, C., Preston, M.D., Duffy, C.W., Nair, M.B., Adroub, S.A., Kadir, K.A., Goldberg, J.M., Neafsey, D.E., Divis, P., 2015. Population genomic structure and adaptation in the zoonotic malaria parasite *Plasmodium knowlesi*. Proc. Natl. Acad. Sci. U. S. A. 112, 13027–13032.

Aung, N.M., Kaung, M., Kyi, T.T., Kyaw, M.P., Min, M., Htet, Z.W., Anstey, N.M., Kyi, M.M., Hanson, J., 2015. The safety of a conservative fluid replacement strategy in adults hospitalised with malaria. PLoS One 10, e0143062.

Aung, N.M., Nyein, P.P., Htut, T.Y., Htet, Z.W., Kyi, T.T., Anstey, N.M., Kyi, M.M., Hanson, J., 2018. Antibiotic therapy in adults with malaria (ANTHEM): high rate of clinically significant bacteremia in hospitalized adults diagnosed with falciparum malaria. Am. J. Trop. Med. Hyg. 99, 688–696.

Barber, B.E., William, T., Jikal, M., Jilip, J., Dhararaj, P., Menon, J., Yeo, T.W., Anstey, N.M., 2011. *Plasmodium knowlesi* malaria in children. Emerg. Infect. Dis. 17, 814–820.

Barber, B.E., William, T., Grigg, M.J., Menon, J., Auburn, S., Marfurt, J., Anstey, N.M., Yeo, T.W., 2013a. A prospective comparative study of knowlesi, falciparum and vivax malaria in Sabah, Malaysia: high proportion with severe disease from *Plasmodium knowlesi* and *P. vivax* but no mortality with early referral and artesunate therapy. Clin. Infect. Dis. 56, 383–397.

Barber, B.E., William, T., Grigg, M.J., Piera, K., Yeo, T.W., Anstey, N.M., 2013b. Evaluation of the sensitivity of a pLDH-based and an aldolase-based rapid diagnostic test for the diagnosis of uncomplicated and severe malaria caused by PCR-confirmed *Plasmodium knowlesi, Plasmodium falciparum* and *Plasmodium vivax*. J. Clin. Microbiol. 51, 1118–1123.

Barber, B.E., William, T., Grigg, M.J., Yeo, T.W., Anstey, N.M., 2013c. Limitations of microscopy to differentiate *Plasmodium* species in a region co-endemic for *Plasmodium falciparum*, *Plasmodium vivax* and *Plasmodium knowlesi*. Malar. J. 12, 8.

Barber, B.E., Bird, E., Wilkes, C.S., William, T., Grigg, M.J., Paramaswaran, U., Menon, J., Jelip, J., Yeo, T.W., Anstey, N.M., 2014. *Plasmodium knowlesi* malaria in pregnancy. J. Infect. Dis. 211, 1104–1110.

Barber, B.E., Grigg, M.J., William, T., Yeo, T.W., Anstey, N.M., 2016a. The treatment of *Plasmodium knowlesi* malaria. Trends Parasitol. 33, 242–253.

Barber, B.E., Grigg, M.J., William, T., Yeo, T.W., Anstey, N.M., 2016b. Intravascular haemolysis with haemoglobinuria in a splenectomized patient with severe Plasmodium knowlesi malaria. Malaria J 15, 462.

Barber, B.E., Grigg, M.J., Piera, K., William, T., Boyle, M.J., Yeo, T.W., Anstey, N.M., 2017. Effects of aging on parasite biomass, inflammation, endothelial activation and microvascular dysfunction in *plasmodium knowlesi* and *P. falciparum* malaria. J. Infect. Dis. 215, 1908–1917.

Barber, B.E., Grigg, M.J., Piera, K., William, T., Cooper, D.J., Plewes, K., Dondorp, A., Yeo, T.W., N.M, A., 2018. Intravascular haemolysis in severe *Plasmodium knowlesi* malaria: association with endothelial activation, microvascular dysfunction, and acute kidney injury. Emerg. Microbes & Infect. 7, 106.

Burns, A.L., Sleebs, B.E., Siddiqui, G., De Paoli, A.E., Anderson, D., Liffner, B., Harvey, R., Beeson, J.G., Creek, D.J., Goodman, C.D., 2020. Retargeting azithromycin analogues to have dual-modality antimalarial activity. BMC Biol. 18, 1–23.

Cooper, D.J., Plewes, K., Grigg, M.J., Rajahram, G.S., Piera, K.A., William, T., Chatfield, M.D., Yeo, T.W., Dondorp, A.M., Anstey, N.M., 2018a. The effect of regularly dosed paracetamol versus no paracetamol on renal function in *plasmodium knowlesi* malaria (PACKNOW): study protocol for a randomised controlled trial. Trials 19, 250.

Cooper, D.J., Grigg, M.J., Plewes, K., Rajahram, G.S., Piera, K.A., William, T., Barzi, F., Menon, J., Koleth, J., Patel, A., Yeo, T.W., Dondorp, A., Anstey, N.M., Barber, B.E., 2018b. A randomised controlled trial of regularly dosed paracetamol (acetaminophen) to reduce renal dysfunction in Plasmodium knowlesi malaria via reduction of cell free haemoglobin-mediated oxidative damage: (PACKNOW). In: American Society of Tropical Medicine and Hygiene 67th Annual Meeting, New Orleans.

Cooper, D.J., Rajahram, G.S., William, T., Jelip, J., Mohammad, R., Benedict, J., Alaza, D.A., Malacova, E., Yeo, T.W., Grigg, M.J., 2019. *Plasmodium knowlesi* malaria in Sabah, Malaysia, 2015-2017: ongoing increase in incidence despite near-elimination of the human-only *Plasmodium* species. Clin. Infect. Dis. 70, 361–367.

Coutrier, F.N., Tirta, Y.K., Cotter, C., Zarlinda, I., González, I.J., Schwartz, A., Maneh, C., Marfurt, J., Murphy, M., Herdiana, H., 2018. Laboratory challenges of Plasmodium species identification in Aceh Province, Indonesia, a malaria elimination setting with newly discovered *P. knowlesi*. PLoS Negl. Trop. Dis. 12, e0006924.

Cox-Singh, J., Davis, T.M., Lee, K.S., Shamsul, S.S., Matusop, A., Ratnam, S., Rahman, H.A., Conway, D.J., Singh, B., 2008. *Plasmodium knowlesi* malaria in humans is widely distributed and potentially life threatening. Clin. Infect. Dis. 46, 165–171.

Cuenca, P.R., Key, S., Jumail, A., Surendra, H., Ferguson, H.M., Drakely, C., Fornace, K., 2021. Epidemiology of the zoonotic malaria *Plasmodium knowlesi* in changing landscapes. Adv. Parasitol. 113, 225–286.

Daneshvar, C., Davis, T.M., Cox-Singh, J., Rafa'ee, M., Zakaria, S., Divis, P., Singh, B., 2009. Clinical and laboratory features of human *Plasmodium knowlesi* infection. Clin. Infect. Dis. 49, 852–860.

Daneshvar, C., Davis, T.M., Cox-Singh, J., Rafa'ee, M., Zakaria, S., Divis, P., Singh, B., 2010. Clinical and parasitological response to oral chloroquine and primaquine in uncomplicated human *Plasmodium knowlesi* infections. Malar. J. 9, 238.

Dellicour, S., Desai, M., Aol, G., Oneko, M., Ouma, P., Bigogo, G., Burton, D.C., Breiman, R.F., Hamel, M.J., Slutsker, L., 2015. Risks of miscarriage and inadvertent exposure to artemisinin derivatives in the first trimester of pregnancy: a prospective cohort study in western Kenya. Malar. J. 14, 1–9.

Dondorp, A., Nosten, F., Stepniewska, K., Day, N., White, N., South East Asian Quinine Artesunate Malaria Trial (Seaquamat) Group, 2005. Artesunate versus quinine for treatment of severe falciparum malaria: a randomised trial. Lancet 366, 717–725.

Dondorp, A.M., Fanello, C.I., Hendriksen, I.C., Gomes, E., Seni, A., Chhaganlal, K.D., Bojang, K., Olaosebikan, R., Anunobi, N., Maitland, K., 2010. Artesunate versus quinine in the treatment of severe falciparum malaria in African children (AQUAMAT): an open-label, randomised trial. Lancet 376, 1647–1657.

Douglas, N.M., Lampah, D.A., Kenangalem, E., Simpson, J.A., Poespoprodjo, J.R., Sugiarto, P., Anstey, N.M., Price, R.N., 2013. Major burden of severe anemia from non-falciparum malaria species in southern Papua: a hospital-based surveillance study. PLoS Med. 10, e1001575.

Ehrhardt, J., Trein, A., Kremsner, P.G., Frank, M., 2013. *Plasmodium knowlesi* and HIV co-infection in a German traveller to Thailand. Malar. J. 12, 283.

Fanello, C., Onyamboko, M., Lee, S., Woodrow, C., Setaphan, S., Chotivanich, K., Buffet, P., Jauréguiberry, S., Rockett, K., Stepniewska, K., 2017. Post-treatment haemolysis in African children with hyperparasitaemic falciparum malaria; a randomized comparison of artesunate and quinine. BMC Infect. Dis. 17, 1–8.

Fatih, F.A., Siner, A., Ahmed, A., Woon, L.C., Craig, A.G., Singh, B., Krishna, S., Cox-Singh, J., 2012. Cytoadherence and virulence–the case of *Plasmodium knowlesi* malaria. Malar. J. 11, 33.

Fatih, F.A., Staines, H.M., Siner, A., Ahmed, M.A., Woon, L.C., Pasini, E.M., Kocken, C., Singh, B., Cox-Singh, J., Krishna, S., 2013. Susceptibility of human *Plasmodium knowlesi* infections to anti-malarials. Malar. J. 12, 1186.

Figtree, M., Lee, R., Bain, L., Kennedy, T., Mackertich, S., Urban, M., Cheng, Q., Hudson, B.J., 2010. *Plasmodium knowlesi* in human, Indonesian Borneo. Emerg. Infect. Dis. 16, 672.

Gilson, P.R., Nguyen, W., Poole, W.A., Teixeira, J.E., Thompson, J.K., Guo, K., Stewart, R.J., Ashton, T.D., White, K.L., Sanz, L.M., Gamo, F.-J., Charman, S.A., Wittlin, S., Duffy, J., Tonkin, C.J., Tham, W.-H., Crabb, B.S., Cooke, B.M., Huston, C.D., Cowman, A.F., Sleebs, B.E., 2019. Evaluation of 4-amino 2-anilinoquinazolines against *Plasmodium* and other apicomplexan parasites in vitro and in a *P. falciparum* humanized NOD-SCID Il2Rγnull mouse model of malaria. Antimicrob. Agents Chemother. 63, e01804-18.

Gómez-Junyent, J., Ruiz-Panales, P., Calvo-Cano, A., Gascón, J., Muñoz, J., 2015. Delayed haemolysis after artesunate therapy in a cohort of patients with severe imported malaria due to *Plasmodium falciparum*. Enferm. Infecc. Microbiol. Clin. 35, 516–519. pii: S0213-005X(15)00393-6.

Grigg, M.J., William, T., Barber, B.E., Paramaswaran, U., Bird, E., Piera, K., Aziz, A., Dhanaraj, P., Yeo, T.W., Anstey, N.M., 2014. Combining parasite lactate dehydrogenase-based rapid tests to improve specificity for the diagnosis of malaria due to *Plasmodium knowlesi* and other *Plasmodium* species in Sabah, Malaysia. J. Clin. Microbiol. 52, 2053–2060.

Grigg, M.J., William, T., Menon, J., Dhanaraj, P., Barber, B.E., Wilkes, C.S., Von Seidlein, L., Rajahram, G.S., Pasay, C., McCarthy, J.S., 2016a. Artesunate–mefloquine versus chloroquine for treatment of uncomplicated *Plasmodium knowlesi* malaria in Malaysia (ACTKNOW): an open-label, randomised controlled trial. Lancet Infect. Dis. 16, 180–188.

Grigg, M.J., Barber, B.E., Marfurt, J., Imwong, M., William, T., Bird, E., Piera, K.A., Aziz, A., Drakeley, C.J., Cox, J., 2016b. Dihydrofolate-reductase mutations in *Plasmodium knowlesi* appear unrelated to selective drug pressure from putative human-to-human transmission in Sabah, Malaysia. PLoS One 11, e0149519.

Grigg, M.J., William, T., Menon, J., Barber, B.E., Wilkes, C.S., Rajahram, G., Edstein, M., Auburn, S., Price, R.N., Yeo, T.W., Anstey, N.M., 2016c. Efficacy of artesunate-mefloquine against high-grade chloroquine-resistant *Plasmodium vivax* malaria in Malaysia: an open-label randomised controlled trial. Clin. Infect. Dis. 62, 1403–1411.

Grigg, M.J., William, T., Barber, B.E., Rajahram, G.S., Menon, J., Schimann, E., Piera, K., Wilkes, C.S., Patal, K., Chandra, A., Drakely, C., Yeo, T.W., Anstey, N.A., 2018a. Age-related clinical spectrum of *Plasmodium knowlesi* malaria and predictors of severity. Clin. Infect. Dis. 67, 350–359.

Grigg, M.J., William, T., Barber, B.E., Rajahram, G.S., Menon, J., Schimann, E., Wilkes, C.S., Patel, K., Chandna, A., Price, R.N., 2018b. Artemether–lumefantrine versus chloroquine for the treatment of uncomplicated *Plasmodium knowlesi* malaria: an open-label randomized controlled trial can know. Clin. Infect. Dis. 66, 229–236.

Grigg, M.J., Lubis, I.N., Tetteh, K.K., Britton, S., Barber, B.E., William, T., Rajahram, G.S., Tan, A.F., Drakely, C.J., Sutherland, C.J., Noviyanti, R., Anstey, N.M., 2021. *Plasmodium knowlesi* detection methods: diagnosis and surveillance. Adv. Parasitol. 113, 77–130.

Grüring, C., Moon, R.W., Lim, C., Holder, A.A., Blackman, M.J., Duraisingh, M.T., 2014. Human red blood cell-adapted *Plasmodium knowlesi* parasites: a new model system for malaria research. Cell. Microbiol. 16, 612–620.

Hanson, J.P., Lam, S.W., Mohanty, S., Alam, S., Pattnaik, R., Mahanta, K.C., Hasan, M.U., Charunwatthana, P., Mishra, S.K., Day, N.P., 2013. Fluid resuscitation of adults with severe falciparum malaria: effects on acid-base status, renal function, and extravascular lung water. Crit. Care Med. 41, 972–981.

Hanson, J., Anstey, N.M., Bihari, D., White, N.J., Day, N.P., Dondorp, A.M., 2014. The fluid management of adults with severe malaria. Crit. Care 18, 1–9.

Hoosen, A., Shaw, M., 2011. *Plasmodium knowlesi* in a traveller returning to New Zealand. Travel Med. Infect. Dis. 9, 144–148.

Imai, N., White, M.T., Ghani, A.C., Drakeley, C.J., 2014. Transmission and control of *Plasmodium knowlesi*: a mathematical modelling study. PLoS Negl. Trop. Dis. 8, e2978.

Ishioka, H., Plewes, K., Pattnaik, R., Kingston, H.W., Leopold, S.J., Herdman, M.T., Mahanta, K., Mohanty, A., Dey, C., Alam, S., 2020. Associations between restrictive fluid management and renal function and tissue perfusion in adults with severe falciparum malaria: a prospective observational study. J. Infect. Dis. 221, 285–292.

Jauréguiberry, S., Ndour, P.A., Roussel, C., Ader, F., Safeukui, I., Nguyen, M., Biligui, S., Ciceron, L., Mouri, O., Kendjo, E., 2014. Postartesunate delayed hemolysis is a predictable event related to the lifesaving effect of artemisinins. Blood 124, 167–175.

Kerlin, D.H., Boyce, K., Marfurt, J., Simpson, J.A., Kenangalem, E., Cheng, Q., Price, R.N., Gatton, M.L., 2012. An analytical method for assessing stage-specific drug activity in *plasmodium vivax* malaria: implications for ex vivo drug susceptibility testing. PLoS Negl. Trop. Dis. 6, e1772.

Lee, K.-S., Cox-Singh, J., Singh, B., 2009. Morphological features and differential counts of *Plasmodium knowlesi* parasites in naturally acquired human infections. Malar. J. 8, 73.

Lee, C.E., Adeeba, K., Freigang, G., 2010. Human *Plasmodium knowlesi* infections in Klang Valley, peninsular Malaysia: a case series. Med J Malaysia 65, 63–65.

Lee, K.-S., Divis, P.C.S., Zakaria, S.K., Matusop, A., Julin, R.A., Conway, D.J., Cox-Singh, J., Singh, B., 2011. *Plasmodium knowlesi*: reservoir hosts and tracking the emergence in humans and macaques. PLoS Pathog. 7, e1002105.

Lim, C., Hansen, E., Desimone, T.M., Moreno, Y., Junker, K., Bei, A., Brugnara, C., Buckee, C.O., Duraisingh, M.T., 2013. Expansion of host cellular niche can drive adaptation of a zoonotic malaria parasite to humans. Nat. Commun. 4, 1638.

Llanos-Cuentas, A., Casapia, M., Chuquiyauri, R., Hinojosa, J.-C., Kerr, N., Rosario, M., Toovey, S., Arch, R.H., Phillips, M.A., Rozenberg, F.D., 2018. Antimalarial activity of single-dose DSM265, a novel plasmodium dihydroorotate dehydrogenase inhibitor, in patients with uncomplicated *Plasmodium falciparum* or *Plasmodium vivax* malaria infection: a proof-of-concept, open-label, phase 2a study. Lancet Infect. Dis. 18, 874–883.

Loy, D.E., Liu, W., Li, Y., Learn, G.H., Plenderleith, L.J., Sundararaman, S.A., Sharp, P.M., Hahn, B.H., 2017. Out of Africa: origins and evolution of the human malaria parasites *Plasmodium falciparum* and *Plasmodium vivax*. Int. J. Parasitol. 47, 87–97.

Mackroth, M.S., Tappe, D., Tannich, E., Addo, M., Rothe, C., 2016. Rapid-antigen test negative malaria in a traveler returning from Thailand, molecularly diagnosed as *Plasmodium knowlesi*. Open Forum Infect. Dis. 3, ofw039.

Mcgready, R., Lee, S., Wiladphaingern, J., Ashley, E., Rijken, M., Boel, M., Simpson, J., Paw, M., Pimanpanarak, M., Mu, O., 2012. Adverse effects of falciparum and vivax malaria and the safety of antimalarial treatment in early pregnancy: a population-based study. Lancet Infect. Dis. 12, 388–396.

Ministry Of Health Malaysia, 2014. Management Guidelines of Malaria in Malaysia. Vector Borne Disease Sector, Disease Control Division, Ministry of Health, Malaysia.

Moon, R.W., Hall, J., Rangkuti, F., Ho, Y.S., Almond, N., Mitchell, G.H., Pain, A., Holder, A.A., Blackman, M.J., 2013. Adaptation of the genetically tractable malaria pathogen *Plasmodium knowlesi* to continuous culture in human erythrocytes. Proc. Natl. Acad. Sci. U. S. A. 110, 531–536.

Moore, K.A., Simpson, J.A., Paw, M.K., Pimanpanarak, M., Wiladphaingern, J., Rijken, M.J., Jittamala, P., White, N.J., Fowkes, F.J., Nosten, F., 2016. Safety of artemisinins in first trimester of prospectively followed pregnancies: an observational study. Lancet Infect. Dis. 16, 576–583.

Mosha, D., Mazuguni, F., Mrema, S., Sevene, E., Abdulla, S., Genton, B., 2014. Safety of artemether-lumefantrine exposure in first trimester of pregnancy: an observational cohort. Malar. J. 13, 1–8.

Ninan, T., Nalees, K., Newin, M., Sultan, Q., Than, M.M., Shinde, S., Habana, A.V.F., Yusof, N.M., 2012. *Plasmodium knowlesi* malaria infection in human. Brunei Int. Med. J. 8, 358–361.

Phillips, M.A., White, K.L., Kokkonda, S., Deng, X., White, J., El Mazouni, F., Marsh, K., Tomchick, D.R., Manjalanagara, K., Rudra, K.R., 2016. A triazolopyrimidine-based dihydroorotate dehydrogenase inhibitor with improved drug-like properties for treatment and prevention of malaria. ACS Infect. Dis. 2, 945–957.

Pinheiro, M.M., Ahmed, M.A., Millar, S.B., Sanderson, T., Otto, T.D., Lu, W.C., Krishna, S., Rayner, J.C., Cox-Singh, J., 2015. *Plasmodium knowlesi* genome sequences from clinical isolates reveal extensive genomic dimorphism. PLoS One 10, e0121303.

Plewes, K., Kingston, H.W., Ghose, A., Maude, R.J., Herdman, M.T., Leopold, S.J., Ishioka, H., Hasan, M.M.U., Haider, M.S., Alam, S., 2017. Cell-free hemoglobin mediated oxidative stress is associated with acute kidney injury and renal replacement therapy in severe falciparum malaria: an observational study. BMC Infect. Dis. 17, 313.

Plewes, K., Kingston, H., Ghose, A., Wattanakul, T., Hassan, M., Dutta, P., Islam, M., Alam, S., Jahangir, S., Zahed, A., Sattar, M., Chowdhury, M., Herdman, M., Leopold, S., Ishioka, H., Piera, K., Charunwatthana, P., Silamut, K., Yeo, T.W., Lee, S., Mukaka, M., Maude, R.J., Turner, G., Faiz, M.A., Tarning, J., Oates, J.A., Anstey, N.M., White, N., Day, N., Hossain, M.A., Roberts, L., Dondorp, A., 2018.

Acetaminophen as a renoprotective adjunctive treatment in patients with severe and moderately severe falciparum malaria: a randomized, controlled, open-label trial. Clin. Infect. Dis. 67, 991–999.

Price, R.N., Von Seidlein, L., Valecha, N., Nosten, F., Baird, J.K., White, N.J., 2014. Global extent of chloroquine-resistant *plasmodium vivax*: a systematic review and meta-analysis. Lancet Infect. Dis. 14, 982–991.

Rajahram, G.S., Barber, B.E., William, T., Menon, J., Anstey, N.M., Yeo, T.W., 2012. Deaths due to *Plasmodium knowlesi* malaria in Sabah, Malaysia: association with reporting as *P. malariae* and delayed parenteral artesunate. Malaria J. 11, 284.

Rajahram, G.S., Barber, B.E., William, T., Grigg, M.J., Menon, J., Yeo, T.W., Anstey, N.M., 2016. Falling *Plasmodium knowlesi* malaria death rate among adults despite rising incidence, Sabah, Malaysia, 2010–2014. Emerg. Infect. Dis. 22, 41–48.

Rajahram, G.S., Cooper, D.J., William, T., Grigg, M.J., Anstey, N.M., Barber, B.E., 2019. Deaths from *Plasmodium knowlesi* malaria: case series and systematic review. Clin. Infect. Dis. 69, 1–36.

Russell, B., Chalfein, F., Prasetyorini, B., Kenangalem, E., Piera, K., Suwanarusk, R., Brockman, A., Prayoga, P., Sugiarto, P., Cheng, Q., 2008. Determinants of in vitro drug susceptibility testing of *Plasmodium vivax*. Antimicrob. Agents Chemother. 52, 1040–1045.

Setiadi, W., Sudoyo, H., Trimarsanto, H., Sihite, B.A., Saragih, R.J., Juliawaty, R., Wangsamuda, S., Asih, P.B.S., Syafruddin, D., 2016. A zoonotic human infection with simian malaria, *Plasmodium knowlesi*, in Central Kalimantan, Indonesia. Malar. J. 15, 1.

Sinclair, D., Donegan, S., Isba, R., Lalloo, D.G., 2012. Artesunate versus quinine for treating severe malaria. Cochrane Database Syst. Rev. 2012, CD005967.

Singh, B., Daneshvar, C., 2013. Human infections and detection of *Plasmodium knowlesi*. Clin. Microbiol. Rev. 26, 165–184.

Singh, B., Sung, L.K., Matusop, A., Radhakrishnan, A., Shamsul, S.S.G., Cox-Singh, J., Thomas, A., Conway, D.J., 2004. A large focus of naturally acquired *Plasmodium knowlesi* infections in human beings. Lancet 363, 1017–1024.

Temple, R., 2006. Hy's law: predicting serious hepatotoxicity. Pharmacoepidemiol. Drug Saf. 15, 241–243.

Tyagi, R.K., Das, M.K., Singh, S.S., Sharma, Y.D., 2013. Discordance in drug resistance-associated mutation patterns in marker genes of *Plasmodium falciparum* and *Plasmodium knowlesi* during coinfections. J. Antimicrob. Chemother. 68, 1081–1088.

van Schalkwyk, D.A., Moon, R.W., Blasco, B., Sutherland, C.J., 2017. Comparison of the susceptibility of *Plasmodium knowlesi* and *plasmodium falciparum* to antimalarial agents. J. Antimicrob. Chemother. 72, 3051–3058.

van Schalkwyk, D.A., Blasco, B., Nuñez, R.D., Liew, J.W., Amir, A., Lau, Y.L., Leroy, D., Moon, R.W., Sutherland, C.J., 2019. *Plasmodium knowlesi* exhibits distinct in vitro drug susceptibility profiles from those of *Plasmodium falciparum*. Int. J. Parasitol. Drugs Drug Resist. 9, 93–99.

van Schalkwyk, D.A., Riscoe, M.K., Pou, S., Winter, R.W., Nilsen, A., Duffey, M., Moon, R.W., Sutherland, C.J., 2020. Novel endochin-like quinolones exhibit potent in vitro activity against *Plasmodium knowlesi* but do not synergize with proguanil. Antimicrob. Agents Chemother. 64, e02549-19.

William, T., Menon, J., Rajahram, G., Chan, L., Ma, G., Donaldson, S., Khoo, S., Fredrick, C., Jilip, J., Anstey, N.M., Yeo, T.W., 2011. Severe *Plasmodium knowlesi* malaria in a tertiary hospital, Sabah, Malaysia. Emerg. Infect. Dis. 17, 1248–1255.

Willmann, M., Ahmed, A., Siner, A., Wong, I., Woon, L., Singh, B., Krishna, S., Cox-Singh, J., 2012. Laboratory markers of disease severity in *Plasmodium knowlesi* infection: a case control study. Malar. J. 11, 363.

World Health Organization, 2014. Severe malaria. Trop. Med. Int. Health 19, 7–131.

World Health Organization, 2020. World Malaria Report 2020. World Health Organisation, Geneva.

World Health Organization, 2021. Who Guidelines for Malaria. World Health Organisation, Geneva.

World Health Organization & Regional Office for the Western Pacific, 2017. Expert Consultation on *Plasmodium knowlesi* Malaria to Guide Malaria Elimination Strategies, Kota Kinabalu, Malaysia, 1–2 March 2017: Meeting Report. WHO Regional Office for the Western, Manila.

> CHAPTER THREE

Plasmodium knowlesi detection methods for human infections—Diagnosis and surveillance

Matthew J. Grigg[a,b,*], Inke N. Lubis[c], Kevin K.A. Tetteh[d], Bridget E. Barber[a,b,e], Timothy William[b,f,g], Giri S. Rajahram[b,f,h], Angelica F. Tan[a,b], Colin J. Sutherland[d], Rintis Noviyanti[i], Chris J. Drakeley[d], Sumudu Britton[e], and Nicholas M. Anstey[a,b]

[a]Menzies School of Health Research, Charles Darwin University, Darwin, NT, Australia
[b]Infectious Diseases Society Sabah-Menzies School of Health Research Clinical Research Unit, Kota Kinabalu, Sabah, Malaysia
[c]Faculty of Medicine, Universitas Sumatera Utara, Medan, Sumatera Utara, Indonesia
[d]Faculty of Infectious and Tropical Diseases, London School of Hygiene and Tropical Medicine, London, United Kingdom
[e]QIMR Berghofer Medical Research Institute, Brisbane, QLD, Australia
[f]Clinical Research Centre, Queen Elizabeth Hospital 1, Kota Kinabalu, Malaysia
[g]Gleneagles Medical Centre, Kota Kinabalu, Malaysia
[h]Queen Elizabeth Hospital 2, Kota Kinabalu, Malaysia
[i]Eijkman Institute for Molecular Biology, Jakarta, Indonesia
*Corresponding author: e-mail address: matthew.grigg@menzies.edu.au

Contents

1.	Introduction	78
2.	Point-of-care diagnosis	81
	2.1 Microscopy	81
	2.2 Rapid diagnostic tests	86
3.	Molecular detection	94
	3.1 PCR assays	94
	3.2 Loop-mediated isothermal amplification (LAMP)	107
4.	Serology	110
	4.1 Importance of serology for malaria surveillance	110
	4.2 Development of serologic assays for *P. knowlesi* detection	111
	4.3 Potential use case scenarios for *P. knowlesi* serologic tools	113
5.	Conclusion	117
	Acknowledgements	117
	References	117

Advances in Parasitology, Volume 113
ISSN 0065-308X
https://doi.org/10.1016/bs.apar.2021.08.002

Copyright © 2021 Elsevier Ltd
All rights reserved.

77

Abstract

Within the overlapping geographical ranges of *P. knowlesi* monkey hosts and vectors in Southeast Asia, an estimated 1.5 billion people are considered at risk of infection. *P. knowlesi* can cause severe disease and death, the latter associated with delayed treatment occurring from misdiagnosis. Although microscopy is a sufficiently sensitive first-line tool for *P. knowlesi* detection for most low-level symptomatic infections, misdiagnosis as other *Plasmodium* species is common, and the majority of asymptomatic infections remain undetected. Current point-of-care rapid diagnostic tests demonstrate insufficient sensitivity and poor specificity for differentiating *P. knowlesi* from other *Plasmodium* species. Molecular tools including nested, real-time, and single-step PCR, and loop-mediated isothermal amplification (LAMP), are sensitive for *P. knowlesi* detection. However, higher cost and inability to provide the timely point-of-care diagnosis needed to guide appropriate clinical management has limited their routine use in most endemic clinical settings. *P. knowlesi* is likely underdiagnosed across the region, and improved diagnostic and surveillance tools are required. Reference laboratory molecular testing of malaria cases for both zoonotic and non-zoonotic *Plasmodium* species needs to be more widely implemented by National Malaria Control Programs across Southeast Asia to accurately identify the burden of zoonotic malaria and more precisely monitor the success of human-only malaria elimination programs. The implementation of specific serological tools for *P. knowlesi* would assist in determining the prevalence and distribution of asymptomatic and submicroscopic infections, the absence of transmission in certain areas, and associations with underlying land use change for future spatially targeted interventions.

1. Introduction

The recent increase in zoonotic transmission of the Cercopithecinae Old World monkey malaria parasite *Plasmodium knowlesi*, endemic to Southeast Asia, exemplifies how intensive anthropogenic land–use change is driving emerging disease spill–over to humans (Brock et al., 2019). Although a single presumed anomalous human *P. knowlesi* infection was first reported in the 1960s in Peninsular Malaysia (Chin et al., 1965), it was not until 2004 that Singh and colleagues using molecular detection methods identified a large number of naturally acquired human knowlesi malaria cases in Sarawak, East Malaysia (Singh et al., 2004). Molecular analysis of archival samples in Sarawak (Lee et al., 2009a) and Thailand (Jongwutiwes et al., 2011) demonstrated that in this region *P. knowlesi* had been misreported on routine microscopy at least as far back as the mid–1990s. Regional under–reporting of *P. knowlesi* infections is likely occurring, with PCR confirmed infections now documented from all countries in Southeast Asia where its major natural macaque hosts (*Macaca fascicularis* and

M. nemestrina) and *Anopheles* Leucosphyrus group vectors are present (Herdiana et al., 2016; Iwagami et al., 2018; Lubis et al., 2017; Moyes et al., 2014; Singh and Daneshvar, 2013).

Changes in human land use are thought to play a major role in driving the increase in *P. knowlesi* exposure to humans, with the relative influence of associated environmental factors such as forest fragmentation varying at different spatial scales (Brock et al., 2019; Fornace et al., 2019b). Increased interaction between humans, vectors and the monkey parasite reservoir results from adaptive behaviours in response to these changing landscapes (Fornace et al., 2019a; Stark et al., 2019). Differences in monkey and human host biting preferences between *An.* leucosphyrus group species may also influence spatial variation in *P. knowlesi* transmission patterns (Vythilingam, 2010). Vector adaptation includes features such as earlier outside peak biting times in the evening for *An. balabacensis*, an incriminated *P. knowlesi* vector in Sabah (Wong et al., 2015). Adaptation to human-to-human transmission as a potential underlying driver of the emergence of *P. knowlesi* has not been evident in studies to date comparing parasite genetic lineages between macaque and human hosts (Divis et al., 2015; Jeslyn et al., 2011; Jongwutiwes et al., 2011; Lee et al., 2011). However, vector competence for this transmission mode has been experimentally proven (Chin et al., 1968), with incriminated *P. knowlesi* vectors such as *An. dirus* and *An. balabacensis* also being the primary vector for non-zoonotic *Plasmodium* species in certain areas (Marchand et al., 2011; Vythilingam, 2010). A decrease in cross-protective human immunity from the reduction of malaria transmission due to *P. vivax* may also be contributing to the prevalence of symptomatic disease or patent *P. knowlesi* infections detectable by microscopy in endemic areas (Muh et al., 2020).

Technological advances in malaria detection methods, specifically the advent of highly sensitive and specific molecular tools, have allowed accurate confirmation of *P. knowlesi* human infections across Southeast Asia (Singh and Daneshvar, 2013). However, first-line point-of-care testing for suspected malaria in most co-endemic settings in Southeast Asia primarily involves microscopy, which is inherently unreliable for diagnosing *P. knowlesi* due to morphological similarities with *P. malariae* and *P. falciparum*. Further complicating microscopic diagnosis, *P. knowlesi* co-infections particularly with *P. vivax* are common in endemic areas (Singh and Daneshvar, 2013). Current lateral flow malaria rapid diagnostic assays designed for non-zoonotic malaria species have shown poor sensitivity and specificity for *P. knowlesi* detection, particularly at the low parasite counts often seen even in symptomatic infections (Barber et al., 2013b; Grigg et al., 2014). Molecular tools including nested, real-time, and single-step PCR, and loop-mediated isothermal amplification (LAMP), have now been designed for *P. knowlesi* detection (Singh and Daneshvar, 2013). However, higher cost and inability to provide the timely point-of-care diagnosis needed to guide appropriate clinical management has limited their routine use in most endemic clinical settings.

Molecular tools used for research surveillance purposes, including in monkey hosts and mosquito vectors, have highlighted key knowledge gaps in estimating regional variation in the transmission and disease burden of *P. knowlesi* (Shearer et al., 2016). This includes the detection of underreported asymptomatic or submicroscopic infections (Fornace et al., 2016b; Grignard et al., 2019; Imwong et al., 2019; Jongwutiwes et al., 2011; Lubis et al., 2017; Marchand et al., 2011). In this context, understanding of *P. knowlesi* transmission has been further enhanced by the recent development of serological surveillance tools for *P. knowlesi* indicating past exposure. These multiplex sero-surveillance platforms also offer the potential for more detailed understanding of factors associated with exposure to *P. knowlesi* and other malaria species over time (Herman et al., 2018). Use of these sero-surveillance tools has already provided important insights into *P. knowlesi* transmission and specific environmental associations, including identifying infection exposure in demographic groups such as children and women thought to be at lower risk (Fornace et al., 2019b).

The emergence of *P. knowlesi* in Southeast Asia, with an intractable monkey parasite reservoir and ongoing misidentification with other *Plasmodium* species, threatens regional malaria elimination goals (Chin et al., 2020; Cox-Singh and Singh, 2008). In Malaysia, implementation of routine PCR for species confirmation of all malaria cases since 2012 has enabled public health authorities to demonstrate the near-elimination of *P. falciparum* and *P. vivax* malaria, alongside a concurrent increase in *P. knowlesi* cases in high-risk groups such as adult males with a history of forest exposure or agricultural work (Chin et al., 2020; Hussin et al., 2020; WHO, 2020). Molecular tools have also allowed accurate descriptions of the disease spectrum of *P. knowlesi*, ranging from asymptomatic infections, to severe malaria in 6%–9% (Grigg et al., 2018a; Singh and Daneshvar, 2013), and fatalities in 2.5 per 1000 cases (Rajahram et al., 2019). However, routine molecular confirmation of cases is not possible in many resource constrained settings, and WHO do not specifically include PCR-confirmed *P. knowlesi* case notifications in global yearly reporting

(Barber et al., 2017b; WHO, 2020). Thus, the true regional prevalence and disease burden of *P. knowlesi* infections remains poorly understood, with limited use of accurate detection methods outside research settings.

In 2017 the WHO convened an evidence review group to guide research priorities in response to the public health threat posed by the emergence of *P. knowlesi*, which included a major recommendation to develop and improve laboratory detection methods (WHO, 2017). The following sections review current detection methods for both point-of-care diagnosis and surveillance of *P. knowlesi* human infections.

2. Point-of-care diagnosis

2.1 Microscopy

Microscopy remains the gold standard for malaria diagnosis in most endemic countries, as it is inexpensive, fast, sensitive and allows parasite quantification. Microscopy does however require trained laboratory technicians and equipment, an electricity supply and ongoing quality assurance procedures (WHO, 2015a). Older malaria microscopy teaching or reference tools generally in routine use in Southeast Asia do not include descriptions of *P. knowlesi* or comment on similarities with *P. malariae* or *P. falciparum*. Formal public health malaria reporting by microscopy in most countries outside Malaysia have not yet added provisions for suspected *P. knowlesi*. *P. malariae* remains the conventional reporting default, further limiting accurate regional estimates on the true burden of disease (Barber et al., 2013; Cox-Singh et al., 2008). Morphological similarities between *P. knowlesi* and *P. malariae* have allowed the existence of human *P. knowlesi* cases to previously remain undiagnosed. Misdiagnosis of *P. knowlesi* as the more benign *P. malariae* has also contributed to a lack of recognition of severe disease, with important adverse clinical and treatment outcomes (Rajahram et al., 2012; William et al., 2011), including case-fatalities (Rajahram et al., 2019). In contrast to *P. knowlesi*, *P. malariae* preferentially infects older senescent red blood cells (RBCs), which in addition to a slow 72-h replication cycle and host immunity results in chronic infections with low parasite counts (Collins and Jeffery, 2007). In *P. knowlesi* endemic areas, infections appearing morphologically similar to *P. malariae*, particularly with higher parasite counts, should be reported and treated as *P. knowlesi* with PCR confirmation for final reporting purposes where possible (Barber et al., 2017a,b).

2.1.1 P. knowlesi *morphology in human infections*

The first descriptions of the morphology of *P. knowlesi* in experimental inoculated human infections by Knowles and Das Gupta in 1932 commented on the similarity with *P. malariae*, including little or no amoeboid activity, and normal size of infected red blood cells (Knowles and Gupta, 1932). Sinton and Mulligan more extensively detailed the 24-h life-cycle of the parasite, the distinctive stippling occasionally observed in schizont-infected cells (different from that seen in *P. vivax*) and the presence of an accessory chromatin dot (Sinton and Mulligan, 1933), originally thought to be diagnostic for *P. knowlesi* but subsequently found to be present in other simian *Plasmodium* species (Coatney et al., 1971).

More recently, Lee et al. in 2009 described detailed microscopy findings in 10 human *P. knowlesi* cases from Sarawak, Malaysia (as in Fig. 1). Early trophozoites resembled those of *P. falciparum*, with a ring-like cytoplasm, and double chromatin dots, multiply infected red blood cells and applique forms were all seen. Late trophozoites were almost indistinguishable from *P. malariae*, with dense irregular cytoplasm and band-like forms often present. Schizonts were noted on average to contain 10 merozoites, and up to 16, in contrast to *P. malariae*, which has a maximum of 12 and are more regularly arranged (Lee et al., 2009b). Stippling was not observed in this study, although has been described in other case reports (Figtree et al., 2010; Jongwutiwes et al., 2004). Gametocytes have been described as being rare, spherical, and develop over 48h. Resembling *P. malariae* sexual stages, the mature female macrogametocyte stains blue and contains a small eccentrically placed nucleus, compared to the pink staining male microgametocyte with a nucleus making up about half of the body of the parasite (Coatney et al., 1971).

2.1.2 P. knowlesi *parasite count measurements*

The majority of symptomatic *P. knowlesi* human infections consist of patent low-level asexual parasites when quantified on peripheral blood films. A large prospective study of 481 knowlesi malaria cases presenting to primary health facilities in Sabah, Malaysia demonstrated a median parasite count of 2480/μL (IQR 538–8481/μL; range 20–263,772/μL). Median parasitemia was lower than that seen in falciparum or vivax malaria in both adults and children. Children less than 12 years of age with *P. knowlesi* infections had a lower median parasitemia of 1722/μL (IQR 386–4830/μL) compared to adults (Grigg et al., 2018a).

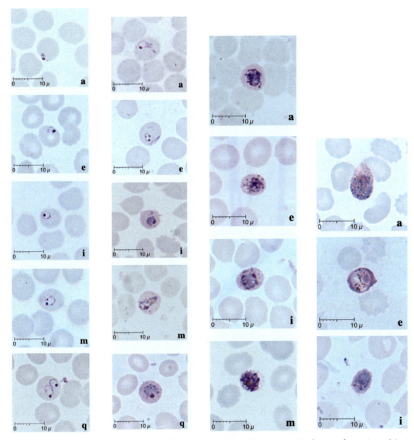

Fig. 1 Morphology of *P. knowlesi* life-stages. L-R columns: 1. Early trophozoites (rings): note normal sized RBC, multiply infected RBCs, double chromatin dots; 2. Late trophozoites (including band forms); 3. Schizonts; 4. Gametocytes (a) macrogametocyte, (e) microgametocyte, (i) young gametocyte. *Adapted from Lee, K.S., Cox-Singh, J., Singh, B., 2009b. Morphological features and differential counts of Plasmodium knowlesi parasites in naturally acquired human infections. Malaria J. 8, 73. https:/doi.org/10.1186/1475-2875-8-73.*

Extremely high parasite counts of greater than 500,000 parasites/μL (10% of infected red blood cells) can occur, in part attributed to the fast 24-h parasite life-cycle, although more definitely linked to alternative red blood cell invasion pathways such as the presence of *P. knowlesi* normocyte binding proteins (Ahmed et al., 2014). A lower parasite count threshold of 100,000/μL to define hyperparasitemia compared to falciparum malaria was determined from severe knowlesi malaria cases in Malaysia (Barber et al., 2013a) and subsequently adopted as the WHO epidemiological and definition for hyperparasitemia defining severe malaria for *P. knowlesi* (WHO, 2014). These guidelines defined a parasitemia >20,000/μL as the clinical definition requiring treatment as severe malaria in those in whom other laboratory measures of severe malaria cannot be measured (WHO, 2014).

2.1.3 P. knowlesi *life stages in human infections*

Similar to *P. malariae* and *P. vivax*, the majority of *P. knowlesi* infections (86%) are asynchronous in data from Sabah, with a mean proportion of early trophozoite ring stages relative to other parasite life stages of 44%, compared to late trophozoites at 54% and schizonts comprising on average 2% (Grigg et al., 2018a), consistent with other prospective tertiary hospital data (Barber et al., 2013a). In contrast to *P. falciparum* infections, which due to microvascular cytoadherence demonstrate almost exclusively synchronous ring stage infections in peripheral blood films, *P. knowlesi* synchronous ring stage-only infections were seen in a small proportion (5%) of cases (Grigg et al., 2018a). *P. knowlesi* asynchronous infections had a higher median parasite count of 2177/μL, compared to synchronous ring-stage infections of 461/μL. Schizonts were present in 38% (95% CI 33%–42%) of *P. knowlesi* infections in this study overall, with a schizont proportion >10% relative to other life-stages found to be associated with higher parasite counts and severe disease (Barber et al., 2013a; Grigg et al., 2018a). Gametocytes were noted to be present by microscopy in 14% (95% CI 11%–18%) of patients (Grigg et al., 2018a), lower than in Lee et al. where detailed research microscopy demonstrated four (40%) patients had gametocytes, although also at very low levels of up to ~3% of infected red blood cells (Lee et al., 2009b).

2.1.4 *Diagnostic performance of routine malaria microscopy for* P. knowlesi *infections*

Studies involving reference PCR diagnostics have consistently demonstrated the poor utility of thick blood film microscopy to correctly identify symptomatic *P. knowlesi* infections (Mahittikorn et al., 2021). In addition to misidentification with *P. malariae*, *P. knowlesi* is often misreported as both *P. falciparum* and *P. vivax*, and vice versa, despite the latter having distinct morphological differences including enlargement of infected red blood cells (Barber et al., 2013; Coutrier et al., 2018). In countries north of Malaysia, *P. knowlesi* has been most commonly detected as co-infections with *P. falciparum* or *P. vivax*, creating further challenges for the use of microscopy for accurate diagnosis and reporting (Jongwutiwes et al., 2011; Marchand et al., 2011). Co-infections also highlight the shared mosquito vectors between zoonotic and human-only *Plasmodium* species in co-endemic areas (Marchand et al., 2011). Implications of these findings for co-endemic settings in Southeast Asia include the lack of anti-relapse therapy for *P. vivax* and, historically, the inappropriate treatment of *P. falciparum* with chloroquine.

In Malaysia, Barber et al. described the limitations of microscopy to reliably distinguish between *Plasmodium* species in a co-endemic region of Malaysia in a prospective evaluation of PCR-confirmed *Plasmodium* infections (Barber et al., 2013a). In routine hospital-based microscopy of 130 malaria patients, only 72% of PCR confirmed *P. knowlesi* monoinfections were identified as '*P. malariae/P. knowlesi*', 13% as *P. falciparum* and 10% as *P. vivax* (Barber et al., 2013a). More recently in state-wide malaria notifications from Sabah over the period 2015–2017, despite nearing elimination of *P. falciparum* and *P. vivax*, the specificity of microscopy to correctly identify *P. knowlesi* remained low for at 68% (95% CI 62%–73%) against reference malaria PCR (Cooper et al., 2020).

In other countries where research studies have used appropriate PCR methods to detect *P. knowlesi* infections, routine microscopy has been shown to perform poorly in terms of differentiating all *Plasmodium* species. In Aceh Province, Indonesia, in 2014–2015, a small study of 41 microscopy positive malaria cases, including 3 cases reported as *P. malariae*, found 19 *P. knowlesi* monoinfections using PCR, with routine microscopy misidentifying 56% of all infections (Coutrier et al., 2018). In a study from North Sumatra, Indonesia, of 1169 participants with PCR confirmed *Plasmodium* species infections, 377 were found to be positive for *P. knowlesi* (including around half with mixed *P. vivax* infections) on PCR, with none of the 34 with patent microscopic infections reported as *P. knowlesi* (Lubis et al., 2017). In Thailand in a study conducted in 2008–2009, there were 3300 febrile patients with PCR confirmed malaria, nearly all of whom were diagnosed with either *P. falciparum* (52%) or *P. vivax* (48%) by microscopy. Of these patients 23 were subsequently confirmed as *P. knowlesi* (8 monoinfections, and 15 mixed infections) (Jongwutiwes et al., 2011). The monkey malaria species *P. cynomolgi*, also known to infect humans in Southeast Asia albeit more rarely, resembles *P. vivax* morphologically on microscopy, further complicating accurate diagnosis and reporting (Grignard et al., 2019; Imwong et al., 2019).

2.1.5 *Automated visualisation of blood films for detecting* P. knowlesi *infections*

Novel diagnostic devices based on automated visualization of malaria microscopy blood films using machine learning approaches are increasingly being validated for detection of *Plasmodium* species infections (Torres et al., 2018). These approaches hold promise, with a recent malaria microscopy scanner device evaluating laboratory cultured *P. knowlesi* and *P. falciparum* parasites demonstrating higher precision than microscopy for parasitemia at a lower limit of 0.1% of infected RBCs, although further development to allow differentiation between species on clinical samples using thick blood films is required (Firdaus et al., 2021).

2.2 Rapid diagnostic tests

Point-of-care diagnostics such as immunochromatographic rapid diagnostic tests (RDTs) play an important role in parasite-based malaria diagnosis world-wide, as they can be performed by people with minimal training in areas where good quality microscopy cannot be maintained (WHO, 2021). Other advantages, particularly compared to molecular detection tools, include the limited amount of time needed to conduct the RDT and receive a result (usually less than 20 min) and relatively low cost. Commercially available sensitive RDTs to detect *Plasmodium* genus and/or species–specific tests for *P. falciparum* and *P. vivax* are widely used, including in returned travellers from endemic settings (WHO, 2020). Of the most commonly used RDTs, many utilise antigen capture for parasite lactate dehydrogenase (pLDH), with a variety of monoclonal antibodies targeting different epitopes associated with *P. falciparum* and *P. vivax* pLDH isoforms allowing species specific identification (McCutchan et al., 2008). Although no specific *P. knowlesi* RDTs have been designed to date, cross–reactivity between certain pLDH epitopes for *P. falciparum* and *P. vivax* with a subset of *P. knowlesi* parasites also expressing these epitopes allows their detection, with sensitivity associated with the degree of binding affinity. In addition, tests targeting non-specific *Plasmodium* species pLDH or aldolase enzyme are able to detect *P. knowlesi* (McCutchan et al., 2008); Table 1.

Importantly, *P. knowlesi* does not appear to cross-react with the highly specific *P. falciparum* histidine-rich protein-2 (HRP2), used in the most sensitive *P. falciparum*-based RDTs. The extensive use of *P. falciparum*-HRP2 based RDTs has resulted in selection of parasites with deletions in the *pfhrp2* and *pfhrp3* genes, rendering *P. falciparum* infections with these deletions undetectable. However, *pfhrp2/3* deletions have been reported only in

Table 1 Sensitivity of individual antigen/antibody targets in commercially available RDTs evaluated to date for detecting *P. knowlesi*.

RDT name (manufacturer; product code)	WHO RDT testing round/ product code	Target antibody (epitope)	Target *Plasmodium* species	Sensitivity for *P. knowlesi*, n/N, % (95% CI)	Parasitaemia Median parasites/µL, (IQR) [range]	Lowest parasite count/µL detected	Location	Year	References
First Response Malaria Antigen pLDH/HRP2 Combo Card Test Premier Medical Corporation Ltd., Mumbai, India	1, 2 I16FRC25	Pan-pLDH	*P. genus*	30/34, 88 (73–95)	7493 [907–584,018]	907	Kota Kinabalu, Sabah, Malaysia	2013	Barber et al. (2013)
		Pf-HRP2	*P. falciparum*	0/34, 0 (0)					
ParaHIT Total Dipstick SPAN Diagnostics, Ltd., Surat, India	1, 2 55IC204-10	Pan-aldolase	*P. genus*	22/96, 23 (16–32)	50,794 [395–340,954]	4412	Kota Kinabalu, Sabah, Malaysia	2013	Barber et al. (2013)
		Pf-HRP2	*P. falciparum*	0/96, 0 (0)					
BinaxNOW Malaria Inverness Medical Innovations, Inc., FL, USA	1, 2 IN660050	Pan-aldolase	*P. genus*	8/28, 29 (12–26)	9131 [159–911,616]	1/12 for <500/µL	Sarikei, Sarawak, Malaysia	2014	Foster et al. (2014)
		Pf-HRP2	*P. falciparum*	0/28, 0 (0)	9131 [159–911,616]	NA			
Paramax-3 Rapid Test for Malaria Pan/ Pv/Pf Zephyr Biomedicals, India	1, 2 50320025	Pan-pLDH	*P. genus*	10/25, 40 (21–59)	9131 [159–911,616]	2/6 for <5000/µL	Sarikei, Sarawak, Malaysia	2014	Foster et al. (2014)
		Pv-pLDH	*P. vivax*	8/25, 32 (15–54)	9131 [159–911,616]	1/8 for <500/µL			
		Pf-HRP2	*P. falciparum*	1/25[a], 4 (0–20)	9131 [159–911,616]	—			

Continued

Table 1 Sensitivity of individual antigen/antibody targets in commercially available RDTs evaluated to date for detecting *P. knowlesi.*—cont'd

RDT name (manufacturer; product code)	WHO RDT testing round/ product code	Target antibody (epitope)	Target *Plasmodium* species	Sensitivity for *P. knowlesi*, n/N, % (95% CI)	Parasitaemia Median parasites/μL, (IQR) [range]	Lowest parasite count/μL detected	Location	Year	References
OptiMAL-IT DiaMed, CA, USA	1, 3 710024	Pf-pLDH (17E4)	*P. falciparum*	18/28, 64 (44–81)	9131 [159–911,616]	1/3 for <500/μL	Sarikei, Sarawak, Malaysia	2014	Foster et al. (2014)
				55/190, 29 (22–35)	2301 [30–641,464]	30 parasites/μL	Kota Kinabalu, Sabah, Malaysia	2014	Grigg et al. (2014)
		Pan-pLDH (19G4)	*P. genus*	20/28, 71 (54–88)	9131 [159–911,616]	1/3 for <500/μL	Sarikei, Sarawak, Malaysia	2014	Foster et al. (2014)
				57/189, 30 (24–37)	2301 [30–641,464]	30 parasites/μL	Kota Kinabalu, Sabah, Malaysia	2014	Grigg et al. (2014)
CareStart™ Malaria HRP2/pLDH (Pf/ VOM) Combo Access Bio, Inc. NJ, USA	2, 4 G0171	VOM-pLDH	*P. vivax, P. ovale, P. malariae*	77/178, 43 (36–51)	2301 [30–641,464]	50 parasites/μL	Kota Kinabalu, Sabah, Malaysia	2014	Grigg et al. (2014)
		Pf-HRP2	*P. falciparum*	4/183[a], 2 (0–4)	2301 [30–641,464]	—			

[a]False positive Pf-HRP2 result.
Systematic evaluations, pre-treatment, fresh whole blood samples only.

countries outside Southeast Asia, and non-expression of pLDH or aldolase targets has not been documented. WHO recommends ongoing use of *P. falciparum*-HRP2 based tests in areas where <5% false negative rates for *P. falciparum* detection are present (WHO, 2021).

2.2.1 Pan-pLDH based RDTs

The best performing RDT published to date for detecting *P. knowlesi* was the First Response Malaria pLDH/HRP2 Combo™ test (Premier Medical Ltd., India). Barber et al. demonstrated a sensitivity of the pan-pLDH component of 74% (95% CI 65%–80%) for detecting *P. knowlesi* infections, with a positive result in 95/129 patients. For samples tested prior to antimalarial treatment the sensitivity increased to 88% (95% CI 73%–95%), although with a higher median parasite count of 7493/μL (IQR 3823–19,895/μL) among those tested. Within this group, for those with parasite counts greater than 1000/μL sensitivity further increased to 97% (95% CI 83%–99%), although had a corresponding low sensitivity of 25% below this parasite count cut-off. Sensitivity in severe malaria with higher parasitemias was 95% (36/38; 95% CI, 83–99), however the pLDH target failed to detect two moderately high individual parasite counts of 3486 and 48,833 parasites/μL. All *P. knowlesi* samples tested negative for the concurrent *P. falciparum* HRP2 target (Barber et al., 2013b).

The OptiMAL-IT™ malaria RDT (DiaMed, USA) includes a pan-pLDH based component and was evaluated by Foster et al., with positive tests reported in 18 freshly collected *P. knowlesi* samples, resulting in a sensitivity of 64% (95% CI 44%–81%). The median parasite count of samples tested was 9131/μL, however sensitivity was markedly reduced in those with lower parasitemias, with a single positive result in the small number of three total samples tested with parasite counts below 500/μL (Foster et al., 2014). The poor performance of the pan-pLDH component in the OptiMAL-IT™ test was consistent with a separate larger study of 190 *P. knowlesi* clinical samples, which comprised a lower median parasite count of 2301/μL among those tested. A poorer sensitivity of 29% (95% CI 22%–35%) for the OptiMAL-IT™ pan-pLDH target was demonstrated, despite a low minimum detectable parasite count of 30 parasites/μL (Grigg et al., 2014).

The Paramax-3 Rapid Test for Malaria Pan/Pv/Pf™ (Zephyr Biomedicals, India) was evaluated by Foster et al., who reported a poor sensitivity of the pan-pLDH test component of 32% (95% CI 17%–46%) in fresh *P. knowlesi* infected samples (Foster et al., 2014). Grigg et al. evaluated the

CareStart™ Malaria HRP2/pLDH (Pf/VOM) Combo RDT (Access Bio Inc., USA), with the VOM pLDH component targeting non-falciparum species (*P. vivax*, *P. ovale* and *P. malariae*). This pLDH based target was also relatively poor for detecting *P. knowlesi*, with 77/178 clinical samples positive, resulting in a low sensitivity of 43% (95% CI 36–51) (Grigg et al., 2014). For the studies evaluating the Paramax-3™ and CareStart™ RDTs which also contain a *P. falciparum*-HRP2 test, a small number of false positive results, less than 0.04%, were recorded for *P. knowlesi* samples read by research staff blinded to the underlying PCR-confirmed *Plasmodium* species result (Foster et al., 2014; Grigg et al., 2014).

2.2.2 *P. falciparum* and *P. vivax*–*pLDH* antibody cross-reactivity with *P. knowlesi*

The known *P. knowlesi* cross-reactivity with certain *P. falciparum* and *P. vivax*-pLDH epitopes has been exploited to evaluate RDTs containing these test components for detection of *P. knowlesi* infections. For *P. knowlesi* a high homology of 96.8% has been found with the pLDH ortholog for *P. vivax*, and over 90% for *P. falciparum*, *P. malariae* and *P. ovale* (Singh et al., 2012). Despite the inherent lack of specificity in this approach, cross-reactivity against *P. knowlesi* in clinical samples has been demonstrated. A *P. falciparum*-pLDH (rather than HRP2) target in the OptiMAL-IT™ RDT demonstrated positive test results in 18/28 *P. knowlesi* samples in Sarawak, Malaysia with a sensitivity of 64% (95% CI 44%–81%) (Foster et al., 2014). Positive results for *P. falciparum*-pLDH were also recorded among 190 patients with comparatively lower overall *P. knowlesi* parasite counts, resulting in a sensitivity of 29% (95% CI 22%–35%) in Sabah, Malaysia (Grigg et al., 2014). A *P. vivax*-pLDH target was evaluated in the Paramax-3™ RDT, with a lower sensitivity of 32% (95 %CI 15%–54%) for detecting *P. knowlesi* compared to the pan-pLDH component (Foster et al., 2014). The Core Malaria Pan/Pv/Pf™ malaria RDT (Core Diagnostics Ltd., USA) demonstrated a positive *P. vivax*-pLDH result for a single returned traveller with PCR confirmed knowlesi malaria and a parasite count of 40,000/μL (Berry et al., 2011). The addition of the *P. falciparum*-pLDH or *P. vivax*-pLDH tests in the OptiMAL-IT™ and Paramax-3™ RDTs respectively did not confer any improvement in overall sensitivity when results were combined with the pan–pLDH test components for *P. knowlesi* diagnosis.

2.2.3 Pan-aldolase based RDTs

The BinaxNOW Malaria RDT™ (Inverness Medical Innovations Inc., USA) contains a pan-aldolase target validated for conventional major human *Plasmodium* species (*P. falciparum*, *P. vivax*, *P. malariae* and *P. ovale*), in addition to a *P. falciparum* HRP2 test component. The pan-aldolase test performed poorly when conducted on *P. knowlesi* samples, with a reported sensitivity of 29% (95% CI 12%–26%), including negative results for all 10 *P. knowlesi* samples tested with a parasite count of less than 5000/μL (Foster et al., 2014). The ParaHIT Total Dipstick™ RDT was evaluated by Barber et al, which also contains a pan-aldolase target and *P. falciparum* HRP2 target. *P. knowlesi* detection was also poor, with the pan-aldolase target demonstrating a sensitivity of 23% (95% CI 16%–32%) and the lowest parasite count detected was 4412/μL (Barber et al., 2013b).

2.2.4 RDT use in returned travellers from endemic countries

Published case reports from returned travellers with *P. knowlesi* malaria who visited endemic countries in Southeast Asia including from the Netherlands, Sweden, Spain, Australia, France, Japan, Germany, and Italy most commonly described the use of the BinaxNOW™ RDT as a primary point-of-care diagnostic tool. The pan-aldolase test strip for *Plasmodium* species detection was positive in thtree case reports in patients with moderate to high parasite counts of 84,000/μL (van Hellemond et al., 2009), 40,000/μL (Berry et al., 2011) and 7700/μL (Ong et al., 2009), with the remainder negative. A number of *P. knowlesi* case reports from various non-endemic countries after the BinaxNOW™ evaluation was published in 2014 highlights the ongoing use of this RDT as a first line point of care malaria diagnostic tool in returned travellers. This is despite the poor performance demonstrated for detecting *P. knowlesi*, in addition to that seen for *P. vivax* at lower parasite counts in previous WHO malaria RDT product testing (WHO, 2015b). The OptiMAL-IT™ RDT has also been reported as having positive *P. falciparum*-pLDH results when conducted in Netherlands (van Hellemond et al., 2009) and Singapore (Ong et al., 2009) for *P. knowlesi* confirmed symptomatic infections. The Core Malaria Pan/Pv/Pf™ malaria RDT used in a single *P. knowlesi* case report demonstrated a positive pan-pLDH and negative *P. falciparum*-HRP2 test in addition to the positive *P. vivax*-pLDH result previously mentioned (Berry et al., 2011).

2.2.5 RDT detection for Plasmodium species in monkey hosts

Kawai et al. evaluated two malaria RDTs for the detection of different simian malaria species infections in non-natural Japanese macaque hosts. The study macaques were separately inoculated with *P. knowlesi* Hackeri strain, *P. gonderi*, *P. cynomolgi* B strain, and *P. coatneyi* CDC strain and monitored over the ensuing course of infection (Kawai et al., 2009). The Entebe Malaria Casette™ (Laboritorium Hepatika, Indonesia) was evaluated, which contains a *P. vivax*-pLDH target found to be initially negative for the *P. knowlesi* infected macaque at a parasitemia of 0.04%, and subsequently positive at later higher parasitemias of 11.2% and 28.8% of infected red blood cells. The OptiMAL-IT™ RDT was also concurrently evaluated with positive *P. falciparum*-pLDH and pan-pLDH results at the same parasite count levels. Serial dilutions of the quantified *P. knowlesi* sample were used to demonstrate weakly positive results remaining present at a minimum of 100 parasites/µL for both RDTs. Both the *P. vivax*-pLDH target for the Entebe Malaria Cassette™ and the OptiMAL-IT™ pan-pLDH test demonstrated positivity when tested on other Old World non-human primate malaria species infections including *P. gonderi*, *P. cynomolgi* and *P. coatneyi*. The *P. falciparum*-pLDH test component for OptiMAL-IT™ was positive for *P. gonderi*, however negative for *P. cynomolgi* and *P. coatneyi* (Kawai et al., 2009).

2.2.6 Summary and recommendations for RDT use

Commercially available RDTs evaluated to date have limited utility in accurately detecting *P. knowlesi* clinical infections and should not replace microscopy as an existing first line malaria diagnostic tool in endemic areas, or PCR detection methods for accurate final *Plasmodium* species reporting. Neither pan-pLDH or pan-aldolase based tests have demonstrated sufficient sensitivity for detecting *P. knowlesi*, particularly with low parasite counts of less than 1000/µL which are seen in around 33% (95% CI 32%–34%) of over 8000 *P. knowlesi* malaria cases in endemic areas such as Sabah, Malaysia over recent years (*unpublished data, Sabah Ministry of Health*). Cross-reactivity of *P. knowlesi* with *P. falciparum*-pLDH and *P. vivax*-pLDH test components are also insufficiently sensitive to diagnose *P. knowlesi* reliably. In co-endemic areas specificity for the original *P. falciparum* and *P. vivax* pLDH targets is potentially less than manufacturer's report (Grigg et al., 2014).

Point-of-care malaria RDT use in returned travellers from *P. knowlesi* endemic areas requires the concurrent use of microscopy for initial diagnosis and clinical management, and validated PCR detection methods for accurate final *Plasmodium* species reporting.

RDTs remain a major point-of-care malaria diagnostic tool in Southeast Asia, with over 12.7 million distributed in the WHO regions encompassing *P. knowlesi* endemic areas in 2019 (WHO, 2020). Consistent with current WHO recommendations, in malaria endemic areas in Southeast Asia (or in returned travellers) where RDTs are used as a first line tool, a *P. falciparum*-HRP2 based test should be preferentially used to distinguish falciparum versus non-falciparum malaria. An additional pan-pLDH and *P. falciparum*-pLDH test component which cross-reacts with *P. knowlesi*, or a *P. vivax*-pLDH test utilising a specific epitope which has been definitively shown to lack any cross-reactivity with *P. knowlesi* (McCutchan et al., 2008), may theoretically assist in identifying *P. vivax* infections. However, in general current RDTs remain unable to distinguish mixed *P. vivax/ P. knowlesi* infections, and the poor sensitivities demonstrated to date limit the possible use of any current combination of target antigens to accurately diagnose *P. knowlesi* monoinfections (Grigg et al., 2014).

Commercial appeal for developing and including *P. knowlesi* specific targets in malaria RDTs is constrained in part by the relatively low reported regional incidence of human infections, which in turn is underestimated by the lack of accurate point-of-care diagnostic tools. Current epitopes particularly for pLDH based tests are usually undisclosed by commercial manufacturers, with reported specificity for the major *P. falciparum* and *P. vivax* RDT targets not known to be determined against *P. knowlesi* or other simian malaria species able to cause human infections, such as *P. cynomolgi* or *P. simium*, for which cross-reactivity may also exist. WHO malaria RDT product testing also report rigorously conducted panel detection scores only against *P. falciparum* and *P. vivax* (WHO, 2018), and ideally would expand validation protocols to encompass *P. knowlesi* and other clinically relevant human or simian malaria species. Future novel RDTs such as magneto-optical detection of hemozoin, an intrinsic by product of *Plasmodium* species haemoglobin digestion, hold promise for sensitive *P. knowlesi* detection at low parasite counts, although also need to be able to reliably differentiate major *Plasmodium* species (Arndt, 2021) (Box 1).

BOX 1 Point-of-care summary and diagnostic reporting recommendations

These summary guidelines refer to *P. knowlesi* endemic areas in Southeast Asia.

Microscopy
- Microscopy remains a sufficiently sensitive first-line tool for *P. knowlesi* detection for the majority of low-level symptomatic infections.
- Routine microscopy is unable to differentiate *P. knowlesi* infections from *P. malariae*, or early ring stage infections with *P. falciparum*, and misidentification with *P. vivax* also occurs.
- In knowlesi-endemic areas where microscopy is used as a first-line tool, blood films in which parasite morphology appears similar to *P. malariae* and the parasite count is less than 5000/μL should be reported as '*P. knowlesi/ P. malariae*' (or 'suspected *P. knowlesi*' in relevant national guidelines).
- Blood films in which parasite morphology appears similar to *P. malariae* and the parasite count is greater than 5000/μL should be reported as *P. knowlesi*, and for any infections with a parasite count greater than 15,000/μL consider early administration of intravenous artesunate due to the high risk of severe disease.

Rapid diagnostic tests
- Current RDTs (pLDH or aldolase-based) remain insufficiently sensitive to detect low-level *P. knowlesi* infections and should not replace microscopy as a first-line diagnostic tool where possible.
- Cross-reactivity of *P. knowlesi* with *P. falciparum* and *P. vivax*-pLDH based test components occurs, however is insufficiently sensitive and specific for diagnostic purposes.
- Where RDTs are used as a first-line diagnostic tool, they should include a *P. falciparum*-specific HRP2 test component.
- RDTs should additionally include the highest performing pan-pLDH test possible to detect non-falciparum malaria.
- RDTs containing a pan-aldolase test component should not preferentially be used.
- Positive RDT results should where possible have subsequent PCR conducted for final *Plasmodium* species confirmation.

3. Molecular detection

3.1 PCR assays

3.1.1 Background

The development of molecular detection assays for *P. knowlesi* has delivered enhanced sensitivity and specificity compared to microscopy. A number of assays utilizing different gene targets and methods have been developed, including the use of nested PCR, real-time PCR, single-step PCR; summarized in Table 2.

SSU rRNA has been used as the most common target for all *Plasmodium* species identification as most *Plasmodium* parasites have two to three distinct genes that are differentially expressed during the parasite's life cycle (Waters, 1994). The first *P. knowlesi* oligonucleotide primers, Pmk8-Pmkr9, developed by Singh et al. targeted the ssu rRNA-S gene expressed during the sexual stages (Singh et al., 2004). This PCR assay enables simultaneous examination for other *Plasmodium* infections using initial well-established genus-specific primers (rPLU6 with either rPLU1 or rPLU5) in the primary PCR followed by species-specific detection (Snounou and Singh, 2002). In conjunction with initial confirmatory sequencing of part of the *P. knowlesi* ssu rRNA and csp genes, this PCR assay was instrumental in demonstrating that the majority of malaria cases in the Kapit division of Sarawak, Malaysia, were actually single-species or mixed *P. knowlesi* infections (Singh et al., 2004).

Further study in Thailand however subsequently confirmed the possibility of cross-reactivity of these primers with *P. vivax* isolates. When the *P. knowlesi* and *P. vivax* ssu rRNA-S gene sequences were aligned, they showed identical sequences corresponding to the Pmkr9 primer and also similarities in the first 19 bases of the Pmk8 primer despite the differences at the 3′ end. Therefore, Pmk8-Pmkr9 primers may cause false amplification of *P. vivax* ssu rRNA under certain amplification conditions (Imwong et al., 2009). In addition, these 18S rRNA gene primers were also reported to cross-react with four other malaria parasites present in forest macaques of SE Asia: *P. inui, P. hylobati, P. cynomolgi,* and *P. coatneyi* (Lucchi et al., 2012). New primers using a fragment of the *P. knowlesi* ssu rRNA gene expressed during the asexual stages were subsequently designed. The PkF1160, PkF1140 and PkR1150 primers were shown to be specific for *P. knowlesi* with a level of detection of 1 to 10 parasite genomes per sample (Imwong et al., 2009). Updated ssu rRNA gene primers (Kn1f and Kn3r) were also developed in Sarawak, with specificity validated against other endemic simian *Plasmodium* species (Lee et al., 2011).

The Pmk8 and Pmk9 primers initially developed for *P. knowlesi* have now been updated or superseded with alternative primer pairs in routine practice in Malaysia at state reference laboratories (Divis et al., 2010; Nuin et al., 2020). Cross-reactivity of *P. knowlesi* infections with older *P. vivax*-designed primers amplifying parts of the ssu rRNA gene (Kimura et al., 1997) and the mitochondrial Cox1 gene (Tham et al., 1999) have also

Table 2 Molecular detection methods for *P. knowlesi*.

Type of assay	Gene target	Primers or probe(s) sequence	Limit of detection	Advantages	Disadvantages	References
Nested PCR	SSU rRNA	Pmk8 Pmkr9	1–6 parasites/μL	Highly conserved; can be combined with nested non-zoonotic malaria	Can spuriously amplify *P. vivax*	Singh et al. (2004)
		PKF1160 PKR1150 PKF1140	1–10 parasite genomes/sample	Sensitive/specific; can be combined with nested non-zoonotic malaria	Lengthy amplification rounds (105 mins each nest)	Imwong et al. (2009)
		Kn1f Kn3r	1–6 parasites/μL	Sensitive/specific; can be combined with nested non-zoonotic malaria		Lee et al. (2011)
		PK18SF PK18SRc	NR			Jongwutiwes et al. (2011)
	DHFR-thymidylate synthase	Pk-Lin-F Pk-Lin-R	Not reported	1 μL of genomic DNA; 0.4 U Taq; heminested; amplification efficiency and specificity less prone to genetic variations within species or cross-hybridization between species	Lengthy amplification rounds (90 and 105 mins)	Tanomsing et al. (2010)

	Mitochondrial cytochrome B	PKCBF PKCFR	1–10 copies/μL	Detected on saliva and urine; highly sensitive - more copies in the mtDNA than 18S rRNA; highly conserved with limited variation; Cytb saliva detection better than microscopy	Secondary PCR has to be performed separately for each species	Putaporntip et al. (2011)
		PKCBF PkCBR-ed	Not reported			Tanizaki et al. (2013)
		PKCBF PkCBR-ed	Not reported	1 μL DNA; *Pk* DNA from urine and faeces is detected for a longer period than from blood	*P. knowlesi* only	Kawai et al. (2014)
	SICAvar	SICAf1 SICAf2 SICAr1	0.1 parasites/μL	Sensitive	*P. knowlesi* only; specificity not cross-checked using *P. vivax* PCR on clinical samples	Lubis et al. (2017)
Real-time PCR	SSU rRNA	Pk1 probe Pk2 probe	10 copies/μL	Simultaneous detection of all *Plasmodium* species; no cross-reactivity with other pathogens	Cannot differentiate mixed *P. vivax* and *P. knowlesi*; four probes; expensive	Babady et al. (2009)

Continued

Table 2 Molecular detection methods for *P. knowlesi.*—cont'd

Type of assay	Gene target	Primers or probe(s) sequence	Limit of detection	Advantages	Disadvantages	References
		NVPK–F NVPK–R NVPK–Probe	5 copies/reaction (<1 parasites/µL)	Sensitive	*P. knowlesi* only	Link et al. (2012)
		Pke'F Pkg'R	100 copies/µL	Detects all species; low cost compared to other RT-PCR	Still expensive; two probes; different melting temperatures	Oddoux et al. (2011)
		Pk probe	10 copies/µL (<3 parasites/µL on clinical samples)	Rapid results; low contamination risk; high throughput; quantification of parasites No cross-reactivity-including *P. cynomolgi* and *P. inui;* needs Plasmo1 and 2 primers	Standard 5 µL DNA used	Divis et al. (2010)
Plasmepsin	Pk (probe)	1–6 parasites/µL	Five species High reported sensitivity and specificity 4.5 h from DNA preparation to PCR amplification 96-well (for 5 species)	Limited to BioRad iQ5 multicolor RT PCR; no lower limit of detection tested with clinical samples	Reller et al. (2013)

Single step PCR	SSU rRNA		0.25 parasites/µL	1.5 µL DNA; faster, less labour intensive; Detects all species; very sensitive; can detect co-infections; less expensive	Inconsistent results due to primers and DNA competition effects; minimal samples of *P. ovale* and *P. malariae*	Chew et al. (2012)
	[a]Consensus repeat sequences	Pkr140	1 parasite/µL	Non-nested; 1 µL DNA; sensitive	*P. knowlesi* only; specificity not well validated with lack of clinical samples tested; bioinformatics approach to sequence target selection	Lucchi et al. (2012)
	Cytochrome c oxidase subunit 1	PlasmoCOI (FDB + RDB)	Not reported		Validated on a single *P. knowlesi* sample	Setiadi et al. (2016)
LAMP	β-tubulin	F3, B3, FIP, BIP, FLP, BLP	100 plasmid copies/sample			Iseki et al. (2010)
	AMA-1	F3, B3, FIP, BIP, FLP, BLP	10 plasmid copies/sample			Lau et al. (2011)
	18S rRNA	F3, B3, FIP, BIP, FLP, BLP	10 plasmid copies/sample			Lau et al. (2016)
	Mitochondrial	Pk 101	0.2 parasites/µL			Britton et al. (2016)

[a]Consensus repeat sequences: chromosome ends and interiors; not protein-encoding.
Adapted from Singh, B., Daneshvar, C., 2013. Human infections and detection of Plasmodium knowlesi. Clin. Microbiol. Rev. 26, 165–184. https://doi.org/10.1128/cmr.00079-12.

been demonstrated in returned travellers (Berry et al., 2011; Tanizaki et al., 2013). Other *P. vivax* ssu rRNA gene primers (Perandin et al., 2004) have also been demonstrated to show cross-reactivity with the closely genetically related zoonotic monkey parasite *P. cynomolgi* in Cambodia (Imwong et al., 2019). The routine use of newer PCR assays where specificity against *P. knowlesi* and other simian *Plasmodium* species has been tested is highly recommended.

3.1.2 Alternative target genes for P. knowlesi *identification*

Target genes of *Plasmodium* species that provide an alternative to the ssu rRNA gene include circumsporozoite surface protein (csp), a nuclear gene encoding a cysteine protease, cytochrome *b* (Conway, 2007), and dihydrofolate reductase (Tanomsing et al., 2010). More recently, the high copy number gene family encoding SICAvar antigens has been used as an alternative target (Lubis et al., 2017).

The use of mitochondrial-encoded cytochrome *b* is well established for diagnostics and species-discrimination in *Plasmodium* (Conway, 2007). It is highly conserved and possesses multiple copy numbers (20–150) in each parasite (Feagin, 1992; Mercereau-Puijalon et al., 2002), compared to 4–8 copies of the 18S rRNA (Vaidya and Mather, 2005). It has also been used to determine the evolutionary history of parasites (Escalante et al., 1998).

Dihydrofolate reductase (DHFR) and thymidylate synthase (TS) of *Plasmodium* species are enzymes with an essential role in the intra-erythrocytic life-cycle. They are relatively conserved between different isolates of the same species. Amplification of these genes has been used to investigate point mutations implicated in parasite antifolate resistance (Grigg et al., 2016a,b). The sensitivity and specificity to detect *P. knowlesi* has been reported to be similar to those detected by ssu rRNA assays. Other advantages are the ability to detect mixed-species infections, as these loci are less prone to genetic variation than the non-protein coding ribosomal genes (Tanomsing et al., 2010).

The schizont-infected cell agglutination variant antigens (SICavar) genes encode an antigen family unique to *P. knowlesi*, with an estimated number of more than 100 members, including both multiexon and truncated forms randomly distributed across all 14 chromosomes (Pain et al., 2008). SICAvar was designed to address potential cross-reactivity between *P. vivax* and *P. knowlesi*, with higher sensitivity also reported in one study compared to ssu rRNA and cytb amplification (Lubis et al., 2017).

3.1.3 Comparative performance of PCR assays

PCR based amplification assays for identification of malaria parasites to the species level have been developed in various formats, including nested PCR, heminested, multiplex PCR, and real-time PCR. The nested PCR is time-consuming, labour-intensive, and requires a large number of reagents and disposable consumables. It also has high risk of cross-contamination, although this can be minimised by training of laboratory staff and well-designed laboratory layout. Real-time PCR has the advantage of a rapid result, minimal contamination risk (as it is a sealed system) and also allows parasite quantification. However, it is more expensive due to the costs of fluorescent reagents and specialized assay platforms. A single-step multiplex PCR reduces the time needed for PCR amplification and reactions, therefore saving on costs. It allows simultaneous identification of all human-infecting *Plasmodium* species, however the primer design and optimisation steps are challenging to ensure a highly sensitive and specific assay (Chew et al., 2012).

Since its introduction in the 1990s, nested PCR targeting the ssu rRNA gene has been considered the gold standard method for malaria detection (Snounou et al., 1993). The nested Kn1f and Kn3r (Lee et al., 2011) and the heminested PkF1160, PkF1140 and PkR1150 (Imwong et al., 2009) PCR assays were developed with improved specificity against other zoonotic and non-zoonotic species, targeting the sexual and asexual stages of *P. knowlesi* ssu rRNA, respectively. Either primer set can be used as a nested reaction following primary amplification with broad genus-specific *Plasmodium* primers (Snounou et al., 1993), and have a reported level of detection of 1–6 parasites/µL. However, it takes six PCR amplifications to enable the identification of *P. knowlesi* and the four major human-only *Plasmodium* species, with further PCR amplifications required if necessary to distinguish other co-endemic macaque *Plasmodium* species such as *P. cynomolgi*, *P. coatneyi*, *P. inui* and *P. fieldi* (Lee et al., 2011). The latter macaque *Plasmodium* species have recently been described to naturally infect humans in Malaysia (Yap et al., 2021), with *P. inui*, *P. inui*-like, *P. coatneyi*, and also *P. simiovale* able to be described with the use of nested PCR (Lee et al., 2011) and additional sequencing of the ssu rRNA and COX1 genes (Yap et al., 2021).

In contrast to nested PCR, a significant advantage of qPCR is the straightforward *Plasmodium* species detection analysis through the use of fluorophores, without the need for gel electrophoresis. Several assays for *P. knowlesi* detection using qPCR targeting either S-type (Babady et al., 2009;

Divis et al., 2010; Link et al., 2012) or A-type (Oddoux et al., 2011) ssu loci have also been developed. Two of these incorporated a *P. knowlesi*-specific probe (Divis et al., 2010; Link et al., 2012), with the remaining assays using a multiplexed *P. knowlesi*-probe with the human-only *Plasmodium* probes to allow detection of all *Plasmodium* species in a single reaction (Babady et al., 2009; Oddoux et al., 2011). Babady et al. used four FRET probes to enable simultaneous detection of five *Plasmodium* species at two reading channels. Although this assay has the advantages of a qPCR assay and maintains the sensitivity and specificity for all *Plasmodium* species identification, the four probes used increased the cost of the reaction and remains of limited value for field deployment (Babady et al., 2009). Another approach to minimise the cost of all *Plasmodium* species identification by qPCR was the modification of a SYBR Green qPCR protocol to include a *P. knowlesi*-specific probe. However, the sensitivity of this assay is much poorer (100 copies/µL) than that offered by Babady (Oddoux et al., 2011).

These limitations led to the development of a single-step hexaplex PCR assay (Chew et al., 2012). This assay is comprised of a single reverse *Plasmodium* genus-specific and five forward species-specific primers of human malaria parasites (*P. knowlesi, P. falciparum, P. vivax, P. malariae, P. ovale curtisi* and *P. ovale wallikeri*). The single-step hexaplex approach allows detection of single or mixed malaria infections within a shorter laboratory timeframe (~3 h). In addition, the limit of detection for *P. knowlesi* was reported to be lower than previous published PCR assays at 0.25 parasites/µL. Although primers were robustly designed for *Plasmodium* species specificity, when testing specificity against 171 clinical malaria isolates the reference nested PCR assay used to confirm *P. knowlesi* included the original Pmk8 and Pmk9 primers known to falsely amplify a proportion of *P. vivax* monoinfections. Specificity was also not reported against the epidemiologically relevant *P. cynomolgi*. Despite this, with further validation this assay has the potential to provide an ideal and more affordable molecular detection method for malaria diagnosis (Chew et al., 2012).

The cytochrome *b* assay allows the identification of all *Plasmodium* species with high sensitivity and has been used with samples of body fluids other than blood. The first nested PCR developed targeting cytochrome *b* was designed by Putaporntip et al. The *cytb* PCR detected malarial DNA from a higher proportion of blood samples compared to the reference 18S rRNA assay, resulting in an improved sensitivity by 16%, with a reported limit of detection of 10 parasites/µL. When using saliva and urine samples, *cytb* amplification demonstrated marked superiority compared to the ssu rRNA assay, which was not able to identify *P. knowlesi* (Putaporntip et al., 2011). Cytb-targeted primers were further adapted to detect *P. knowlesi* in urine and additional faecal samples. After an inoculation of *P. knowlesi* infected RBCs into a macaque, *P. knowlesi* DNA in urine samples was detected early at day 2 similar to the detection of DNA in blood samples, while the DNA in faecal samples were only detected on day 7. However, the parasite DNA in faecal samples was detected up to 37 days after blood samples were PCR-negative. This may be due to the accumulation of parasite DNA in the gallbladder, from where it is gradually excreted to the faeces. This offers an attractive approach for studies in macaque hosts (Kawai et al., 2014; Putaporntip et al., 2011; Tanizaki et al., 2013).

The SICAvar gene assay was developed as a heminested PCR amplification protocol and was tested against human and simian malaria parasites. It was reported to be specific for *P. knowlesi*, with the limit of detection of 0.2 parasites/μL, lower than most of other reported *P. knowlesi* PCR assays. This assay identified a significant number of sub-microscopic and asymptomatic *P. knowlesi* cases in a malaria endemic area of Indonesia, of which nearly half were co-infected with other *Plasmodium* species, most commonly *P. vivax*. However, the apparent presence of the many *P. knowlesi-P.vivax* co-infections in the study could not be confirmed by performing head-to-head PCR assays using the other target genes due to the limited material available from the samples, which had been collected as dried blood spots (Lubis et al., 2017).

3.1.4 Detection of submicroscopic or asymptomatic infections

The use of highly sensitive PCR assays in research settings has increasingly demonstrated the extent of submicroscopic or asymptomatic *P. knowlesi* infections in population-based surveys across Southeast Asia. This includes a proportion of documented *P. knowlesi* infections from molecular surveys in Thailand (Jongwutiwes et al., 2011), Vietnam (Marchand et al., 2011), East Malaysia (Fornace et al., 2016b; Grignard et al., 2019; Siner et al., 2017), West Malaysia (Jiram et al., 2016; Noordin et al., 2020), Indonesia (Lubis et al., 2017), Myanmar (Ghinai et al., 2017) and Cambodia (Imwong et al., 2019). The potential role of asymptomatic or submicroscopic human *P. knowlesi* infections contributing to ongoing transmission in human or monkey host populations is not established, although these transmission modes have been experimentally demonstrated (Chin et al., 1968). It remains unclear what proportion of these low-level infections either spontaneously resolve, persist at levels sufficient to be transmitted, develop into symptomatic disease resulting in seeking treatment and detection, or progress further to high parasitemia and severe disease.

Different approaches to maximizing the sensitivity of molecular methods to detect very low-level *Plasmodium* species infections have been used. In a cross-sectional community malaria survey conducted in Cambodia, Imwong et al. initially used a previously validated high-volume *P. genus* quantitative assay (uPCR) able to detect to down to 22 genomes/mL of blood (Imwong et al., 2014). Samples positive for malarial DNA on this screening assay were then evaluated using a novel nested PCR amplifying 18S ssu rRNA genes (both A and S type), which encompasses 14 zoonotic malaria species including the endemic macaque parasites *P. knowlesi*, *P. cynomolgi*, *P. coatneyi* and *P. inui*. The PCR products (233–298 bp) were then sequenced and aligned against corresponding individual reference ssu rRNA sequences for final diagnosis. This method was able to detect 8 *P. knowlesi* monoinfections, and 11 *P. cynomolgi infections* (including 2 co-infections with *P. vivax*). The very low-level parasitemia of asymptomatic *P. knowlesi* or *P. cynomolgi* infections seen in this study (geometric mean 52 and 4 parasites/μL respectively) means a large proportion of infections in this area are likely to be below the threshold of ~40 parasites/μL able to be detected using routine microscopy or pan-pLDH based RDTs (Imwong et al., 2019).

A study of household and village members of confirmed *P. knowlesi* cases in Sabah revealed a high proportion of submicroscopic *P. knowlesi* carriage, with an estimated prevalence of 6.9% using latent class analysis of multiple *P. knowlesi* species-specific PCR assays (Fornace et al., 2016a). Findings differed depending on the sensitivity of the molecular *P. knowlesi*-specific assay, with the ssu rRNA nested assay expected to identify 15% of these infections, compared to Cytb nested PCR (59.1%), ssRNA qPCR (87.9%), and Plasmepsin qPCR (81.3%) (Fornace et al., 2016a). A subsequent rigorously designed community cross-sectional survey of 10,100 participants conducted in the same area in Sabah used a pooled 10×10 matrix of samples for DNA extraction and PCR detection for submicroscopic *Plasmodium* species infections (Fornace et al., 2019b). A well-established nested *P. genus* and non-zoonotic species-specific PCR assay targeting the ssu rRNA was initially conducted (Snounou et al., 1993), followed by the SICAvar assay for *P. knowlesi* detection (Lubis et al., 2017), with 9 infections found: 2 *P. knowlesi*, 1 *P. knowles/P. vivax*, with the remainder non-zoonotic *Plasmodium* species. A further analysis using 876 selected high-risk samples from the same survey conducted the nested zoonotic malaria PCR and sequencing method developed previously (Imwong et al., 2019), demonstrating improved sensitivity with 54 (6.2%) submicroscopic *Plasmodium* species infections reported. This included 3 *P. knowlesi* infections, and 2 *P. cynomolgi* infections (previously misdiagnosed as *P. vivax* and mixed *P. knowlesi/P. vivax*), with the remainder non-zoonotic species infections (Grignard et al., 2019).

In a longitudinal molecular malaria survey in Sarawak, Siner et al. used a pooled sample of four individuals dried blood spots for initial nested ssu rRNA PCR *P. genus* screening in 2118 participants, before DNA re-extraction and individual participant screening on those positive with Pmk8-Pmkr9 primers for *P. knowlesi* (Singh et al., 2004), other zoonotic monkey *Plasmodium* species (Lee et al., 2011) and non-zoonotic malaria. A further 884 individuals underwent the same PCR assay protocol without initial pooling of four samples. There were seven *P. knowlesi* infections in total detected, including a single asymptomatic submicroscopic infection, and five asymptomatic infections with parasite counts $<50/\mu L$, with no apparent difference in detection between samples initially pooled vs non-pooled (Siner et al., 2017).

3.1.5 Molecular detection of P. knowlesi *gametocytes*

The 24-h replication cycle of *P. knowlesi* in human host RBCs is known to rapidly produce mature gametocytes within around 48 h (Knowles and Gupta, 1932). A short period of gametocyte infectivity then follows, with the timing hypothesised to increase transmission efficiency by occurring mainly at night during peak blood-feeding of mosquitoes (Hawking et al., 1968), although other mechanisms related to circadian within-host immunity and RBC physiology have been proposed (Mideo et al., 2013). The ability to accurately detect and quantify the level of gametocyte production in human *P. knowlesi* infections would assist in exploring fundamental parasite biology questions related to adaptation and replication in human hosts. This includes more accurately defining the timing and degree of gametocytogenesis relative to asexual parasitemia, infectivity to mosquitoes, and the risk of sustained human-human transmission. Other major applications of sensitive gametocyte detection include the ability to identify or evaluate the effect of future transmission blocking vaccines or treatments.

Molecular methods to detect *P. knowlesi* sexual life-stage stages hold significant advantages over microscopy, with most *P. knowlesi* infections likely to have gametocyte densities below the threshold of microscopic detection (Grigg et al., 2018a). Microscopy is insensitive due to the scarcity of gametocytes present in peripheral blood films (Lee et al., 2009b), and the limited number of fields screened usually in thick films when concurrently quantifying asexual parasite infected RBCs by counting the presence of up to 200 white blood cells (WHO, 2015a). Targets for the design of molecular assays to detect gametocytes are based on the underlying sexual-stage parasite biology. In preparation for gametocyte activation after mosquito ingestion in the midgut, mRNA transcripts encoding stage-specific proteins are produced by gametocytes in the human host in order to repress translation for the subsequent rapid genome replication and nuclear division. For *P. falciparum* this includes *pfs*16 mRNA, present from the earliest gametocyte stage onwards, *pfpeg*3 and *pfpeg*4 present in stage II gametocytes, and *pfs*25 mRNA for which transcription only begins to occur in mature stage IV gametocytes (Bousema and Drakeley, 2011). Other female specific gametocyte surface proteins include *pfs*47, thought to be involved in immune evasion in the mosquito midgut, and their male gametocyte paralogs *pfs*48/45 (Molina-Cruz et al., 2020).

Molecular detection assays for *P. falciparum* gametocyte protein orthologs have been designed and evaluated for *P. knowlesi,* with various primers developed to detect *pks*25 mRNA from mature gametocytes (Armistead et al., 2018; Grigg et al., 2016a,b; Maeno et al., 2017). In a clinical trial of antimalarial treatment for patients with uncomplicated knowlesi malaria in Sabah, Malaysia, Grigg et al. demonstrated the presence of *P. knowlesi pks*25 mRNA transcripts in 85/100 (85%; 95%CI 76%–91%) of participants tested at enrolment (Grigg et al., 2016a,b). Of those positive for *pks*25 mRNA only 16% had gametocytes detected by microscopy (Grigg et al., 2016a,b), consistent with a separate clinical trial where only microscopy was performed and 32/123 (26%) patent infections had gametocytes present (Grigg et al., 2018b). There was an association with higher parasitemia and detectable with a median parasite count of 2140 vs 704 parasites/μL respectively; $P = 0.019$. At day 7, there were 5/97 (5%) patients persistently positive for *pks*25 mRNA: 3 p25 mRNA: 3 patients initially treated with artesunate-mefloquine, and 2 with chloroquine (Grigg et al., 2016a,b).

Maeno et al. conducted a comparative study of gametocyte detection for four species in Khan Hoa Province, Vietnam in both humans and mosquitoes. A nested real-time PCR assay was developed targeting *pks*25 mRNA to detect *P. knowlesi* gametocytes, with 15/32 (47%) of those with *P. knowlesi* confirmed asexual stage infections also positive for *pks*25 transcripts. All *P. knowlesi* samples were co-infections with one or more non-zoonotic *Plasmodium* species. The proportion of *P. knowlesi* infections with detectable *pks*25 mRNA was comparable to that seen for the *P. falciparum* and *P. vivax* gametocyte specific targets. Serial dilution of gametocytes from a *P. knowlesi* infected monkey was used to demonstrate a lower limit of detection of 1 gametocyte/µL for the RT-PCR *pks*25 assay. In this study, 70% of mosquitoes with *P. knowlesi* in their salivary glands also carried human malaria parasites, supporting the possibility that mosquitoes are infected with *P. knowlesi* from human infections (Maeno et al., 2017).

Armistead et al. designed multiple *P. knowlesi* RT-qPCR detection assays across gametocyte developmental stages, including targets for *pks*16, *pks*25, and *pks*47 mRNA. Using *P. knowlesi* H-strain cultured samples, they demonstrated infectivity of *An. dirus* through membrane infected RBC feeders, however none of the quantified transcripts of the 3 targets correlated well with infectivity, and peaks in *pks*25 and *pks*47 transcription were not associated with gametocyte maturation as may have been expected (Armistead et al., 2018).

3.2 Loop-mediated isothermal amplification (LAMP)

More recently LAMP has been evaluated as a potentially simple and sensitive diagnostic tool compared to microscopy as an alternative molecular diagnostic option for *P. knowlesi* infections in resource limited areas without specialized facilities for PCR (Britton et al., 2016). First described by Notomi, briefly, this molecular approach relies on a *Bacillus stearothermophilus* (*Bst*) polymerase to perform DNA strand separation and amplification of target sequences of 300 base pairs, at a single temperature of 65°C for 1 h using a set of four primers that form a stem-and-loop structure that promotes ongoing DNA amplification (Notomi et al., 2000). Magnesium pyrophosphate, a by-product of the LAMP DNA amplification process, forms a white precipitate following successful target amplification that can then be visualized by eye, by turbidimetry (Mori et al., 2001) or colourimetrically using hydroxynaphthol blue (Britton et al., 2016), malachite green (Lucchi et al., 2016b), phenol red (Lai et al., 2020) or SYBR green (Lai et al., 2021) to objectively confirm a positive result.

3.2.1 LAMP platforms

There are two commercially available LAMP platforms. The first, the Eiken Loopamp™ MALARIA detection kit (Eiken chemical company, Japan) offers a *Plasmodium* genus specific assay (panLAMP) for identifying parasites that cause human infection and one able to specifically detect *Plasmodium falciparum* (PfLAMP) infection. When used together to identify non-falciparum infections, this panLAMP platform was able to identify *P. knowlesi* from 50 patients with uncomplicated *P. knowlesi* infections, at a genus level, with 100% sensitivity and specificity for infections with mean parasitemia of 1197 parasites/μL (IQR 300-3920) and a limit of detection of 2 parasites/μL (Piera et al., 2017). However, this platform does not have a *P. knowlesi* species-specific assay currently available. The second commercial platform, *Illumigene* Malaria LAMP (Meridian Biosciences Inc., Cincinnati, OH) has demonstrated good sensitivity and specificity for identifying *Plasmodium* species using undisclosed LAMP primers (Lucchi et al., 2016a; Rypien et al., 2017) but has not been validated using *P. knowlesi* clinical samples. Several non-commercial LAMP platforms have also been published, such as HTP-LAMP (Perera et al., 2017) and RealAMP (Patel et al., 2013) one of which, HtLAMP, has been evaluated in *P. knowlesi* samples (Britton et al., 2016).

3.2.2 P. knowlesi *specific LAMP primers*
Since its first use in identifying *P. falciparum* (Poon et al., 2006), several LAMP primers specific for detecting *P. knowlesi* have been developed (summarised in Table 2), each with different targets, advantages and drawbacks. The first *P. knowlesi*-specific LAMP primers targeting the beta-tubulin gene demonstrated good species specificity and limit of detection of 10^2 copies/μL of target DNA but was only validated in samples from infected macaque monkeys and not human clinical samples (Iseki et al., 2010). Lau et al. published *P. knowlesi* specific LAMP primers targeting the apical membrane antigen 1 (AMA-1) (Lau et al., 2011) followed by genus and species-specific primers targeting the 18S rRNA gene for each of the *Plasmodium* parasites that cause human infection (Lau et al., 2016). These LAMP primers demonstrated a reported 100% sensitivity and specificity on a limited number of clinical samples, n = 13 (Lau et al., 2011), n = 57 (Lau et al., 2016), and n = 71 (Lai et al., 2021), including validation against *P. vivax*, however lacked detail on the limit of detection for these primers. In keeping with other LAMP studies demonstrating superior analytical sensitivity of primers targeting mitochondrial genes (Polley et al., 2010), *P. knowlesi*-specific mitochondrial target LAMP primers have been shown to have a limit of detection of 0.2 parasites/μL (Britton et al., 2016). However, given the 97% sequence homology between *P. vivax* and *P. knowlesi* at the target gene, this assay demonstrated 96% sensitivity, 30% specificity overall, but 100% specificity only if *P. vivax* samples were excluded (Britton et al., 2016).

3.2.3 Challenges for LAMP as a diagnostic tool

The advantages of LAMP include less need for equipment and technical expertise compared with PCR, potential for high specificity and rapid turnaround time. However, the requirement for parasite DNA extraction processes, high potential risk of contamination given the large amount of DNA amplification and cost per sample remain limitations to the widespread use of the LAMP for diagnosis of malaria in primary care settings compared with microscopy.

Much effort has been made to simplify the preparation of DNA template for LAMP. LAMP has been performed on DNA templates generated directly from heat-treated blood samples (Poon et al., 2006), boil and spin method (Hopkins et al., 2013) and closed-circuit PURE extraction technology (Eiken chemical company) (Polley et al., 2013) with the latter two processes showing 97.5% sensitivity compared with nested PCR (Hopkins et al., 2013). A comparison of different volumes of whole blood with chelex or chelex-saponin extraction protocol found lower limit of detection with LAMP with a 20 µL blood volume with chelex-saponin compared with 5 or 10 µL (Britton et al., 2015) confirming that, similar to high volume ultrasensitive PCR (Imwong et al., 2014), blood volume impacts LAMP performance particularly at low parasitemia. Filter paper dried blood spots (DBS) have also been extracted using a multistep Chelex-based process (Han et al., 2007) from symptomatic and asymptomatic patients (Aydin-Schmidt et al., 2017) or sodium dodecyle sulphate (SDS) (Polley et al., 2010). LAMP performed on whole blood extracted by SDS was able to detect 2–5 parasites/µL compared with 10 parasites/µL from DBS extracted with SDS (Polley et al., 2010). Commercial DNA extraction kits with closed systems such as PURE (Eiken Chemical company, Japan) for either small number of samples (Polley et al., 2013) or high throughput (Perera et al., 2017) minimize the risk of potential contamination found in the multistep DNA extraction protocols but with associated increased cost. LAMP performed on blood samples appeared to be more sensitive than when performed on saliva (Singh et al., 2013) or urine (Najafabadi et al., 2014) for identifying *P. falciparum* and *P. vivax*. However, no direct comparison of DBS with different volumes of whole blood or on different sample types has been performed using LAMP in the detection of *P. knowlesi*.

3.2.4 The future of LAMP for P. knowlesi *diagnosis*

Overall, the optimal role for LAMP, as either a point of care diagnostic for case detection or a molecular tool for surveillance, remains unresolved. Platforms such as non–instrumented nucleic acid amplification by LAMP

(NINA-LAMP) (Sema et al., 2015), lateral-flow device LAMP (Mallepaddi et al., 2018) and LAMP MinION nanopore sequencing (Imai et al., 2017) combined with appropriately sensitive species-specific primers may improve its applicability as a point-of-care diagnostic test. However, these technologies remain constrained by need for DNA extraction, risk of contamination, low sample throughput capacity and cost. LAMP also has been incorporated into several lab-on-a-chip platforms such as multiplex microfluidic arrays (Mao et al., 2018) and microchambers on cell microarrays (Ido et al., 2019) which hold much promise for improved field applicability of LAMP technology. However, except for LFD-LAMP, all of these platforms are yet to be fully validated in large numbers of *P. knowlesi* clinical samples.

In terms of surveillance, two high throughput platforms have been published to overcome the limited number of samples and prohibitive costs associated with existing commercial platforms for this application. The colourimetric high-throughput LAMP (HtLAMP) platform based on a 96 well plate required minimal infrastructure, was low cost and was applied in a resource limited setting (Britton et al., 2015). However, this assay required a separate DNA extraction process, whereas an alternative high-throughput LAMP (HTP LAMP) was able to combine a 96 well plate platform with a closed DNA extraction process (Perera et al., 2017) albeit at likely high cost. However, only the HtLAMP platform has been evaluated with *P. knowlesi* specific primers (Britton et al., 2016).

Therefore, the applicability of LAMP for *P. knowlesi* diagnosis remains constrained by two significant challenges: analytical sensitivity to detect sub-microscopic parasitemia without compromising species specificity, and cost-effective applicability in resource limited settings as an alternative to PCR either as a point of care diagnostic tool or for purposes of *P. knowlesi* malaria surveillance.

4. Serology
4.1 Importance of serology for malaria surveillance

The use of serology as a tool to survey and monitor transmission and exposure to infection, in addition to measuring the success of interventions has been well documented for *P. falciparum* (Plucinski et al., 2018; Wu et al., 2020) and *P. vivax* (Edwards et al., 2021; Longley et al., 2020). Measuring antibodies provides a fast and simple means for evaluating transmission intensity (Stewart et al., 2009) and in combination with parasite prevalence data can be used to monitor changes in malaria transmission over time

(Drakeley et al., 2005). In this context serological tools have a major advantage compared to molecular methods, as they can capture exposure from asymptomatic or transient symptomatic infections in those not seeking treatment (Corran et al., 2007). However, to date less focus has been afforded to understanding transmission for the other causes of human malaria including *P. knowlesi* using serological methods, meaning neglected infections from species such as *P. knowlesi* remain excluded from the elimination narrative (Barber et al., 2017b; Chin et al., 2020).

4.2 Development of serologic assays for *P. knowlesi* detection

To complement existing approaches for assessing exposure to infection, species-specific serological reagents are an essential part of the toolbox. The ability to accurately assess the prevalence of each infecting species and monitor the impact of control and intervention approaches on each could help to provide better guidance for country-level programmatic decision-making. Serology has a number of obvious advantages, specifically the ability to accurately measure recent and historical exposure to infection (Edwards et al., 2021; Helb et al., 2015). Increasingly serology assays are also being designed using multiplex platforms (Chan et al., 2021). These platforms have allowed for high-throughput biomarker discovery and evaluation which in turn has led to an expansion in both the number and utility of the protein targets available (Tran and Crompton, 2020). As more serology tools are discovered and developed, the utility of the individual, or panel of, targets need to be properly assessed. Early sero-epidemiological studies aimed at assessing non-specific malaria exposure through cross-reactivity to *P. knowlesi* antigens were conducted using indirect haemaglutination tests (Kagan et al., 1969). This approach was based on crude parasite preparations generated from lysed infected erythrocytes taken from splenectomised rhesus monkeys. The unrefined nature of the antigen preparation would suggest there were antigens conserved across the *Plasmodium* spp. present in the assay, highlighted by the wide geographical distribution of seropositive responses in non-*P. knowlesi* endemic settings seen in military personnel when using this technique (Kagan et al., 1969).

Designing recombinant proteins provides a more focused means for developing specific targets for use in serology assays. However, previous approaches have focused on targeting proteins such as MSP1 and AMA1 that shared moderate to high levels of sequence homology, and or exhibited cross-reactive responses with other *Plasmodium* spp. (Muh et al., 2020;

Narum and Thomas, 1994; Waters et al., 1990). This includes other previous *P. knowlesi* antigens designed mainly to interrogate underlying parasite biology rather than for use as sero-surveillance tools in co-endemic areas such as *Pk*CSP (Sharma and Godson, 1985), *Pk*DPB (Singh et al., 2002), *Pk*SPATR (Mahajan et al., 2005), *Pk*LDH (Singh et al., 2012), *Pk*1-Cys peroxiredoxin (Hakimi et al., 2013), *Pk* knowpains (Prasad et al., 2012), *Pk*MSP1-42 (Cheong et al., 2013a,b), *Pk*MSP1-33 (Cheong et al., 2013a, 2013b), *Pk*MSP1-19 (Lau et al., 2014), *Pk*Trags (Tyagi et al., 2015), *Pk*MSP3 (Silva et al., 2016) and *Pk*SBP1 (Lucky et al., 2016). Such reagents likely would lack the required specificity to accurately define exposure to dissect *P. knowlesi* infections in regions co-endemic for other species, increasing the potential for false positive responses.

In order to facilitate *P. knowlesi* sero-surveillance in areas of Southeast with co-endemic *Plasmodium* species, Herman et al. used an in silico modelling approach to design four novel recombinant *P. knowlesi* antigen constructs from three genes: *Pk*SERA3-antigen 1, *Pk*SERA3-antigen 2, *Pk*SSP2/TRAP, and *Pk*TSERA2-antigen 1 (Herman et al., 2018). Initial target candidate genes were selected from known seroreactive *P. falciparum* orthologues, with protein sequences processed using analytical in silico tools aiming to maximise specificity for *P. knowlesi* against other *Plasmodium* species. This included iterative BlastP interrogation of target sequences against *Plasmodium* specific and other relevant databases, domain prediction, exclusion of signal peptides and transmembrane domains and glutathione-S-transferase tagging to aid expression solubility, and construction of phylogenetic trees to exclude high identity cross-species amino acid alignments. An *Escherichia coli* expression system was used to produce soluble, multimerised and stable antigen products with final yields from 11.9 to 20.5 mg/L. Blood-stage transcription of SERA3 and TSERA2 candidate genes was also confirmed, in contrast to the sporozoite stage SSP/TRAP gene. Finally, non-synonymous SNPs associated with the three known distinct *P. knowlesi* genetic subpopulations were characterized and shown to predominantly exist outside regions covered by the recombinant constructs, highlighting their potential utility for all *P. knowlesi* strains (Herman et al., 2018).

Validation of the four new recombinant antigens was subsequently conducted using ELISA to detect IgG responses for 97 individuals with acute *P. knowlesi* infections at three time points (day 0, day 7 and day 28) following treatment in a clinical trial in Sabah, Malaysia. Negative controls consisted of 26 Ethiopian non-*P. knowlesi* and 29 UK malaria-naïve sera, with cut-off values to define reactivity for *P. knowlesi* antigens taken as the mean OD ($\pm$3 SD) from the latter group. A single weakly positive sample was recorded for both SERA3 ag 1 and SSP2/TRAP in the Ethiopian negative controls. The best performing antigen was the *Pk*SERA3 antigen 2, which was positive in 67% of all time-points in *P. knowlesi* cases, with maximum positivity at day 7 and up to 50-fold increases compared to day 0 recorded. Antibody prevalence for *Pk*SERA3 antigen 1, *Pk*SSP2 and *Pk*TSERA2 antigen 1 also peaked at day 7, however remained relatively low at 18%, 33% and 43% respectively. Using data adaptive boosted tree regression models, the combined ability of all four antigens to classify *P. knowlesi* exposure was 89% (IQR 43%–61%), defined as the cross-validated area under the receiver operating curve, with the highest relative variable importance contributed by *Pk*SERA3 antigen 2 at 50% (Herman et al., 2018).

A separate panel of 9 recombinant *P. knowlesi* antigens was generated by Müller-Sienerth and colleagues, based on the most highly expressed *P. falciparum* and *P. vivax* protein orthologues known to produce high antibody responses in endemic areas: CyRPA, GAMA MSP10, MSP4, MSP5, P12, P38, P41, and P92 (Müller-Sienerth et al., 2020). This study differed in approach by utilizing a mammalian expression system in order to improve the likelihood that appropriate post-translational modifications such as disulfide bonds are present (Crosnier et al., 2013). This in turn allows correct protein folding to recreate the original conformation of epitopes and therefore improve antibody recognition (Forsström et al., 2015). Malaysian sera from PCR confirmed *P. knowlesi* infections initially demonstrated the highest antibody responses in P12, MSP10 and P38 when quantified by ELISA. Cross-species seropositivity of these three *P. knowlesi* antigens was minimal when tested as part of a larger panel including 19 selected antigens for *P. falciparum*, *P. vivax*, *P. malariae* and *P. ovale* using sera from small numbers of European returned travellers with malaria. Cross-reactivity was not shown to be related to the degree of sequence identity between protein orthologues, including for the P12 antigen despite a high sequence identity of 72% between *P. knowlesi* and *P. vivax*. Logistic regression classification models combining the three *P. knowlesi* antigens were then used to demonstrate on a larger dataset of 50 *P. knowlesi* sera and 66 uninfected controls from Malaysia a high AUC of the median ROC curve of 0.91. Using a model score of greater than 0.5 was shown to accurately diagnose 82% of *P. knowlesi* infections with a 3% false positive rate.

4.3 Potential use case scenarios for *P. knowlesi* serologic tools

In 2017 a meeting was convened in Paris to review the state-of-theart with antibody-based assays in the context of malaria surveillance (Greenhouse et al., 2019). A key aim was to define potential use-case scenarios in terms of use and evaluation of serological biomarkers in control and elimination programmes. Although focused on *P. falciparum* and *P. vivax*, many of the use cases could be applied to *P. knowlesi*, including: (i) documenting the absence of transmission over a given geographic space; (ii) stratification of transmission level; (iii) measuring the impact of interventions and monitoring changes in malaria transmission; and (iv) decentralized immediate public health response. The summary provided a detailed understanding of what tests would be required for a given situation/population, establishing target product profiles for the future development of diagnostics and surveillance tools (Greenhouse et al., 2019).

Using recently developed *P. knowlesi* antigens designed as species-specific reagents (Herman et al., 2018). Fornace and colleagues conducted a survey of 2503 participants to determine the level of exposure and infection within case-study communities across Sabah, Malaysia and neighbouring Palawan, Philippines (Fornace et al., 2018). This was the first study to assess *P. knowlesi* infection and associated risk using antibodies, demonstrating a seroprevalence of 7.1% to *Pk*SERA3 antigen 2, including comparable seroreactivity between adult men and women (despite passive case detection of acute infections mainly consisting of men), and 4.2% seroprevalence in children <15 years. Despite a very low acute infection prevalence of 0.2% using PCR, the use of serological tools was able to demonstrate marked spatial heterogeneity in transmission intensity between sites (i.e., higher intensity in Malaysia compared to Philippines), and associations with *P. knowlesi* exposure and agricultural work, high forest cover or clearing around houses (Fornace et al., 2018).

This was followed by a large population-based cross-sectional malaria survey of 10,100 individuals to assess exposure and environmental risk to *P. knowlesi* across Northern Sabah, Malaysia (Fornace et al., 2019b). In this study, a multiplex Luminex platform was used to concurrently evaluate IgG responses for *P. knowlesi* SERA3 ag 2 and SSP2, in addition to 8 other antigens for *P. falciparum* and 5 for *P. vivax*. Classification of seropositive individuals for *P. knowlesi* (exposure in the last year), *P. falciparum*, and *P. vivax* was conducted using a data adaptive meta-learning algorithm (Super Learner, van der Laan et al., 2007). The overall seroprevalence of *P. knowlesi* was 5.1% (95% CI 4.8–5.4), with high antibody responses seen across all age groups. However, individual-level associations with higher *P. knowlesi* exposure risk in the final Bayesian hierarchical model were seen with increasing age and male sex, in addition to macaque contact and forest activities, with personal insecticide use protective. Household-level associations with exposure included raised level house construction, lower geographical elevation and fragmented land types classified at varying spatial scales around the household (intact forest, irrigated farming land, pulpwood and oil-palm plantations). The latter are consistent with separate modelling demonstrating the relative importance of different environmental variables at small scales of <1 km around households (proportion of cleared land, aspect, slope), compared to larger spatial scales of 4-5 km (fragmentation of deforested areas) (Brock et al., 2019).

The implementation of serological tools in national malaria control programmes would result in several potential benefits. Using serological exposure to understand the mechanistic links between land use change and *P. knowlesi* transmission highlights their utility in the possible design of spatially-targeted interventions, particularly for low-resource settings with scarce or absent occurrence data. Future use of serological tools outside highly studied areas in Malaysia are also vital to understand regional differences, including demonstrating the potential absence of transmission in certain areas. However, implementation of serology for *P. knowlesi* will require guidance on validated and consistent data analysis methods to define seropositivity cut-offs (Chan et al., 2021). This is particularly the case in multiplex platforms, which ideally need to take into account known antibody titers and kinetics, regional variation in transmission, and population-level immunity for other human-only *Plasmodium* species that may be providing some cross-protective effect (Muh et al., 2020) (Box 2).

BOX 2 Molecular and serology methods summary and diagnostic reporting recommendations

These summary guidelines refer to *P. knowlesi* endemic areas in Southeast Asia.

PCR and LAMP

- A number of PCR assays have been developed which are highly sensitive and specific for *P. knowlesi* detection.
- A validated *P. knowlesi* species-specific PCR assay should be included routinely as part of any PCR assay conducted for suspected or microscopy positive malaria from Southeast Asia.
- Nested PCR assays targeting the 18S ssu rRNA gene are the most commonly used for *P. knowlesi* detection. Compared to real-time PCR they have lower sensitivity and are more time consuming, although are less expensive.

Continued

BOX 2 Molecular and serology methods summary and diagnostic reporting recommendations—cont'd

- The most well-validated nested PCR assays include an initial *P. genus* amplification round, followed by species specific detection for *P. falciparum*, *P. vivax*, *P. malariae*, *P. ovale* and *P. knowlesi*. Where possible, species-specific detection for *P. cynomolgi* should also be considered.
- Early *P. knowlesi* designed nested primers, Pmk8-Pmkr9, can cross-react with *P. vivax* monoinfections to produce a false-positive mixed *P. vivax/P. knowlesi* result.
- Updated and more specific nested ssu rRNA primers for *P. knowlesi* include PkF1160, PkF1140 and PkR1150, or Kn1f and Kn3r, which have been validated against zoonotic and non-zoonotic *Plasmodium* species.
- Some older nested PCR assays contain *P. vivax* species-specific primers which have been shown to cross-react with *P. knowlesi* and *P. cynomolgi*. The well-established VIV1-VIV2 primers do not.
- PCR has been successfully used in Malaysia, a pre-elimination setting for non-zoonotic malaria, for accurate species reporting of all zoonotic and non-zoonotic malaria cases, and for research surveillance purposes across Southeast Asia including the detection of submicroscopic or asymptomatic infections.
- Reference laboratory molecular testing of malaria cases for both zoonotic and non-zoonotic *Plasmodium* species needs to be more widely implemented by National Malaria Control Programmes across Southeast Asia to accurately identify the burden of zoonotic malaria and to more accurately monitor the success of human-only malaria elimination programmes.
- *P. knowlesi* mature gametocytes are able to be detected by real-time qPCR assays targeting *pks*25 mRNA, with validation and implementation in naturally infected human clinical studies demonstrating much higher sensitivity compared to microscopy.
- LAMP based platforms for *P. knowlesi* diagnosis remain constrained by two main challenges: the ability to detect submicroscopic infections while retaining high species-specificity, and any significant cost benefit compared to PCR for diagnostic species-confirmation or surveillance.

Serology

- Antigenic reagents have been identified that can distinguish exposure to *P. knowlesi* infection from human-only malaria with a reasonable degree of specificity.
- Antibody responses to these antigens can be used at the population-level to assess the degree of exposure, including the absence of exposure.
- Antibody responses can also be used to identify demographic and spatial risk factors which can support targeting of control approaches.
- Population-level evaluation of novel targets would allow the identification of antigens for development of species-specific lateral flow devices to help with rapid case management.

5. Conclusion

P. knowlesi is an emergent public health threat across Southeast Asia. Implementation of improved detection methods and reporting practices for point-of-care diagnostics are vital to understanding the disease burden and distribution of symptomatic human infections and allowing the timely administration of appropriate treatment. Newer lateral flow or novel RDTs with the ability to accurately differentiate *P. knowlesi* and other non-*P. falciparum* species are ideally required for this to occur. Molecular methods incorporating validated PCR assays for *P. knowlesi* can improve accurate regional case reporting to monitor progress towards elimination of other human-only species, with additional utility in detection of low-level infections to understand broader transmission dynamics. However, molecular tools remain expensive in low-resource settings and public health programmes may require further input to understand the background prevalence or predicted transmission risk in order to guide their optimal targeted deployment. The implementation of multiplex serological tools with *Plasmodium* species specific recombinant proteins allows improved understanding of geographically heterogenous *P. knowlesi* transmission intensity and associated underlying environmental drivers, in addition to the ability to guide both the design and evaluation of future spatially targeted interventions.

Acknowledgements

M.J.G., I.N.L., and R.N. are supported by the ZOOMAL project ('Evaluating zoonotic malaria and agricultural land use in Indonesia'; #LS-2019-116), Australian Centre for International Agricultural Research and Department of Foreign Affairs, Australian Government. K.K.A.T. was supported by a Bloomsbury SET Innovation Fellowship ('Development of a suspension bead assay targeting the zoonotic malaria parasite *Plasmodium knowlesi*'; BSA14). This work was also supported by the Australian National Health and Medical Research Council (grant numbers 1037304 and 1045156; fellowships to N.M.A. [1042072], B.E.B. [1088738]; M.J.G. [1138860] and 'Improving Health Outcomes in the Tropical North: A multidisciplinary collaboration "Hot North"', [grant 1131932]). The Sabah Malaria Research Program is supported by the US NIH IRIDA program. We thank Sitti Saimah binti Sakam from the IDSKKS-Menzies Clinical Research Unit, Sabah, Malaysia for input into the microscopic diagnosis section.

References

Ahmed, A.M., Pinheiro, M.M., Divis, P.C., Siner, A., Zainudin, R., Wong, I.T., Lu, C.W., Singh-Khaira, S.K., Millar, S.B., Lynch, S., Willmann, M., Singh, B., Krishna, S., Cox-Singh, J., 2014. Disease progression in *Plasmodium knowlesi* malaria is linked to variation in invasion gene family members. PLoS Negl. Trop. Dis. 8, e3086. https://doi.org/10.1371/journal.pntd.0003086.s017.

Armistead, J.S., Barros, R.R.M., Gibson, T.J., Kite, W.A., Mershon, J.P., Lambert, L.E., Orr-Gonzalez, S.E., Sá, J.M., Adams, J.H., Wellems, T.E., 2018. Infection of mosquitoes from in vitro cultivated *Plasmodium knowlesi* H strain. Int. J. Parasitol. 48, 601–610. https://doi.org/10.1016/j.ijpara.2018.02.004.

Arndt, L., et al., 2021. Magneto-optical diagnosis of symptomatic malaria in Papua New Guinea. Nat. Commun. https://doi.org/10.1038/s41467-021-21110-w.

Aydin-Schmidt, B., Morris, U., Ding, X.C., Jovel, I., Msellem, M.I., Bergman, D., Islam, A., Ali, A.S., Polley, S., Gonzalez, I.J., Mårtensson, A., Björkman, A., 2017. Field evaluation of a high throughput loop mediated isothermal amplification test for the detection of asymptomatic *Plasmodium* infections in Zanzibar. PLos One 12, e0169037. https://doi.org/10.1371/journal.pone.0169037.

Babady, N.E., Sloan, L.M., Rosenblatt, J.E., Pritt, B.S., 2009. Detection of *Plasmodium knowlesi* by real-time polymerase chain reaction. Am. J. Trop. Med. Hyg. 81, 516–518.

Barber, B.E., William, T., Grigg, M.J., Yeo, T.W., Anstey, N.M., 2013. Limitations of microscopy to differentiate *Plasmodium* species in a region co-endemic for *Plasmodium falciparum*, *Plasmodium vivax* and *Plasmodium knowlesi*. Malaria J. 12, 8. https://doi.org/10.1186/1475-2875-12-8.

Barber, B.E., William, T., Grigg, M.J., Menon, J., Auburn, S., Marfurt, J., Anstey, N.M., Yeo, T.W., 2013a. A prospective comparative study of Knowlesi, Falciparum, and Vivax Malaria in Sabah, Malaysia: high proportion with severe disease from *Plasmodium Knowlesi* and *Plasmodium Vivax* but no mortality with early referral and artesunate therapy. Clin. Infect. Dis. 56, 383–397. https://doi.org/10.1093/cid/cis902.

Barber, B.E., William, T., Grigg, M.J., Piera, K., Yeo, T.W., Anstey, N.M., 2013b. Evaluation of the sensitivity of a pLDH-based and an aldolase-based rapid diagnostic test for diagnosis of uncomplicated and severe malaria caused by PCR-confirmed *Plasmodium knowlesi*, *Plasmodium falciparum*, and *Plasmodium vivax*. J. Clin. Microbiol. 51, 1118–1123. https://doi.org/10.1128/jcm.03285-12.

Barber, B.E., Grigg, M.J., William, T., Yeo, T.W., Anstey, N.M., 2017a. The treatment of *Plasmodium knowlesi* malaria. Trends Parasitol. 33, 242–253. https://doi.org/10.1016/j.pt.2016.09.002.

Barber, B.E., Rajahram, G.S., Grigg, M.J., William, T., Anstey, N.M., 2017b. World Malaria report: time to acknowledge *Plasmodium knowlesi* malaria. Malaria J. 16, 135. https://doi.org/10.1186/s12936-017-1787-y.

Berry, A., Iriart, X., Wilhelm, N., Valentin, A., Cassaing, S., Witkowski, B., Benoit-Vical, F., Menard, S., Olagnier, D., Fillaux, J., Sire, S., Coustumier, A.L., Magnaval, J.F., 2011. Imported *Plasmodium knowlesi* malaria in a French tourist returning from Thailand. Am. J. Trop. Med. Hyg. 84, 535–538. https://doi.org/10.4269/ajtmh.2011.10-0622.

Bousema, T., Drakeley, C., 2011. Epidemiology and infectivity of *Plasmodium falciparum* and *Plasmodium vivax* gametocytes in relation to malaria control and elimination. Clin. Microbiol. Rev. 24, 377–410. https://doi.org/10.1128/cmr.00051-10.

Britton, S., Cheng, Q., Sutherland, C.J., McCarthy, J.S., 2015. A simple, high-throughput, colourimetric, field applicable loop-mediated isothermal amplification (HtLAMP) assay for malaria elimination. Malaria J. 14, 335. https://doi.org/10.1186/s12936-015-0848-3.

Britton, S., Cheng, Q., Grigg, M.J., William, T., Anstey, N.M., McCarthy, J.S., 2016. A sensitive, colorimetric, high-throughput loop-mediated isothermal amplification assay for the detection of *Plasmodium knowlesi*. Am. J. Trop. Med. Hyg. 95, 120–122. https://doi.org/10.4269/ajtmh.15-0670.

Brock, P.M., Fornace, K.M., Grigg, M.J., Anstey, N.M., William, T., Cox, J., Drakeley, C.J., Ferguson, H.M., Kao, R.R., 2019. Predictive analysis across spatial scales links zoonotic malaria to deforestation. Proc. R. Soc. B 286, 20182351. https://doi.org/10.1098/rspb.2018.2351.

Chan, Y., Fornace, K., Wu, L., Arnold, B.F., Priest, J.W., Martin, D.L., Chang, M.A., Cook, J., Stresman, G., Drakeley, C., 2021. Determining seropositivity—a review of approaches to define population seroprevalence when using multiplex bead assays to assess burden of tropical diseases. PLos Negl. Trop. D 15, e0009457. https://doi.org/10.1371/journal.pntd.0009457.

Cheong, F.W., Fong, M.Y., Lau, Y.L., Mahmud, R., 2013a. Immunogenicity of bacterial-expressed recombinant *Plasmodium knowlesi* merozoite surface protein-142 (MSP-142). Malaria J. 12, 454. https://doi.org/10.1186/1475-2875-12-454.

Cheong, F.-W., Lau, Y.-L., Fong, M.-Y., Mahmud, R., 2013b. Evaluation of recombinant *Plasmodium knowlesi* merozoite surface protein-1(33) for detection of human malaria. Am. J. Trop. Med. Hyg. 88, 835–840. https://doi.org/10.4269/ajtmh.12-0250.

Chew, C.H., Lim, Y.A.L., Lee, P.C., Mahmud, R., Chua, K.H., 2012. Hexaplex PCR detection system for identification of five human *Plasmodium* species with an internal control. J. Clin. Microbiol. 50, 4012–4019. https://doi.org/10.1128/jcm.06454-11.

Chin, W., Contacos, P.G., Coatney, G.R., Kimball, H.R., 1965. A naturally acquired quotidian-type malaria in man transferable to monkeys. Science 149, 865.

Chin, W., Contacos, P.G., Collins, W.E., Jeter, M.H., Alpert, E., 1968. Experimental mosquito-transmission of *Plasmodium knowlesi* to man and monkey. Am. J. Trop. Med. Hyg. 17, 355–358.

Chin, A.Z., Maluda, M.C.M., Jelip, J., Jeffree, M.S.B., Culleton, R., Ahmed, K., 2020. Malaria elimination in Malaysia and the rising threat of *Plasmodium knowlesi*. J. Physiol. Anthropol. 39, 36. https://doi.org/10.1186/s40101-020-00247-5.

Coatney, G.R., Collins, W.E., Warren, M., Contacos, P.G., 1971. The Primate Malarias. US Government.

Collins, W.E., Jeffery, G.M., 2007. *Plasmodium malariae*: parasite and disease. Clin. Microbiol. Rev. 20, 579–592. https://doi.org/10.1128/cmr.00027-07.

Conway, D.J., 2007. Molecular epidemiology of malaria. Clin. Microbiol. Rev. 20, 188–204. https://doi.org/10.1128/cmr.00021-06.

Cooper, D.J., Rajahram, G.S., William, T., Jelip, J., Mohammad, R., Benedict, J., Alaza, D.A., Malacova, E., Yeo, T.W., Grigg, M.J., Anstey, N.M., Barber, B.E., 2020. *Plasmodium knowlesi* malaria in Sabah, Malaysia, 2015–2017: ongoing increase in incidence despite near-elimination of the human-only *Plasmodium* species. Clin. Infect. Dis. 70. ciz237 https://doi.org/10.1093/cid/ciz237.

Corran, P., Coleman, P., Riley, E., Drakeley, C., 2007. Serology: a robust indicator of malaria transmission intensity? Trends Parasitol. 23, 575–582. https://doi.org/10.1016/j.pt.2007.08.023.

Coutrier, F.N., Tirta, Y.K., Cotter, C., Zarlinda, I., González, I.J., Schwartz, A., Maneh, C., Marfurt, J., Murphy, M., Herdiana, H., Anstey, N.M., Greenhouse, B., Hsiang, M.S., Noviyanti, R., 2018. Laboratory challenges of *Plasmodium* species identification in Aceh Province, Indonesia, a malaria elimination setting with newly discovered *P. knowlesi*. PLoS Negl. Trop. Dis. 12, e0006924. https://doi.org/10.1371/journal.pntd.0006924.

Cox-Singh, J., Singh, B., 2008. Knowlesi malaria: newly emergent and of public health importance? Trends Parasitol. 24, 406–410. https://doi.org/10.1016/j.pt.2008.06.001.

Cox-Singh, J., Davis, T.M., Lee, K.S., Shamsul, S.S., Matusop, A., Ratnam, S., Rahman, H.A., Conway, D.J., Singh, B., 2008. *Plasmodium knowlesi* malaria in humans is widely distributed and potentially life threatening. Clin. Infect. Dis. 46, 165–171. https://doi.org/10.1086/524888.

Crosnier, C., Wanaguru, M., McDade, B., Osier, F.H., Marsh, K., Rayner, J.C., Wright, G.J., 2013. A library of functional recombinant cell-surface and secreted *P. falciparum* merozoite proteins. Mol. Cell Proteomics 12, 3976–3986. https://doi.org/10.1074/mcp.o113.028357.

Divis, P.C., Shokoples, S.E., Singh, B., Yanow, S.K., 2010. A TaqMan real-time PCR assay for the detection and quantitation of *Plasmodium knowlesi*. Malaria J. 9, 344. https://doi.org/10.1186/1475-2875-9-344.

Divis, P.C.S., Singh, B., Anderios, F., Hisam, S., Matusop, A., Kocken, C.H., Assefa, S.A., Duffy, C.W., Conway, D.J., 2015. Admixture in humans of two divergent *Plasmodium knowlesi* populations associated with different macaque host species. PLoS Pathog. 11, e1004888. https://doi.org/10.1371/journal.ppat.1004888.s014.

Drakeley, C.J., Corran, P.H., Coleman, P.G., Tongren, J.E., McDonald, S.L.R., Carneiro, I., Malima, R., Lusingu, J., Manjurano, A., Nkya, W.M.M., Lemnge, M.M., Cox, J., Reyburn, H., Riley, E.M., 2005. Estimating medium- and long-term trends in malaria transmission by using serological markers of malaria exposure. Proc. Natl. Acad. Sci. U. S. A. 102, 5108–5113. https://doi.org/10.1073/pnas.0408725102.

Edwards, H.M., Dixon, R., de Beyl, C.Z., Celhay, O., Rahman, M., Oo, M.M., Lwin, T., Lin, Z., San, T., Han, K.T., Nyunt, M.M., Plowe, C., Stresman, G., Hall, T., Drakeley, C., Hamade, P., Aryal, S., Roca-Feltrer, A., Hlaing, T., Thi, A., 2021. Prevalence and seroprevalence of *Plasmodium* infection in Myanmar reveals highly heterogeneous transmission and a large hidden reservoir of infection. PLos One 16, e0252957. https://doi.org/10.1371/journal.pone.0252957.

Escalante, A.A., Freeland, D.E., Collins, W.E., Lal, A.A., 1998. The evolution of primate malaria parasites based on the gene encoding cytochrome b from the linear mitochondrial genome. Proc. Natl. Acad. Sci. U. S. A. 95, 8124–8129.

Feagin, J.E., 1992. The 6-kb element of *Plasmodium falciparum* encodes mitochondrial cytochrome genes. Mol. Biochem. Parasitol. 52, 145–148. https://doi.org/10.1016/0166-6851(92)90046-m.

Figtree, M., Lee, R., Bain, L., Kennedy, T., Mackertich, S., Urban, M., Cheng, Q., Hudson, B.J., 2010. Plasmodium knowlesi in human, Indonesian Borneo. Emerg. Infect. Dis. 16, 672–674.

Firdaus, E.R., Park, J.-H., Muh, F., Lee, S.-K., Han, J.-H., Lim, C.-S., Na, S.-H., Park, W.S., Park, J.-H., Han, E.-T., 2021. Performance evaluation of biozentech malaria scanner in *Plasmodium knowlesi* and *P. falciparum* as a new diagnostic tool. Korean J. Parasitol. 59, 113–119. https://doi.org/10.3347/kjp.2021.59.2.113.

Fornace, K.M., Abidin, T.R., Alexander, N., Brock, P., Grigg, M.J., Murphy, A., William, T., Menon, J., Drakeley, C.J., Cox, J., 2016a. Association between landscape factors and spatial patterns of *Plasmodium knowlesi* infections in Sabah, Malaysia. Emerg. Infect. Dis. 22, 201–209. https://doi.org/10.3201/eid2202.150656.

Fornace, K.M., Nuin, N.A., Betson, M., Grigg, M.J., William, T., Anstey, N.M., Yeo, T.W., Cox, J., Ying, L.T., Drakeley, C.J., 2016b. Asymptomatic and submicroscopic carriage of *Plasmodium knowlesi* malaria in household and community members of clinical cases in Sabah, Malaysia. J. Infect. Dis. 213, 784–787. https://doi.org/10.1093/infdis/jiv475.

Fornace, K.M., Herman, L.S., Abidin, T.R., Chua, T.H., Daim, S., Lorenzo, P.J., Grignard, L., Nuin, N.A., Ying, L.T., Grigg, M.J., William, T., Espino, F., Cox, J., Tetteh, K.K.A., Drakeley, C.J., 2018. Exposure and infection to *Plasmodium knowlesi* in case study communities in Northern Sabah, Malaysia and Palawan, The Philippines. PLos Negl. Trop. D 12, e0006432. https://doi.org/10.1371/journal.pntd.0006432.

Fornace, K.M., Alexander, N., Abidin, T.R., Brock, P.M., Chua, T.H., Vythilingam, I., Ferguson, H.M., Manin, B.O., Wong, M.L., Ng, S.H., Cox, J., Drakeley, C., 2019a. Local human movement patterns and land use impact exposure to zoonotic malaria in Malaysian Borneo. eLife 8, 327. https://doi.org/10.7554/elife.47602.

Fornace, K.M., Brock, P.M., Abidin, T.R., Grignard, L., Herman, L.S., Chua, T.H., Daim, S., William, T., Patterson, C.L.E.B., Hall, T., Grigg, M.J., Anstey, N.M.,

Tetteh, K.K.A., Cox, J., Drakeley, C.J., 2019b. Environmental risk factors and exposure to the zoonotic malaria parasite Plasmodium knowlesi across northern Sabah, Malaysia: a population-based cross-sectional survey. Lancet Planet. Heal. 3, e179–e186. https://doi.org/10.1016/s2542-5196(19)30045-2.

Forsström, B., Axnäs, B.B., Rockberg, J., Danielsson, H., Bohlin, A., Uhlen, M., 2015. Dissecting antibodies with regards to linear and conformational epitopes. PLos One 10, e0121673. https://doi.org/10.1371/journal.pone.0121673.

Foster, D., Cox-Singh, J., Mohamad, D.S., Krishna, S., Chin, P.P., Singh, B., 2014. Evaluation of three rapid diagnostic tests for the detection of human infections with *Plasmodium knowlesi*. Malaria J. 13, 1–7.

Ghinai, I., Cook, J., Hla, T.T.W., Htet, H.M.T., Hall, T., Lubis, I.N., Ghinai, R., Hesketh, T., Naung, Y., Lwin, M.M., Latt, T.S., Heymann, D.L., Sutherland, C.J., Drakeley, C., Field, N., 2017. Malaria epidemiology in central Myanmar: identification of a multi-species asymptomatic reservoir of infection. Malaria J. 16, 16. https://doi.org/10.1186/s12936-016-1651-5.

Greenhouse, B., Daily, J., Guinovart, C., Goncalves, B., Beeson, J., Bell, D., Chang, M.A., Cohen, J.M., Ding, X., Domingo, G., Eisele, T.P., Lammie, P.J., Mayor, A., Merienne, N., Monteiro, W., Painter, J., Rodriguez, I., White, M., Drakeley, C., Müeller, I., Convening, M.S., 2019. Priority use cases for antibody-detecting assays of recent malaria exposure as tools to achieve and sustain malaria elimination. Gates Open Res. 3, 131. https://doi.org/10.12688/gatesopenres.12897.1.

Grigg, M.J., William, T., Barber, B.E., Parameswaran, U., Bird, E., Piera, K., Aziz, A., Dhanaraj, P., Yeo, T.W., Anstey, N.M., 2014. Combining parasite lactate dehydrogenase-based and histidine-rich protein 2-based rapid tests to improve specificity for diagnosis of malaria due to *Plasmodium knowlesi* and other *Plasmodium* species in Sabah, Malaysia. J. Clin. Microbiol. 52, 2053–2060. https://doi.org/10.1128/jcm.00181-14.

Grigg, M.J., Barber, B.E., Marfurt, J., Imwong, M., William, T., Bird, E., Piera, K.A., Aziz, A., Boonyuen, U., Drakeley, C.J., Cox, J., White, N.J., Cheng, Q., Yeo, T.W., Auburn, S., Anstey, N.M., 2016a. Dihydrofolate-reductase mutations in *Plasmodium knowlesi* appear unrelated to selective drug pressure from putative human-to-human transmission in Sabah, Malaysia. PLos One 11, e0149519. https://doi.org/10.1371/journal.pone.0149519.

Grigg, M.J., William, T., Menon, J., Dhanaraj, P., Barber, B.E., Wilkes, C.S., von Seidlein, L., Rajahram, G.S., Pasay, C., McCarthy, J.S., Price, R.N., Anstey, N.M., Yeo, T.W., 2016b. Artesunate–mefloquine versus chloroquine for treatment of uncomplicated Plasmodium knowlesi malaria in Malaysia (ACT KNOW): an open-label, randomised controlled trial. Lancet Infect. Dis. 16, 180–188. https://doi.org/10.1016/s1473-3099(15)00415-6.

Grigg, M.J., William, T., Barber, B.E., Rajahram, G.S., Menon, J., Schimann, E., Piera, K., Wilkes, C.S., Patel, K., Chandna, A., Drakeley, C.J., Yeo, T.W., Anstey, N.M., 2018a. Age-related clinical spectrum of *Plasmodium knowlesi* Malaria and predictors of severity. Clin. Infect. Dis. 67, 350–359. https://doi.org/10.1093/cid/ciy065.

Grigg, M.J., William, T., Barber, B.E., Rajahram, G.S., Menon, J., Schimann, E., Wilkes, C.S., Patel, K., Chandna, A., Price, R.N., Yeo, T.W., Anstey, N.M., 2018b. Artemether-lumefantrine versus chloroquine for the treatment of uncomplicated *Plasmodium knowlesi* Malaria: an open-label randomized controlled trial CAN KNOW. Clin. Infect. Dis. 66, 229–236. https://doi.org/10.1093/cid/cix779.

Grignard, L., Shah, S., Chua, T.H., William, T., Drakeley, C.J., Fornace, K.M., 2019. Natural human infections with *Plasmodium cynomolgi* and other malaria species in an elimination setting in Sabah, Malaysia. J. Infect. Dis. 220, 1946–1949. https://doi.org/10.1093/infdis/jiz397.

Hakimi, H., Asada, M., Angeles, J.M.M., Kawai, S., Inoue, N., Kawazu, S., 2013. *Plasmodium vivax* and *Plasmodium knowlesi*: cloning, expression and functional analysis of 1-Cys peroxiredoxin. Exp. Parasitol. 133, 101–105. https://doi.org/10.1016/j.exppara.2012.10.018.

Han, E.-T., Watanabe, R., Sattabongkot, J., Khuntirat, B., Sirichaisinthop, J., Iriko, H., Jin, L., Takeo, S., Tsuboi, T., 2007. Detection of four plasmodium species by genus- and species-specific loop-mediated isothermal amplification for clinical diagnosis. J. Clin. Microbiol. 45, 2521–2528. https://doi.org/10.1128/jcm.02117-06.

Hawking, F., Worms, M.J., Gammage, K., 1968. Host temperature and control of 24-hour and 48-hour cycles in malaria parasites. Lancet 291, 506–509. https://doi.org/10.1016/s0140-6736(68)91469-4.

Helb, D.A., Tetteh, K.K.A., Felgner, P.L., Skinner, J., Hubbard, A., Arinaitwe, E., Mayanja-Kizza, H., Ssewanyana, I., Kamya, M.R., Beeson, J.G., Tappero, J., Smith, D.L., Crompton, P.D., Rosenthal, P.J., Dorsey, G., Drakeley, C.J., Greenhouse, B., 2015. Novel serologic biomarkers provide accurate estimates of recent *Plasmodium falciparum* exposure for individuals and communities. Proc. Natl. Acad. Sci. U. S. A. 112, E4438–E4447. https://doi.org/10.1073/pnas.1501705112.

Herdiana, H., Cotter, C., Coutrier, F.N., Zarlinda, I., Zelman, B.W., Tirta, Y.K., Greenhouse, B., Gosling, R.D., Baker, P., Whittaker, M., Hsiang, M.S., 2016. Malaria risk factor assessment using active and passive surveillance data from Aceh Besar, Indonesia, a low endemic, malaria elimination setting with *Plasmodium knowlesi*, *Plasmodium vivax*, and *Plasmodium falciparum*. Malaria J. 15, 468. https://doi.org/10.1186/s12936-016-1523-z.

Herman, L.S., Fornace, K., Phelan, J., Grigg, M.J., Anstey, N.M., William, T., Moon, R.W., Blackman, M.J., Drakeley, C.J., Tetteh, K.K.A., 2018. Identification and validation of a novel panel of *Plasmodium knowlesi* biomarkers of serological exposure. PLos Negl. Trop. D 12, e0006457. https://doi.org/10.1371/journal.pntd.0006457.

Hopkins, H., González, I.J., Polley, S.D., Angutoko, P., Ategeka, J., Asiimwe, C., Agaba, B., Kyabayinze, D.J., Sutherland, C.J., Perkins, M.D., Bell, D., 2013. Highly sensitive detection of malaria parasitemia in a malaria-endemic setting: performance of a new loop-mediated isothermal amplification kit in a remote clinic in Uganda. J. Infect. Dis. 208, 645–652.

Hussin, N., Lim, Y.A.-L., Goh, P.P., William, T., Jelip, J., Mudin, R.N., 2020. Updates on malaria incidence and profile in Malaysia from 2013 to 2017. Malaria J. 19. 55–14 https://doi.org/10.1186/s12936-020-3135-x.

Ido, Y., Hashimoto, M., Yatsushiro, S., Tanaka, M., Yokota, K., Kajimoto, K., Kataoka, M., 2019. Loop-mediated isothermal amplification in microchambers on a cell microarray chip for identification of *Plasmodium* species. J. Parasitol. 105, 69–74. https://doi.org/10.1645/18-107.

Imai, K., Tarumoto, N., Misawa, K., Runtuwene, L.R., Sakai, J., Hayashida, K., Eshita, Y., Maeda, R., Tuda, J., Murakami, T., Maesaki, S., Suzuki, Y., Yamagishi, J., Maeda, T., 2017. A novel diagnostic method for malaria using loop-mediated isothermal amplification (LAMP) and MinION^{TM} nanopore sequencer. BMC Infect. Dis. 17, 621. https://doi.org/10.1186/s12879-017-2718-9.

Imwong, M., Tanomsing, N., Pukrittayakamee, S., Day, N.P.J., White, N.J., Snounou, G., 2009. Spurious amplification of a *Plasmodium vivax* small-subunit RNA gene by use of primers currently used to detect *P. knowlesi*. J. Clin. Microbiol. 47, 4173–4175. https://doi.org/10.1128/jcm.00811-09.

Imwong, M., Hanchana, S., Malleret, B., Renia, L., Day, N.P.J., Dondorp, A., Nosten, F., Snounou, G., White, N.J., 2014. High-throughput ultrasensitive molecular techniques for quantifying low-density malaria parasitemias. J. Clin. Microbiol. 52, 3303–3309. https://doi.org/10.1128/jcm.01057-14.

Imwong, M., Madmanee, W., Suwannasin, K., Kunasol, C., Peto, T.J., Tripura, R., von Seidlein, L., Nguon, C., Davoeung, C., Day, N.P.J., Dondorp, A.M., White, N.J., 2019. Asymptomatic natural human infections with the simian malaria parasites *Plasmodium cynomolgi* and *Plasmodium knowlesi*. J Infect Dis 219, 695–702. https://doi.org/10.1093/infdis/jiy519.

Iseki, H., Kawai, S., Takahashi, N., Hirai, M., Tanabe, K., Yokoyama, N., Igarashi, I., 2010. Evaluation of a loop-mediated isothermal amplification method as a tool for diagnosis of infection by the zoonotic simian malaria parasite *Plasmodium knowlesi*. J. Clin. Microbiol. 48, 2509–2514. https://doi.org/10.1128/jcm.00331-10.

Iwagami, M., Nakatsu, M., Khattignavong, P., Soundala, P., Lorphachan, L., Keomalaphet, S., Xangsayalath, P., Kawai, S., Hongvanthong, B., Brey, P.T., Kano, S., 2018. First case of human infection with *Plasmodium knowlesi* in Laos. PLoS Negl. Trop. Dis. 12, e0006244. https://doi.org/10.1371/journal.pntd.0006244.

Jeslyn, W.P.S., Huat, T.C., Vernon, L., Irene, L.M.Z., Sung, L.K., Jarrod, L.P., Singh, B., Ching, N.L., 2011. Molecular epidemiological investigation of *Plasmodium knowlesi* in humans and macaques in Singapore. Vector Borne Zoon. Dis. 11, 131–135. https://doi.org/10.1089/vbz.2010.0024.

Jiram, A., Hisam, S., Reuben, H., Husin, S.Z., Roslan, A., Ismail, W.R.W., 2016. Submicroscopic evidence of the simian malaria parasite, *Plasmodium knowlesi*, in an Orang Asli community. Southeast Asian J. Trop. Med. Public Health 47, 591–599.

Jongwutiwes, S., Putaporntip, C., Iwasaki, T., Sata, T., Kanbara, H., 2004. Naturally acquired *Plasmodium knowlesi* malaria in human, Thailand. Emerg. Infect. Dis. 10, 2211–2213. https://doi.org/10.3201/eid1012.040293.

Jongwutiwes, S., Buppan, P., Kosuvin, R., Seethamchai, S., Pattanawong, U., Sirichaisinthop, J., Putaporntip, C., 2011. *Plasmodium knowlesi* malaria in humans and macaques, Thailand. Emerg. Infect. Dis. 17, 1799–1806.

Kagan, I.G., Mathews, H.M., Rogers, W.A., Fried, J., 1969. Seroepidemiological studies by indirect haemagglutination tests for malaria. Military recruit collections from Argentina, Brazil, Colombia, and the United States of America. Bull. World Heal. Organ. 41, 825–841.

Kawai, S., Hirai, M., Haruki, K., Tanabe, K., Chigusa, Y., 2009. Cross-reactivity in rapid diagnostic tests between human malaria and zoonotic simian malaria parasite *Plasmodium knowlesi* infections. Parasitol. Int. 58, 300–302. https://doi.org/10.1016/j.parint.2009.06.004.

Kawai, S., Sato, M., Kato-Hayashi, N., Kishi, H., Huffman, M.A., Maeno, Y., Culleton, R., Nakazawa, S., 2014. Detection of *Plasmodium knowlesi* DNA in the urine and faeces of a Japanese macaque (Macaca fuscata) over the course of an experimentally induced infection. Malaria J. 13, 1–9. https://doi.org/10.1186/1475-2875-13-373.

Kimura, M., Kaneko, O., Liu, Q., Zhou, M., Kawamoto, F., Wataya, Y., Otani, S., Yamaguchi, Y., Tanabe, K., 1997. Identification of the four species of human malaria parasites by nested PCR that targets variant sequences in the small subunit rRNA gene. Parasitol. Int. 46, 91–95. https://doi.org/10.1016/s1383-5769(97)00013-5.

Knowles, R., Gupta, B.M.D., 1932. A study of monkey-malaria and its experimental transmission to man. Indian Med. Gaz., 246–249.

Lai, M.Y., Ooi, C.H., Jaimin, J.J., Lau, Y.L., 2020. Evaluation of warmstart colorimetric loop-mediated isothermal amplification assay for diagnosis of malaria. Am. J. Trop. Med. Hyg. 102, 1370–1372. https://doi.org/10.4269/ajtmh.20-0001.

Lai, M.Y., Ooi, C.H., Lau, Y.L., 2021. Validation of SYBR green I based closed-tube loop-mediated isothermal amplification (LAMP) assay for diagnosis of knowlesi malaria. Malaria J. 20, 166. https://doi.org/10.1186/s12936-021-03707-0.

Lau, Y.-L., Fong, M.-Y., Mahmud, R., Chang, P.-Y., Palaeya, V., Cheong, F.-W., Chin, L.-C., Anthony, C.N., Al-Mekhlafi, A.M., Chen, Y., 2011. Specific, sensitive and rapid detection of human plasmodium knowlesi infection by loop-mediated isothermal amplification (LAMP) in blood samples. Malaria J. 10, 197. https://doi.org/10.1186/1475-2875-10-197.

Lau, Y.L., Cheong, F.W., Chin, L.C., Mahmud, R., Chen, Y., Fong, M.Y., 2014. Evaluation of codon optimized recombinant *Plasmodium knowlesi* merozoite surface protein-119 (pkMSP-119) expressed in *Pichia pastoris*. Trop. Biomed. 31, 749–759.

Lau, Y.-L., Lai, M.-Y., Fong, M.-Y., Jelip, J., Mahmud, R., 2016. Loop-mediated isothermal amplification assay for identification of five human *Plasmodium* species in Malaysia. Am. J. Trop. Med. Hyg. 94, 336–339. https://doi.org/10.4269/ajtmh.15-0569.

Lee, K.S., Cox-Singh, J., Brooke, G., Matusop, A., Singh, B., 2009a. *Plasmodium knowlesi* from archival blood films: further evidence that human infections are widely distributed and not newly emergent in Malaysian Borneo. Int. J. Parasitol. 39, 1125–1128. https://doi.org/10.1016/j.ijpara.2009.03.003.

Lee, K.S., Cox-Singh, J., Singh, B., 2009b. Morphological features and differential counts of *Plasmodium knowlesi* parasites in naturally acquired human infections. Malaria J. 8, 73. https://doi.org/10.1186/1475-2875-8-73.

Lee, K.S., Divis, P.C.S., Zakaria, S.K., Matusop, A., Julin, R.A., Conway, D.J., Cox-Singh, J., Singh, B., 2011. *Plasmodium knowlesi*: reservoir hosts and tracking the emergence in humans and macaques. PLoS Pathog. 7, e1002015. https://doi.org/10.1371/journal.ppat.1002015.

Link, L., Bart, A., Verhaar, N., van Gool, T., Pronk, M., Scharnhorst, V., 2012. Molecular detection of *Plasmodium knowlesi* in a Dutch traveler by real-time PCR. J. Clin. Microbiol. 50, 2523–2524. https://doi.org/10.1128/jcm.06859-11.

Longley, R.J., White, M.T., Takashima, E., Brewster, J., Morita, M., Harbers, M., Obadia, T., Robinson, L.J., Matsuura, F., Liu, Z.S.J., Li-Wai-Suen, C.S.N., Tham, W.-H., Healer, J., Huon, C., Chitnis, C.E., Nguitragool, W., Monteiro, W., Proietti, C., Doolan, D.L., Siqueira, A.M., Ding, X.C., González, I.J., Kazura, J., Lacerda, M., Sattabongkot, J., Tsuboi, T., Müeller, I., 2020. Development and validation of serological markers for detecting recent *Plasmodium vivax* infection. Nat. Med. 26, 1–19. https://doi.org/10.1038/s41591-020-0841-4.

Lubis, I.N.D., Wijaya, H., Lubis, M., Lubis, C.P., Divis, P.C.S., Beshir, K.B., Sutherland, C.J., 2017. Contribution of *Plasmodium knowlesi* to multispecies human malaria infections in North Sumatera, Indonesia. J. Infect. Dis. 215, 1148–1155. https://doi.org/10.1093/infdis/jix091.

Lucchi, N.W., Poorak, M., Oberstaller, J., DeBarry, J., Srinivasamoorthy, G., Goldman, I., Xayavong, M., da Silva, A.J., Peterson, D.S., Barnwell, J.W., Kissinger, J., Udhayakumar, V., 2012. A new single-step PCR assay for the detection of the zoonotic malaria parasite *Plasmodium knowlesi*. PLoS One 7, e31848. https://doi.org/10.1371/journal.pone.0031848.

Lucchi, N.W., Gaye, M., Diallo, M.A., Goldman, I.F., Ljolje, D., Deme, A.B., Badiane, A., Ndiaye, Y.D., Barnwell, J.W., Udhayakumar, V., Ndiaye, D., 2016a. Evaluation of the Illumigene malaria LAMP: a robust molecular diagnostic tool for malaria parasites. Sci. Rep. UK 6, 36808. https://doi.org/10.1038/srep36808.

Lucchi, N.W., Ljolje, D., Silva-Flannery, L., Udhayakumar, V., 2016b. Use of malachite green-loop mediated isothermal amplification for detection of *Plasmodium spp.* Parasites. PLos One 11, e0151437. https://doi.org/10.1371/journal.pone.0151437.

Lucky, A.B., Sakaguchi, M., Katakai, Y., Kawai, S., Yahata, K., Templeton, T.J., Kaneko, O., 2016. *Plasmodium knowlesi* skeleton-binding protein 1 localizes to the 'Sinton and Mulligan' stipplings in the cytoplasm of monkey and human erythrocytes. PLos One 11, e0164272. https://doi.org/10.1371/journal.pone.0164272.

Maeno, Y., Culleton, R., Quang, N.T., Kawai, S., Marchand, R.P., Nakazawa, S., 2017. *Plasmodium knowlesi* and human malaria parasites in Khan Phu, Vietnam: gametocyte production in humans and frequent co-infection of mosquitoes. Parasitology 144, 527–535. https://doi.org/10.1017/s0031182016002110.

Mahajan, B., Jani, D., Chattopadhyay, R., Nagarkatti, R., Zheng, H., Majam, V., Weiss, W., Kumar, S., Rathore, D., 2005. Identification, cloning, expression, and characterization of the gene for *Plasmodium knowlesi* surface protein containing an altered thrombospondin repeat domain. Infect. Immun. 73, 5402–5409. https://doi.org/10.1128/iai.73.9.5402-5409.2005.

Mahittikorn, A., Masangkay, F.R., Kotepui, K.U., Milanez, G.D.J., Kotepui, M., 2021. Quantification of the misidentification of *Plasmodium knowlesi* as *Plasmodium malariae* by microscopy: an analysis of 1569 P. knowlesi cases. Malaria J. 20, 179. https://doi.org/10.1186/s12936-021-03714-1.

Mallepaddi, P.C., Lai, M.-Y., Lau, Y.-L., Liew, J.W.-K., Polavarapu, R., Podha, S., Ooi, C.-H., 2018. Development of loop-mediated isothermal amplification–based lateral flow device method for the detection of malaria. Am. J. Trop. Med. Hyg. 99, 704–708. https://doi.org/10.4269/ajtmh.18-0177.

Mao, R., Ge, G., Wang, Z., Hao, R., Zhang, G., Yang, Z., Lin, B., Ma, Y., Liu, H., Du, Y., 2018. A multiplex microfluidic loop-mediated isothermal amplification array for detection of malaria-related parasites and vectors. Acta Trop. 178, 86–92. https://doi.org/10.1016/j.actatropica.2017.10.025.

Marchand, R.P., Culleton, R., Maeno, Y., Quang, N.T., Nakazawa, S., 2011. Co-infections of *Plasmodium knowlesi*, *P. falciparum*, and *P. vivax* among humans and anopheles dirus mosquitoes, Southern Vietnam. Emerg. Infect. Dis. 17, 1232–1239. https://doi.org/10.3201/eid1707.101551.

McCutchan, T.F., McCutchan, T.F., Piper, R.C., Piper, R.C., Makler, M.T., Makler, M.T., 2008. Use of malaria rapid diagnostic test to identify *Plasmodium knowlesi* infection. Emerg. Infect. Dis. 14, 1750–1752. https://doi.org/10.3201/eid1411.080480.

Mercereau-Puijalon, O., Barale, J.-C., Bischoff, E., 2002. Three multigene families in *Plasmodium* parasites: facts and questions. Int. J. Parasitol. 32, 1323–1344. https://doi.org/10.1016/s0020-7519(02)00111-x.

Mideo, N., Reece, S.E., Smith, A.L., Metcalf, C.J.E., 2013. The Cinderella syndrome: why do malaria-infected cells burst at midnight? Trends Parasitol. 29, 10–16. https://doi.org/10.1016/j.pt.2012.10.006.

Molina-Cruz, A., Canepa, G.E., Silva, T.L.A.E., Williams, A.E., Nagyal, S., Yenkoidiok-Douti, L., Nagata, B.M., Calvo, E., Andersen, J., Boulanger, M.J., Barillas-Mury, C., 2020. *Plasmodium falciparum* evades immunity of anopheline mosquitoes by interacting with a Pfs47 midgut receptor. Proc. Natl. Acad. Sci. U. S. A. 117, 2597–2605. https://doi.org/10.1073/pnas.1917042117.

Mori, Y., Nagamine, K., Tomita, N., Notomi, T., 2001. Detection of loop-mediated isothermal amplification reaction by turbidity derived from magnesium pyrophosphate formation. Biochem. Biophys. Res. Commun. 289, 150–154. https://doi.org/10.1006/bbrc.2001.5921.

Moyes, C.L., Henry, A.J., Golding, N., Huang, Z., Singh, B., Baird, J.K., Newton, P.N., Huffman, M., Duda, K.A., Drakeley, C.J., Elyazar, I.R.F., Anstey, N.M., Chen, Q., Zommers, Z., Bhatt, S., Gething, P.W., Hay, S.I., 2014. Defining the geographical range of the *Plasmodium knowlesi* reservoir. PLoS Negl. Trop. Dis. 8, e2780. https://doi.org/10.1371/journal.pntd.0002780.s004.

Muh, F., Kim, N., Nyunt, M.H., Firdaus, E.R., Han, J.-H., Hoque, M.R., Lee, S.-K., Park, J.-H., Moon, R.W., Lau, Y.-L., Kaneko, O., Han, E.T., 2020. Cross-species reactivity of antibodies against *Plasmodium vivax* blood-stage antigens to *Plasmodium knowlesi*. PLoS Negl. Trop. Dis. 14. e0008323-21 https://doi.org/10.1371/journal.pntd.0008323.

Müller-Sienerth, N., Shilts, J., Kadir, K.A., Yman, V., Homann, M.V., Asghar, M., Ngasala, B., Singh, B., Färnert, A., Wright, G.J., 2020. A panel of recombinant proteins from human-infective *Plasmodium* species for serological surveillance. Malaria J. 19, 31. https://doi.org/10.1186/s12936-020-3111-5.

Najafabadi, Z.G., Oormazdi, H., Akhlaghi, L., Meamar, A.R., Nateghpour, M., Farivar, L., Razmjou, E., 2014. Detection of *Plasmodium vivax* and *Plasmodium falciparum* DNA in human saliva and urine: loop-mediated isothermal amplification for malaria diagnosis. Acta Trop. 136, 44–49. https://doi.org/10.1016/j.actatropica.2014.03.029.

Narum, D.L., Thomas, A.W., 1994. Differential localization of full-length and processed forms of PF83/AMA-1 an apical membrane antigen of *Plasmodium falciparum* merozoites. Mol. Biochem. Parasitol. 67, 59–68. https://doi.org/10.1016/0166-6851(94)90096-5.

Noordin, N.R., Lee, P.Y., Bukhari, F.D.M., Fong, M.Y., Hamid, M.H.A., Jelip, J., Mudin, R.N., Lau, Y.L., 2020. Prevalence of asymptomatic and/or low-density malaria infection among high-risk groups in Peninsular Malaysia. Am. J. Trop. Med. Hyg. 103, 1107–1110. https://doi.org/10.4269/ajtmh.20-0268.

Notomi, T., Okayama, H., Masubuchi, H., Yonekawa, T., Watanabe, K., Amino, N., Hase, T., 2000. Loop-mediated isothermal amplification of DNA. Nucl. Acids Res. 28, e63. https://doi.org/10.1093/nar/28.12.e63.

Nuin, N.A., Tan, A.F., Lew, Y.L., Piera, K.A., William, T., Rajahram, G.S., Jelip, J., Dony, J.F., Mohammad, R., Cooper, D.J., Barber, B.E., Anstey, N.M., Chua, T.H., Grigg, M.J., 2020. Comparative evaluation of two commercial real-time PCR kits (QuantiFast^{TM} and abTES^{TM}) for the detection of *Plasmodium knowlesi* and other *Plasmodium* species in Sabah, Malaysia. Malaria J. 19, 306. https://doi.org/10.1186/s12936-020-03379-2.

Oddoux, O., Debourgogne, A., Kantele, A., Kocken, C.H., Jokiranta, T.S., Vedy, S., Puyhardy, J.M., Machouart, M., 2011. Identification of the five human Plasmodium species including P. knowlesi by real-time polymerase chain reaction. Eur. J. Clin. Microbiol. Infect. Dis. Off. Publ. Eur. Soc. Clin. Microbiol. 30, 597–601. https://doi.org/10.1007/s10096-010-1126-5.

Ong, C.W.M., Lee, S.Y., Koh, W.H., Ooi, E.E., Tambyah, P.A., 2009. Monkey malaria in humans: a diagnostic dilemma with conflicting laboratory data. Am. J. Trop. Med. Hyg. 80, 927–928.

Pain, A., Bohme, U., Berry, A.E., Mungall, K., Finn, R.D., Jackson, A.P., Mourier, T., Mistry, J., Pasini, E.M., Aslett, M.A., Balasubrammaniam, S., Borgwardt, K., Brooks, K., Carret, C., Carver, T.J., Cherevach, I., Chillingworth, T., Clark, T.G., Galinski, M.R., Hall, N., Harper, D., Harris, D., Hauser, H., Ivens, A., Janssen, C.S., Keane, T., Larke, N., Lapp, S., Marti, M., Moule, S., Meyer, I.M., Ormond, D., Peters, N., Sanders, M., Sanders, S., Sargeant, T.J., Simmonds, M., Smith, F., Squares, R., Thurston, S., Tivey, A.R., Walker, D., White, B., Zuiderwijk, E., Churcher, C., Quail, M.A., Cowman, A.F., Turner, C.M.R., Rajandream, M.A., Kocken, C.H.M., Thomas, A.W., Newbold, C.I., Barrell, B.G., Berriman, M., 2008. The genome of the simian and human malaria parasite *Plasmodium knowlesi*. Nature 455, 799–803. https://doi.org/10.1038/nature07306.

Patel, J.C., Oberstaller, J., Xayavong, M., Narayanan, J., DeBarry, J.D., Srinivasamoorthy, G., Villegas, L., Escalante, A.A., DaSilva, A., Peterson, D.S., Barnwell, J.W., Kissinger, J.C., Udhayakumar, V., Lucchi, N.W., 2013. Real-time loop-mediated isothermal amplification (RealAmp) for the species-specific identification of *Plasmodium vivax*. PLoS One 8, e54986. https://doi.org/10.1371/journal.pone.0054986.

Perandin, F., Manca, N., Calderaro, A., Piccolo, G., Galati, L., Ricci, L., Medici, M.C., Arcangeletti, M.C., Snounou, G., Dettori, G., Chezzi, C., 2004. Development of a real-time PCR assay for detection of *Plasmodium falciparum*, *Plasmodium vivax*, and *Plasmodium ovale* for routine clinical diagnosis. J. Clin. Microbiol. 42, 1214. https://doi.org/10.1128/jcm.42.3.1214-1219.2004.

Perera, R.S., Ding, X.C., Tully, F., Oliver, J., Bright, N., Bell, D., Chiodini, P.L., Gonzalez, I.J., Polley, S.D., 2017. Development and clinical performance of high throughput loop-mediated isothermal amplification for detection of malaria. PLos One 12, e0171126. https://doi.org/10.1371/journal.pone.0171126.

Piera, K.A., Aziz, A., William, T., Bell, D., González, I.J., Barber, B.E., Anstey, N.M., Grigg, M.J., 2017. Detection of *Plasmodium knowlesi*, *Plasmodium falciparum* and *Plasmodium vivax* using loop-mediated isothermal amplification (LAMP) in a co-endemic area in Malaysia. Malaria J. 16, 29. https://doi.org/10.1186/s12936-016-1676-9.

Plucinski, M.M., Candrinho, B., Chambe, G., Muchanga, J., Muguande, O., Matsinhe, G., Mathe, G., Rogier, E., Doyle, T., Zulliger, R., Colborn, J., Saifodine, A., Lammie, P., Priest, J.W., 2018. Multiplex serology for impact evaluation of bed net distribution on burden of lymphatic filariasis and four species of human malaria in northern Mozambique. PLos Negl. Trop. D 12, e0006278. https://doi.org/10.1371/journal.pntd.0006278.

Polley, S.D., Mori, Y., Watson, J., Perkins, M.D., Gonzalez, I.J., Notomi, T., Chiodini, P.L., Sutherland, C.J., 2010. Mitochondrial DNA targets increase sensitivity of malaria detection using loop-mediated isothermal amplification. J. Clin. Microbiol. 48, 2866–2871. https://doi.org/10.1128/jcm.00355-10.

Polley, S.D., González, I.J., Mohamed, D., Daly, R., Bowers, K., Watson, J., Mewse, E., Armstrong, M., Gray, C., Perkins, M.D., Bell, D., Kanda, H., Tomita, N., Kubota, Y., Mori, Y., Chiodini, P.L., Sutherland, C.J., 2013. Clinical evaluation of a loop-mediated amplification kit for diagnosis of imported malaria. J. Infect. Dis. 208, 637–644. https://doi.org/10.1093/infdis/jit183.

Poon, L.L.M., Wong, B.W.Y., Ma, E.H.T., Chan, K.H., Chow, L.M.C., Abeyewickreme, W., Tangpukdee, N., Yuen, K.Y., Guan, Y., Looareesuwan, S., Peiris, J.S.M., 2006. Sensitive and inexpensive molecular test for falciparum malaria: detecting *Plasmodium falciparum* DNA directly from heat-treated blood by loop-mediated isothermal amplification. Clin. Chem. 52, 303–306. https://doi.org/10.1373/clinchem.2005.057901.

Prasad, R., Atul, Soni, A., Puri, S.K., Sijwali, P.S., 2012. Expression, characterization, and cellular localization of knowpains, papain-like cysteine proteases of the *Plasmodium knowlesi* malaria parasite. PLos One 7, e51619. https://doi.org/10.1371/journal.pone.0051619.

Putaporntip, C., Buppan, P., Jongwutiwes, S., 2011. Improved performance with saliva and urine as alternative DNA sources for malaria diagnosis by mitochondrial DNA-based PCR assays. Clin. Microbiol. Infect. 17, 1484–1491. https://doi.org/10.1111/j.1469-0691.2011.03507.x.

Rajahram, G.S., Barber, B.E., William, T., Menon, J., Anstey, N.M., Yeo, T.W., 2012. Deaths due to *Plasmodium knowlesi* malaria in Sabah, Malaysia: association with reporting as *Plasmodium malariae* and delayed parenteral artesunate. Malaria J. 11, 284. https://doi.org/10.1186/1475-2875-11-284.

Rajahram, G.S., Cooper, D.J., William, T., Grigg, M.J., Anstey, N.M., Barber, B.E., 2019. Deaths from *Plasmodium knowlesi* malaria: case series and systematic review. Clin. Infect. Dis. 69, ciz011. https://doi.org/10.1093/cid/ciz011.

Reller, M.E., et al., 2013. Multiplex 5′ nuclease quantitative real-time PCR for clinical diagnosis of malaria and species-level identification and epidemiologic evaluation of malaria-causing parasites, including *Plasmodium knowlesi*. J. Clin. Microbiol. 9 (51).

Rypien, C., Chow, B., Chan, W.W., Church, D.L., Pillai, D.R., 2017. Detection of plasmodium infection by the illumigene malaria assay compared to reference microscopy and real-time PCR. J. Clin. Microbiol. 55, 3037–3045. https://doi.org/10.1128/jcm.00806-17.

Sema, M., Alemu, A., Bayih, A.G., Getie, S., Getnet, G., Guelig, D., Burton, R., LaBarre, P., Pillai, D.R., 2015. Evaluation of non-instrumented nucleic acid amplification by loop-mediated isothermal amplification (NINA-LAMP) for the diagnosis of malaria in Northwest Ethiopia. Malaria J. 14, 44. https://doi.org/10.1186/s12936-015-0559-9.

Setiadi, W., et al., 2016. A zoonotic human infection with simian malaria, *Plasmodium knowlesi*, in Central Kalimantan, Indonesia. Malaria J. 15, 218. https://doi.org/10.1186/s12936-016-1272-z.

Sharma, S., Godson, G., 1985. Expression of the major surface antigen of *Plasmodium knowlesi* sporozoites in yeast. Science 228, 879–882. https://doi.org/10.1126/science.3890178.

Shearer, F.M., Huang, Z., Weiss, D.J., Wiebe, A., Gibson, H.S., Battle, K.E., Pigott, D.M., Brady, O.J., Putaporntip, C., Jongwutiwes, S., Lau, Y.-L., Manske, M., Amato, R., Elyazar, I.R.F., Vythilingam, I., Bhatt, S., Gething, P.W., Singh, B., Golding, N., Hay, S.I., Moyes, C.L., 2016. Estimating geographical variation in the risk of zoonotic *Plasmodium knowlesi* infection in countries eliminating malaria. PLoS Negl. Trop. Dis. 10, e0004915. https://doi.org/10.1371/journal.pntd.0004915.

Silva, J.R.D., Lau, Y.-L., Fong, M.-Y., 2016. Expression and evaluation of recombinant *Plasmodium knowlesi* merozoite surface protein-3 (MSP-3) for detection of human malaria. PLoS One 11, e0158998. https://doi.org/10.1371/journal.pone.0158998.

Siner, A., Liew, S.-T., Kadir, K.A., Mohamad, D.S.A., Thomas, F.K., Zulkarnaen, M., Singh, B., 2017. Absence of *Plasmodium inui* and *Plasmodium cynomolgi*, but detection of *Plasmodium knowlesi* and *Plasmodium vivax* infections in asymptomatic humans in the Betong division of Sarawak, Malaysian Borneo. Malaria J. 16, 1–11. https://doi.org/10.1186/s12936-017-2064-9.

Singh, B., Daneshvar, C., 2013. Human infections and detection of *Plasmodium knowlesi*. Clin. Microbiol. Rev. 26, 165–184. https://doi.org/10.1128/cmr.00079-12.

Singh, A.P., Puri, S.K., Chitnis, C.E., 2002. Antibodies raised against receptor-binding domain of *Plasmodium knowlesi* Duffy binding protein inhibit erythrocyte invasion. Mol. Biochem. Parasitol. 121, 21–31. https://doi.org/10.1016/s0166-6851(02)00017-8.

Singh, B., Sung, L.K., Matusop, A., Radhakrishnan, A., Shamsul, S.S., Cox-Singh, J., Thomas, A., Conway, D.J., 2004. A large focus of naturally acquired *Plasmodium knowlesi* infections in human beings. Lancet 363, 1017–1024. https://doi.org/10.1016/s0140-6736(04)15836-4.

Singh, V., Kaushal, D.C., Rathaur, S., Kumar, N., Kaushal, N.A., 2012. Cloning, over-expression, purification and characterization of *Plasmodium knowlesi* lactate dehydrogenase. Prot. Exp. Purif. 84, 195–203. https://doi.org/10.1016/j.pep.2012.05.008.

Singh, R., Savargaonkar, D., Bhatt, R., Valecha, N., 2013. Rapid detection of *Plasmodium vivax* in saliva and blood using loop mediated isothermal amplification (LAMP) assay. J. Infect. 67, 245–247. https://doi.org/10.1016/j.jinf.2013.04.016.

Sinton, J.A., Mulligan, H.W., 1933. A critical review of the literature relating to the identification of the malarial parasites recorded from monkeys of the families Cercopithecidae and Colobidae. Rec. Malaria Surv. Ind. 3, 381–444.

Snounou, G., Singh, B., 2002. Nested PCR analysis of *Plasmodium* parasites. Meth. Mol. Med. 72, 189–203. https://doi.org/10.1385/1-59259-271-6:189.

Snounou, G., Viriyakosol, S., Jarra, W., Thaithong, S., Brown, K.N., 1993. Identification of the four human malaria parasite species in field samples by the polymerase chain reaction and detection of a high prevalence of mixed infections. Mol. Biochem. Parasitol. 58, 283–292. https://doi.org/10.1016/0166-6851(93)90050-8.

Stark, D.J., Fornace, K.M., Brock, P.M., Abidin, T.R., Gilhooly, L., Jalius, C., Goossens, B., Drakeley, C.J., Salgado-Lynn, M., 2019. Long-tailed macaque response to deforestation in a *Plasmodium knowlesi*-endemic area. EcoHealth 6, e14592–e14599. https://doi.org/10.1007/s10393-019-01403-9.

Stewart, L., Gosling, R., Griffin, J., Gesase, S., Campo, J., Hashim, R., Masika, P., Mosha, J., Bousema, T., Shekalaghe, S., Cook, J., Corran, P., Ghani, A., Riley, E.M., Drakeley, C., 2009. Rapid assessment of malaria transmission using age-specific sero-conversion rates. PLoS One 4, e6083. https://doi.org/10.1371/journal.pone.0006083.

Tanizaki, R., Ujiie, M., Kato, Y., Iwagami, M., Hashimoto, A., Kutsuna, S., Takeshita, N., Hayakawa, K., Kanagawa, S., Kano, S., Ohmagari, N., 2013. First case of *Plasmodium knowlesi* infection in a Japanese traveller returning from Malaysia. Malaria J. 12, 128. https://doi.org/10.1186/1475-2875-12-128.

Tanomsing, N., Imwong, M., Theppabutr, S., Pukrittayakamee, S., Day, N.P.J., White, N.J., Snounou, G., 2010. Accurate and sensitive detection of plasmodium species in humans by use of the dihydrofolate reductase-thymidylate synthase linker region. J. Clin. Microbiol. 48, 3735–3737. https://doi.org/10.1128/jcm.00898-10.

Tham, J.M., Lee, S.H., Tan, T.M., Ting, R.C., Kara, U.A., 1999. Detection and species determination of malaria parasites by PCR: comparison with microscopy and with ParaSight-F and ICT malaria Pf tests in a clinical environment. J. Clin. Microbiol. 37, 1269–1273.

Torres, K., Bachman, C.M., Delahunt, C.B., Baldeon, J.A., Alava, F., Vilela, D.G., Proux, S., Mehanian, C., McGuire, S.K., Thompson, C.M., Ostbye, T., Hu, L., Jaiswal, M.S., Hunt, V.M., Bell, D., 2018. Automated microscopy for routine malaria diagnosis: a field comparison on Giemsa-stained blood films in Peru. Malaria J. 17, 339. https://doi.org/10.1186/s12936-018-2493-0.

Tran, T.M., Crompton, P.D., 2020. Decoding the complexities of human malaria through systems immunology. Immunol. Rev. 293, 144–162. https://doi.org/10.1111/imr.12817.

Tyagi, K., Gupta, D., Saini, E., Choudhary, S., Jamwal, A., Alam, M.S., Zeeshan, M., Tyagi, R.K., Sharma, Y.D., 2015. Recognition of human erythrocyte receptors by the tryptophan-rich antigens of monkey malaria parasite *Plasmodium knowlesi*. PLoS One 10, e0138691.

Vaidya, A.B., Mather, M.W., 2005. A post-genomic view of the mitochondrion in malaria parasites. Curr. Top. Microbiol. 295, 233–250. https://doi.org/10.1007/3-540-29088-5_9.

van der Laan, M.J., Polley, E.C., Hubbard, A.E., 2007. Super learner. Stat. Appl. Genet. Mol. Biol. 6. Article 25 https://doi.org/10.2202/1544-6115.1309.

van Hellemond, J.J., Rutten, M., Koelewijn, R., Zeeman, A.M., Verweij, J.J., Wismans, P.J., Kocken, C.H., van Genderen, P.J.J., 2009. Human *Plasmodium knowlesi* infection detected by rapid diagnostic tests for malaria. Emerg. Infect. Dis. 15, 1478–1480. https://doi.org/10.3201/eid1509.090358.

Vythilingam, I., 2010. Plasmodium knowlesi in humans: a review on the role of its vectors in Malaysia. Trop. Biomed. 27, 1–12.

Waters, A.P., 1994. The ribosomal RNA genes of *Plasmodium*. Adv. Parasitol. 34, 33–79. https://doi.org/10.1016/s0065-308x(08)60136-0.

Waters, A.P., Thomas, A.W., Deans, J.A., Mitchell, G.H., Hudson, D.E., Miller, L.H., McCutchan, T.F., Cohen, S., 1990. A merozoite receptor protein from *Plasmodium knowlesi* is highly conserved and distributed throughout Plasmodium. J. Biol. Chem. 265, 17974–17979.

WHO, 2014. Severe malaria. Trop. Med. Int. Heal. 19 (Suppl. 1), 7–131. https://doi.org/10.1111/tmi.12313_2.

WHO, 2015a. Microscopy for the Detection, Identification and Quantification of Malaria Parasites on Stained Thick and Thin Blood Films in Research Settings. World Health Organisation.

WHO, 2015b. Summary results of WHO product testing of malaria RDTs: round 1-6 (2008–2015). http://apps.who.int/iris/bitstream/10665/204119/1/9789241510042_eng.pdf. (Accessed 3 August 2016).

WHO, M.P.A.C., 2017. Outcomes From the Evidence Review Group on *Plasmodium knowlesi*.

WHO, 2018. Malaria Rapid Diagnostic Test Performance (Round 8).

WHO, 2020. WHO|World Malaria Report 2020.

WHO, 2021. WHO Guidelines for Malaria.

William, T., Menon, J., Rajahram, G., Chan, L., Ma, G., Donaldson, S., Khoo, S., Frederick, C., Jelip, J., Anstey, N.M., Yeo, T.W., 2011. Severe *Plasmodium knowlesi* malaria in a tertiary care hospital, Sabah, Malaysia. Emerg. Infect. Dis. 17, 1248–1255. https://doi.org/10.3201/eid1707.101017.

Wong, M.L., Chua, T.H., Leong, C.S., Khaw, L.T., Fornace, K., Wan-Sulaiman, W.-Y., William, T., Drakeley, C., Ferguson, H.M., Vythilingam, I., 2015. Seasonal and spatial dynamics of the primary vector of Plasmodium knowlesi within a major transmission focus in Sabah, Malaysia. PLoS Negl. Trop. Dis. 9, e0004135. https://doi.org/10.1371/journal.pntd.0004135.t004.

Wu, L., Mwesigwa, J., Affara, M., Bah, M., Correa, S., Hall, T., Singh, S.K., Beeson, J.G., Tetteh, K.K.A., Kleinschmidt, I., D'Alessandro, U., Drakeley, C., 2020. Antibody responses to a suite of novel serological markers for malaria surveillance demonstrate strong correlation with clinical and parasitological infection across seasons and transmission settings in The Gambia. BMC Med. 18, 304. https://doi.org/10.1186/s12916-020-01724-5.

Yap, N.J., Hossain, H., Nada-Raja, T., Ngui, R., Muslim, A., Hoh, B.-P., Khaw, L.T., Kadir, K.A., Divis, P.C.S., Vythilingam, I., Singh, B., Lim, Y.A.-L., 2021. Natural human infections with *Plasmodium cynomolgi*, *P. inui*, and 4 other simian malaria parasites, Malaysia. Emerg. Infect. Dis. 27, 2187–2191. https://doi.org/10.3201/eid2708.204502.

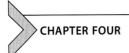

CHAPTER FOUR

The vectors of *Plasmodium knowlesi* and other simian malarias Southeast Asia: challenges in malaria elimination

Indra Vythilingam[a,*], Tock Hing Chua[b,*], Jonathan Wee Kent Liew[a,c], Benny O. Manin[b], and Heather M. Ferguson[d]

[a]Department of Parasitology, University of Malaya, Kuala Lumpur, Malaysia
[b]Department of Pathobiology and Microbiology, Faculty of Medicine and Health Sciences, Universiti Sabah Malaysia, Kota Kinabalu, Sabah, Malaysia
[c]Environmental Health Institute, National Environment Agency, Singapore, Singapore
[d]Institute of Biodiversity, Animal Health and Comparative Medicine, University of Glasgow, Glasgow, Scotland, United Kingdom
*Corresponding authors: e-mail address: indrav@um.edu.my; chuath@gmail.com

Contents

1. Introduction	132
2. Simian malaria parasites in natural vector mosquitoes	134
2.1 Phylogenetic position of *Plasmodium knowlesi* amongst malaria parasites	134
2.2 Detected simian malaria parasites in vector mosquitoes	138
3. Vectors of *Plasmodium knowlesi*—Leucosphyrus Group of *Anopheles*	139
3.1 Phylogenetic studies of vectors in the Leucosphyrus Group of *Anopheles*	139
3.2 Natural vectors of *Plasmodium knowlesi* in the Leucosphyrous Group of *Anopheles*	140
4. Bionomics of natural vectors of *Plasmodium kowlesi* in the Leucosphyrus Group of *Anopheles*	144
4.1 Larval biology	144
4.2 Biting habits of vectors	145
4.3 Host preferences	145
4.4 Vectorial capacity and life expectancy of knowlesi simian malaria vectors	146
5. Suspected vectors of knowlesi malaria in other *Anopheles* Groups	148
6. Experimental transmissions of *Plasmodium knowlesi* and other simian malaria parasites in mosquitoes	149
6.1 Experimental studies on *Plasmodium knowlesi* in mosquitoes	150
6.2 Implication of experimental studies using vectors on the transmission of *P. knowlesi* and other simian malarias in nature	160
7. Control of vectors of *P. knowlesi* and other simian malarias	167
7.1 Tools for control of simian malaria	167
7.2 Vector control for simian malaria in Southeast Asia	168

Advances in Parasitology, Volume 113
ISSN 0065-308X
https://doi.org/10.1016/bs.apar.2021.08.005

8. Challenges	172
9. Conclusions and the way forward	174
Acknowledgement	174
References	174

Abstract

Plasmodium knowlesi, a simian malaria parasite of great public health concern has been reported from most countries in Southeast Asia and exported to various countries around the world. Currently *P. knowlesi* is the predominant species infecting humans in Malaysia. Besides this species, other simian malaria parasites such as *P. cynomolgi* and *P. inui* are also infecting humans in the region. The vectors of *P. knowlesi* and other Asian simian malarias belong to the Leucosphyrus Group of *Anopheles* mosquitoes which are generally forest dwelling species. Continual deforestation has resulted in these species moving into forest fringes, farms, plantations and human settlements along with their macaque hosts. Limited studies have shown that mosquito vectors are attracted to both humans and macaque hosts, preferring to bite outdoors and in the early part of the night. We here review the current status of simian malaria vectors and their parasites, knowledge of vector competence from experimental infections and discuss possible vector control measures. The challenges encountered in simian malaria elimination are also discussed. We highlight key knowledge gaps on vector distribution and ecology that may impede effective control strategies.

1. Introduction

The first simian malaria parasite demonstrated to successfully infect humans under experimental conditions was *Plasmodium knowlesi* (Knowles and Gupta, 1933). This was done by inoculating infected blood from macaque to man. However, efforts to identify the natural vectors of *P. knowlesi* and other simian malaria parasites at that time were unsuccessful (Coggeshall, 1941; Jaswant et al., 1949; Sinton et al., 1938). Up till 1946, hundreds of attempts to infect four different genera of mosquitoes (*Anopheles, Culex, Aedes* and *Armigeres*) with *P. knowlesi* yielded only a single *Anopheles stephensi* with oocysts, and a single *Aedes reginae* and three *Armigeres obturbans* with the transmissible sporozoite stage (only one of which produced an infection in a monkey). As understanding of the simian malaria parasites and their vectors increases, the prevalence of these parasites in monkey hosts and their transmissibility to humans led Garnham to hypothesize that *P. knowlesi* was a potential zoonosis that could be transmitted to humans in nature. It was further postulated that the absence of infection in people could be attributed to the restricted habitats of the primary mosquito vectors (Garnham, 1959).

In 1965 the first natural infection of *P. knowlesi* in human was reported in an American surveyor who had spent time in the jungles of Pahang, Malaysia (Chin et al., 1965). This led to the commencement of numerous projects investigating the zoonotic potential of simian malaria; with the conclusion that simian malaria would be unlikely to spillover from the macaque reservoir into humans (Warren et al., 1970). This view appeared to be accepted until 2004 when the first large focus of *P. knowlesi* malaria cases in humans was reported in Kapit, Sarawak, Malaysian Borneo (Singh et al., 2004). This was followed by several reports of human cases of *P. knowlesi* in all countries in Southeast Asia except for Timor Leste (Jeyaprakasam et al., 2020). In addition, there were also reports of *P. knowlesi* being exported by travellers to countries outside Southeast Asia (Jeyaprakasam et al., 2020). *Plasmodium knowlesi* is currently the predominant species affecting humans in Malaysia (Chin et al., 2020), with *Plasmodium cynomolgi* also recently been reported infecting humans (Grignard et al., 2019; Hartmeyer et al., 2019; Imwong et al., 2019; Raja et al., 2020; Singh et al., 2018; Ta et al., 2014). Moreover, *Plasmodium inui* has now also been found to infect humans in Malaysia (Liew et al., 2021; Yap et al., 2021). The zoonotic potential of these and other simian malaria parasites could pose serious new public health threats; particularly in areas of Southeast Asia where human malaria parasite species have been eliminated (Jeyaprakasam et al., 2020).

The potential threat of simian malaria to malaria elimination has been recognized since the first Global Malaria Eradication campaign (Coatney, 1963). Of all simian malaria species, *P. knowlesi* is currently the only one posing a significant threat to malaria elimination in Southeast Asia (Barber et al., 2017). This is most pronounced in Malaysia where *P. knowlesi* emergence has reversed decades of progress in reducing malaria cases (Barber et al., 2017). Yet while *P. knowlesi* is the predominant species currently affecting humans in Malaysia (Chin et al., 2020), there is a relative lack of urgency in recognizing and addressing this problem. For example, WHO currently does not include *P. knowlesi* malaria within its global malaria elimination strategy (WHO, 2016). Additionally, ability to tackle *P. knowlesi* is further limited by the lack of prioritization of vector surveillance and expertise in affected countries (Russell et al., 2020). Thus, despite the emphasis on understanding vector ecology, behaviour, and distribution of vectors in the current WHO guidelines (WHO, 2018, 2019), the lack of support for simian vector surveillance may jeopardize global malaria eradication. *Plasmodium knowlesi* poses a peculiar challenge because of the distinct ecology of its vectors compared to those of human malarias; and is unlikely similar control approaches can be instituted.

A better understanding of the vectors responsible for the transmission of P. knowlesi and other simian malarias should be pursued to formulate more effective control measures. In this review we review existing knowledge on the ecology, bionomics and transmission potential of these vectors, and discuss vector control measures that could be implemented to reduce transmission to people living in the affected areas.

2. Simian malaria parasites in natural vector mosquitoes

2.1 Phylogenetic position of *Plasmodium knowlesi* amongst malaria parasites

Plasmodium are haemosporidian parasites infecting both vertebrate and definitive insect hosts. There are more than 250 species of *Plasmodium;* with these species categorized into 16 sub-genera based on their host range and morphology in vertebrate blood (Garnham, 1966). Only three sub-genera (*Laverania, Plasmodium* and *Vinckeia*) are found in the primate hosts; with two (*Laverania* and *Plasmodium*) confirmed in humans.

The genus *Plasmodium* is polyphyletic and it is divided into two main groups namely (1) those infecting birds and lizards, and (2) those that infect mammals and transmitted by mosquitoes of *Anophelinae* sub-family. Those infecting birds and lizards are transmitted by mosquitoes from the sub-family of Culicinae except for the subgenus Paraplasmodium which are transmitted by sand flies (Phlebotominae). Mammalian hosts include humans, chimpanzees/gorillas, monkeys, lemurs, rodents and bats (Escalante and Ayala, 1994; Galen et al., 2018; Hayakawa et al., 2008; Lutz et al., 2016; Martinsen et al., 2008; Pacheco et al., 2018; Perkins and Schall, 2002; Qari et al., 1996). The mammalian parasites are subdivided into two groups namely the primate parasites (sub-genus *Plasmodium* infecting mainly macaques and sub-genus *Laverania* infecting apes) and the rodent parasites (sub-genus *Vinckeia* infecting rodents/bats) (Galen et al., 2018). These two major groups diverged about 26–38 million years ago (MYA), and the ancestors of the mammalian parasites (except buffalo parasites) were possibly derived from chimpanzee/gorilla parasites found in Africa (Pacheco et al., 2018). However, Lutz et al. (2016) suggested that malaria parasites found in mammals (primates and rodents) may have originated from the bat parasites (*Polychromophilus* and *Nycteria*).

Phylogenetic analysis indicated that *P. falciparum* is closely related to *P. praefalciparum* (Prugnolle et al., 2010) which has been infecting wild gorillas before jumping to humans (Boundenga et al., 2015; Liu et al., 2010). Furthermore, there are two lineages for *P. falciparum*, suggesting that *P. falciparum* also originated from bonobos before shifting into a human host (Krief et al., 2010). On the other hand, *P. vivax*, has been thought to have originated from Asian monkeys (Arisue et al., 2012, 2019; Nishimoto et al., 2008; Roy and Irimia, 2008; Rutledge et al., 2017). However genomic studies of *P. vivax*-like in African chimpanzees and gorillas indicated its close relationship with human *P. vivax* (Liu et al., 2014; Loy et al., 2018; Prugnolle et al., 2013), implying that *P. vivax* has experienced an extreme bottleneck event that resulted in a drastically reduced population in the African continent, followed by rapid population expansion outside the African continent (Loy et al., 2018).

The simian malaria parasites as a group are joined with *P. gonderi* (Lutz et al., 2016, Arisue et al., 2019) forming a clade which is placed next to the human malaria parasite grouping (Carlton et al., 2008; Pain et al., 2008; Tachibana et al., 2012). A recent review indicated most cases of simian malaria parasites infecting humans occur in Southeast Asian countries, and predominantly in Malaysia and Indonesia (Jeyaprakasam et al., 2020). To date, the following simian malaria parasites been reported to infect humans naturally, the SE Asian *P. knowlesi, P. cynomolgi, P. inui,* and the American *P. brasilianum* and *P. simium* (Brasil et al., 2017; Lalremruata et al., 2015; Singh et al., 2004; Ta et al., 2014; Yap et al., 2021). However, other simian malaria parasites may have potential to naturally infect humans and should not be overlooked given their potential to generate low levels of parasitaemia that may go undetected because individuals are asymptomatic (Fornace et al., 2016; Grignard et al., 2019; Imwong et al., 2019; Jiram et al., 2019; Singh et al., 2018; Yap et al., 2021).

The phylogeny of simian malaria parasites (sub-genus *Plasmodium*) consists of several main lineages namely *P. cynomolgi*—*P. simian/P. vivax* lineage, *P. fragile*—*P. coatneyi*—*P. knowlesi* lineage, *P. inui*—*P. hylobati* lineage and *P. simiovale*—*P. fieldi* lineage (Arisue et al., 2019; Chua et al., 2017; Lutz et al., 2016). Species in the same lineage group share a close relationship. For example, the genome of *P. cynomolgi* and *P. vivax* have 214 identical genes compared to only 100 identical genes between *P. cynomolgi* and *P. knowlesi* and 17 identical genes between *P. vivax* and *P. knowlesi* (Tachibana et al., 2012). However, Arisue et al. have suggested that *P. vivax* is the basal group for simian malaria parasites rather than sharing the same lineage with *P. cynomolgi* based on phylogenetic analysis of the apicoplast genome (Arisue et al., 2019).

The original hosts of *P. knowlesi* were thought to be the monkeys that inhabited the Asian continent before they migrated and inhabited the area now known as Southeast Asia ~1.8 MYA (Harrison et al., 2006). A phylogenetic study (Lee et al., 2011) of *P. knowlesi* specimens sampled in Sarawak, Malaysia supports the emergence of *P. knowlesi* from existing parasite populations in Asia around 98,000–478,000 years ago. This indicates that *P. knowlesi* is older than *P. falciparum* and *P. vivax,* which are respectively estimated to have an ancestor between 50,000–330,000 (Joy et al., 2003; Krief et al., 2010) and 45,000–265,000 years ago (Escalante et al., 2005; Mu et al., 2005). The population of *P. knowlesi* began to expand about 30,000–40,000 years ago in tandem with the expansion of the human population in Southeast Asia (Lee et al., 2011; O'Connell et al., 2018). However, there is no evidence that the expansion of *P. knowlesi* is closely related to the population expansion of monkeys (Lee et al., 2011).

Plasmodium knowlesi parasites in Malaysia can be divided into three main clusters according to the geographical region and the macaque hosts (long-tailed and pig-tailed) of the parasite (Ahmed et al., 2018; Benavente et al., 2019; Divis et al., 2017; Wong et al., 2019; Yusof et al., 2016). Specimens of *P. knowlesi* from Peninsular Malaysia whether sourced from humans or macaques all belong to one genetic cluster, while those from East Malaysia (Sabah and Sarawak) form two clusters depending on the macaque host; with one cluster derived from long-tailed macaques and another from pig-tailed macaques. However, *P. knowlesi* specimens detected in humans in Sabah and Sarawak are found in both clusters. Furthermore, phylogenetic studies using the non-repeat region of the circumsporozoite protein gene and C-terminus of merozoite surface 1 gene failed to show any distinct geographical differentiation of protein haplotypes in Peninsular Malaysia and Borneo Island (Chong et al., 2020; Fong et al., 2015; Yap et al., 2017).

Phylogenetic analysis of all five simian malaria parasites found in Sabah and four human malaria parasites tree groups them into two main clusters, one containing *P. vivax* and simian malaria parasites, and the second with other human malaria parasites (Chua et al., 2017) (Fig. 1). The high percentage identity of nucleotide sequences between the *P. knowlesi* isolates from the long-tailed macaque, the vector *An. balabacensis* and human patients suggests a close genetic relationship between the parasites from these hosts. (Fig. 2). These data somewhat support the conclusion that the ancestral host of *P. knowlesi* was Asian monkeys, with the spread of *P. knowlesi* occurring about 30,000–40,000 years ago likely to have been driven by the expansion

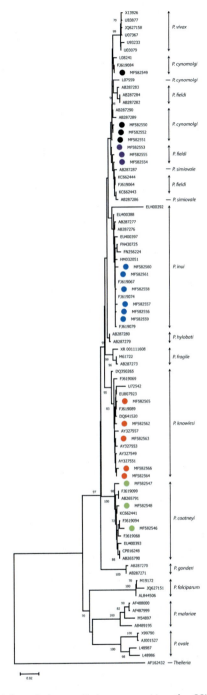

Fig. 1 Neighbour-joining phylogenetic tree comparing the SSU rRNA gene sequences in current study (marked with circle) and with known *Plasmodium* SSU rRNA sequences from the GeneBank data base. The bar below the tree represents distance scale. The evolutionary distances were computed using the maximum composite likelihood method and all positions containing alignment gaps and missing data were eliminated only in the pairwise sequence comparisons. The tree was replicated with 1000 bootstraps and only values > 50% are showed in the tree. The tree was out grouped with *Theileria* spp. (AF162432).

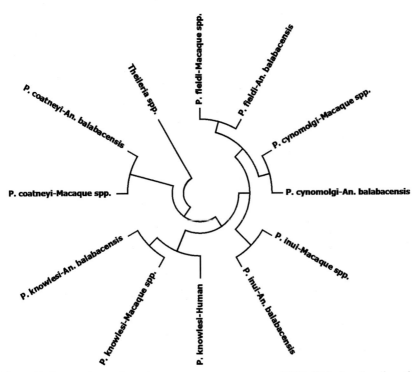

Fig. 2 Phylogenetic tree based on consensus sequences of SSU rRNA showing the relationship between the *Plasmodium* species in Sabah that were found in monkey, *An. balabacensis* and human, constructed using neighbour joining method. The evolutionary distances were computed using the aximum composite likelihood method and all positions containing alignment gaps were eliminated only in the pairwise sequence comparisons. The tree was out grouped with *Theileria* spp.

of the human population in Southeast Asia. The *P. knowlesi* of Malaysia appears to be divided into two geographical clusters representing the specimens from Peninsular Malaysia and the Bornean states, while the latter is again subdivided into two groups based on their reservoir host monkeys. However, more data is required to elucidate and to resolve the ancestry of *P. knowlesi* and other simian malarias in areas where human spillover has occurred.

2.2 Detected simian malaria parasites in vector mosquitoes

The development of molecular techniques has enabled detection of *P. knowlesi* and other simian malaria parasites in wild mosquitoes. Such detection is of crucial importance to incriminate vector species and assessing the potential for zoonotic emergence of other simian malarias. For example, molecular tools were pivotal in the recent confirmation of *P. cynomolgi* and *P. inui* causing infection in humans. Previous studies used molecular techniques to confirm that other simian malaria parasites including *P. inui* and *P. cynomolgi* were present in human-biting mosquitoes in SEA; and often at higher rates of infection or in mixed infections with *P. knowlesi* (Jeyaprakasam et al., 2020). These data highlighted the potential for human exposure to be occurring before human cases were confirmed; thus, indicating molecular surveillance data in mosquitoes could provide a useful early warning of potential spillover. The prevalence of *P. inui* and *P. cynomolgi* in some long-tailed macaque populations are higher than that of *P. knowlesi;* indicating a potentially high force of infection within the reservoir host (Jeyaprakasam et al., 2020). Additionally, a Case-Control carried out in Sabah found that *An. balabacensis* infected with several simian malarias (not *P. knowlesi*) were found in human biting collections both inside and outside of houses (Manin et al., 2016). This highlights the possibility for people in these areas to be regularly exposed to simian malaria both inside and in the peridomestic areas of their homes; as well as when working in farm or forest areas (Chua et al., 2017; Hawkes et al., 2017; Manin et al., 2016; Tan, 2008; Wong et al., 2015). The spillover of these parasites may not have yet resulted in a public health problem, but the risk could be increasing with ongoing deforestation and changes in landscapes (Vythilingam and Hii, 2013).

3. Vectors of *Plasmodium knowlesi*—Leucosphyrus Group of *Anopheles*

3.1 Phylogenetic studies of vectors in the Leucosphyrus Group of *Anopheles*

The recognized vectors of *P. knowlesi* and other simian malaria parasites originate from the Leucosphyrus Group of *Anopheles*. There are 21 *Anopheles* species in the Leucosphyrus Group, which are further divided into 3 Sub-groups (Hackeri Sub-group, Leucosphyrus Sub-group and Riparis Sub-group). The Leucospyrus Sub-group is further divided into Dirus Complex and Leucosphyrus Complex. This Leucosphyrus Group has a wide distribution throughout Southeast Asia, including the islands of Hainan and Taiwan, southern India and Sri Lanka (Sallum et al., 2005b). The Leucosphyrus Group is monophyletic under the Cellia Sub-genus. However, the phylogenetic relationship between these three Sub-groups remains unresolved especially for the Leucosphyrus Sub-group. The Hackeri Sub-group, the Riparis Sub-group and the Dirus Complex are monophyletic (Sallum et al., 2007), although the Hackeri and Riparis Sub-groups were recovered as a sister group of the Dirus Complex and the Leucosphyrus Complex. Furthermore, *An. balabacensis* appears to have a separate lineage from other members of the Leucosphyrus Complex and is closer either to the Hackeri and Riparis Sub-groups or to the Dirus Complex (Sallum et al., 2007). Phylogenetic analysis of *An. balabacensis* from Indonesia based on the ITS2 sequence showed there are at least 2 clades, with specimens from Java and Lombok being in a different clade from those collected from Sebatik Island of Kalimantan (Widiarti et al., 2016). This may also indicate that cryptic species coexist in the population of *An. balabacensis* found in the Philippine Islands (Balabac, Culion, Palawan), Brunei, Malaysian Borneo (Sarawak and Sabah) and Indonesia (Kalimantan, Java, Lombok, Sumbawa and Sumba) (Sinka et al., 2011).

3.2 Natural vectors of *Plasmodium knowlesi* in the Leucosphyrous Group of *Anopheles*

In the 1960s the only method to incriminate a simian malaria vector was to inoculate sporozoites from mosquitoes into macaques and examine whether this led to blood-stage infection. Although this approach can conclusively identify potential vectors; it is currently very expensive to maintain animal facilities for the experiments and is increasingly constrained due to ethical considerations related to the use of non-human primates. Fortunately, there have been advances with molecular tools that enable direct identification of simian parasite species in wild mosquitoes. The gold standard approach for incriminating a new vector species was the demonstration of presence of oocysts and sporozoites in wild caught mosquitoes via dissection (Mueller et al., 2010). However, the current practice is that the dissection should be followed by confirmatory molecular analysis. This approach has been used to incriminate *An. latens*, *An. cracens*, *An. balabacensis* and *An. introlatus* as vectors for *P. knowlesi* (Vythilingam et al., 2018). All mosquitoes belonging to the Leucosphyrus group of *Anopheles* mosquitoes are shown in Table 1.

The vector responsible in the transmission of the first case of *P. knowlesi* in Pahang was not known. However, in the coastal areas of Selangor, studies indicated that *Anopheles hackeri* was the first natural vector incriminated for *P. knowlesi* (Wharton and Eyles, 1961). Further research revealed that *An. hackeri* was positive for the other four species of simian malaria

Table 1 Distribution of Leucosphyrus Group of *Anopheles,* and their important characteristics.

Subgroup	Complex	Species	Vectorial status (*Plasmodium* species)	Peak biting times	Distribution
Leucosphyrus	Leucosphyrus	*An. leucosphyrus*	Pf, Pv, Pm	24.00	Kalimantan, Sumatra, Sulawesi (Sallum et al., 2005b)
		An. latens	Pf, Pv, Pm Pi, Pk,Pcy, Pfi, Pcoat	19.00–20.00	Indonesia, Malaysia, Thailand (Tan, 2008)
		An. introlatus	Pk, Pcy, Pfi, Pi,	20.00–21.00	Indonesia, West Malaysia, Thailand (Wharton et al., 1964)
		An. balabacensis	Pf, Pv,Pk, Pcy, Pi, P coat, Pfi	19.00–20.00	Brunei, Indonesia, East Malaysia, Philippines (Wong et al., 2015, Manin et al., 2016)
		An. baisasi	NA	NA	Philippines (Sallum et al., 2005b)
	Dirus	*An. dirus*	*Pf, Pv, Pk*	19.00–20.00 23.00–24.00	Cambodia, China, Laos, Thailand, Vietnam (Nakazawa et al., 2009)
		An. cracens	*Pk, Pi, Pcy*	20.00–21.00	Indonesia, West Malaysia, Thailand (Jiram et al., 2012)
		An. scanloni	NA	NA	Southern Myanmar, Western & Southern Thailand (Sallum et al., 2005b)
		An. baimaii	Pf, Pv, Pm	22.00–03.00	Bangladesh, India, Thailand, Myanmar, China (Sallum et al., 2005b)
		An. elegans	NA	NA	Southwestern India (Dev and Sharma, 2013)

Continued

Table 1 Distribution of Leucosphyrus Group of *Anopheles*, and their important characteristics.—cont'd

Subgroup	Complex	Species	Vectorial status (*Plasmodium* species)	Peak biting times	Distribution
		An. takasagoensis	Possible vector in Taiwan	NA	China; Taiwan (Sallum et al., 2005b)
		An. nemophilous	NA	18.30–22.00	West Malaysia, Thailand (Sallum et al., 2005b)
Hackeri	—	*An. hackeri*	*Pk, Pcy, Pi, Pcoat Pfi*	NA	East and West Malaysia, Philippines, Thailand (Wharton et al., 1964)
		An. pujutensis	Possible simian malaria vector	NA	Indonesia, East and West Malaysia, Thailand (Warren and Wharton, 1963)
		An. recens	NA	NA	Indonesia (Sallum et al., 2005b)
		An. sulawesi	Human malaria vector		Indonesia (Warren and Wharton, 1963)
		An. mirans	*Pcy, Pi, P. fragile, P. shortti*	NA	India, Sri Lanka (Choudhury et al., 1963; Nelson and Jayasuriya, 1971)
Riparis	—	*An. riparis*	NA	Na	Philippines, (Sallum et al., 2005b)
		An. cristatus	NA	Na	Philippines, (Sallum et al., 2005b)
		An. macarthuri	NA	Na	East and West Malaysia, Thailand (Sallum et al., 2005b)

Pcy, P. cynomolgi; Pi, P. inui; Pf, P. falciparum; Pv, P. vivax; Pm, P. malariae; Pk, P. knowlesi; Pcoat, P. coatneyi; Pfi, P. fieldi.

parasites, i.e., *P. coatneyi, P. cynomolgi, P. fieldi and P. inui* (Wharton et al., 1964). The role of *An. hackeri* in transmission within the macaque reservoir was further confirmed in behavioural experiments that showed this vector predominantly bites macaques and was not attracted to humans (Wharton et al., 1964).

Following the confirmation of a large focus of human *P. knowlesi* cases in Kapit, Sarawak in 2004 (Singh et al., 2004) there was a heightened interest in simian malaria vectors. *Anopheles latens* was incriminated as the primary vector of *P. knowlesi* in the Kapit transmission focus (Vythilingam et al., 2006), followed by incrimination of *An. cracens* as the *P. knowlesi* vector in Pahang (Jiram et al., 2012) and *An. introlatus* in Selangor (Vythilingam et al., 2014). Although only *P. knowlesi* oocysts were initially found in *An. introlatus* (Vythilingam et al., 2014), recent work confirms this vector can develop sporozoite stage infections (unpublished results, Vythilingam, UM). In contrast, numerous studies incriminated another species, *An. balabacensis,* as the primary *P. knowlesi* vector in Sabah (Brown et al., 2020; Hawkes et al., 2019; Wong et al., 2015) and in parts of Sarawak in Malaysian Borneo where there is extensive human spillover (Ang et al., 2020).

In addition to heterogeneity in vector species within Malaysia, there is also considerable variation in *P. knowlesi* vectors between geographical regions in SEA. For example, *An. dirus* was incriminated as the primary vector of both human and simian malaria parasites in Vietnam (Chinh et al., 2019; Maeno et al., 2015; Marchand et al., 2011; Nakazawa et al., 2009), while *An. balabacensis* was found to be positive for oocysts and sporozoites in Palawan in the Philippines (Tsukamoto et al., 1978). Further work demonstrated sporozoites of *P. knowlesi* could develop in this species when fed on infected macaques; leading to the assumption that *An. balabacensis* is the vector in Palawan. Many of the mosquito species that have been confirmed to transmit *P. knowlesi* also harbour other simian malaria parasites including *P. inui, P. cynomologi. P. coatneyi and P. fieldi* (Vythilingam et al., 2018).

In Sri Lanka (formerly known as Ceylon), *An. elegans* (renamed as *An. mirans* and a member of the Leucosphyrus Group) was found to be positive for simian malaria parasites *P. shortti* and *P. fragile* in the forested area of Kandy where the *Macaca sinica* was present (Nelson and Jayasuriya, 1971). Larvae of *An. mirans* were found within wheel track depressions in forested areas, while adults could only be trapped by hanging a net over breeding sites where both newly emerged and gravid mosquitoes were caught. Four of the collected *An. mirans* were positive for sporozoites; with subsequent inoculation into rhesus macaques confirming these parasites to be *P. shortti* and *P. fragile* (Nelson and Jayasuriya, 1971). *Anopheles mirans* (stated as *An. elegans*) was also found to be a vector of simian malaria in the Nilgiris area of South India (Choudhury et al., 1963). Sporozoites from one of the infected mosquitoes was inoculated into *Macaca radiata* and resulted in a dual infection *P. cynomolgi* and *P. inui*.

There is a wide range of confirmed simian malaria vector species in SEA, of which further studies are needed to elucidate their competence for different malaria parasite species and their potential to mediate human spillover.

4. Bionomics of natural vectors of *Plasmodium kowlesi* in the Leucosphyrus Group of *Anopheles*

4.1 Larval biology

The distribution and larval habitats of mosquitoes are of paramount importance for vector control. Vythilingam & Hii presented knowledge on the larval habitats and characteristics of the *An. leucosphyrus* Group (Vythilingam and Hii, 2013). In summary, the immature stages of these forest dwelling species have an affinity for humid, shaded environments and mostly use temporary larval habitats such as pools and puddles. Larvae of *An. latens* are generally found in clear water seepages in swamp forest in peninsular Malaysia (Reid, 1968) and in pools besides forest streams and in swampy patches in hilly areas (Colless, 1956). In Thailand, habitats of larval *An. latens* include ground holes, sand pools, stream margins, seepages, elephant footprints and wheel tracks (Rattanarithkul et al., 2006; Sallum et al., 2005a).

The typical larval habitats of *An. balabacensis* include muddy ground pools, tyre tracks, clear ground pools and swamp water pockets (Ahmad et al., 2018; Byrne et al., 2021). Other rare breeding sites includes swamp edges, rock pools, bamboo stumps, split bamboos, tins, and other artificial containers (Colless, 1956). Recent studies showed that the breeding sites were located within 0.4 Km from the centre of the village (Ahmad et al., 2018). It was also found that *An. balabacensis* was more abundant between December–February and May–July which coincides with Sabah's rainy season (Hawkes et al., 2019). The rain obviously generates temporary aquatic habitats for mosquito larvae. *Anopheles hackeri* was found breeding in inland forest in split bamboo while in coastal areas it was found breeding in the cavities of nipah palm leaves (Wharton and Eyles, 1961). Thus, each species would appear to have its own niche for breeding.

With urbanization, deforestation, environmental changes to landscape and expansion of agricultural plantations; it is likely that that vector distribution in peninsular Malaysia has changed substantially over seven decades. However, there is limited data about the current breeding sites of the vectors apart from those studies done in Sabah, Malaysia.

4.2 Biting habits of vectors

All vectors incriminated to date have peak biting times between 1800 and 2000 h and primarily bite outdoors (Vythilingam et al., 2018). During this time people are generally outdoors or returning home from work. Most of the vector species were predominant in farms followed by forest and village (Vythilingam et al., 2018). However, *An. balabacensis* was predominant in villages in the studied areas (Chua et al., 2019; Wong et al., 2015). The biting behaviour and broad local distribution of *An. balabancensis* presents a challenge to human malaria elimination programmes where residual outdoor transmission is occurring (Hii et al., 2018). Based on epidemiological evidence of knowlesi malaria cases, it seems most likely that people are infected when they visit forested areas or while returning home after working in farms (Fornace et al., 2019; Hawkes et al., 2019; Vythilingam et al., 2018). However, there is evidence that villagers are also infected peri-domestically (Manin et al., 2016).

4.3 Host preferences

Most confirmed simian malaria vectors will bite both macaques and humans, although their relative host preference is often uncertain. In the 1960's the host preference of potential vectors was investigated using monkey baited traps (MBT) and human baited traps (HBT). Wharton and co-workers found that in swamp forest areas of coastal Selangor, *An. hackeri* was found in great numbers in MBT but absent in HBTs, suggesting a strong preference for monkey hosts. In other areas, non Leucosphyrus Anophelines (eg. *An. sundaicus, An. campestris* and *An. sinensis*) were found in greater numbers in HBT compared to MBT (Wharton et al., 1964). In the inland forested areas of Hulu Lui, Selangor, *An. maculatus* (a major human malaria vector) was the predominant species obtained in both MBT and HBT, though overall abundance was much lower in MBT. In the forested areas of Hulu Gombak, Selangor, *An. latens* was the predominant species obtained in both MBT and HBT, closely followed by *An. introlatus* (Wharton et al., 1964). These species preferred to bite monkeys at canopy compared to ground level (Wharton et al., 1964).

More recently, studies in Sarawak, Malaysian Borneo used MBT placed at ground level, and on platforms 3 and 6 m above ground to characterize vector biting behaviour. Here *An. latens* preferred to bite monkeys at 6 m above ground compared to at the ground and 3 m above ground. The ratio of ground:3 m:6 m was 1:10.3:18.4; indicating relative host species preference may vary with ecological setting and host availability. *Anopheles latens* preferred to bite humans compared to monkeys with a ratio of 1:39 (at ground level) (Tan et al., 2008). Conversely, *An. cracens* in Pahang, Peninsular Malaysia preferred human with a biting ratio of monkey to human of 1:4.8 (Jiram et al., 2012). *Anopheles cracens* was attracted to monkeys at ground level and at 3 m height in the early part of the night, and at 6 m height after midnight (Jiram et al., 2012). However, these studies only carried out HBT at ground level. In Sabah Human Landing Catch (HLC) conducted at canopy and ground level found more *An. balabacensis* was caught at ground level compared to canopy (Brant et al., 2016).

A comparative study was carried out in Sabah using the human baited (HENET) and macaque baited (MENET) electrocuting nets against existing trapping methods for these hosts (HLC and MBT respectively) (Hawkes et al., 2017). It found that HLC attracted the most *Anopheles* followed by HENET while macaque baited trap and MENET attracted very few *Anopheles* (Hawkes et al., 2017). The authors report difficulties with MENET and, although the use of conventional MBT is logistically and ethically challenging, it remains one of the best methods to investigate the relative host species preference of simian malaria vectors. The fact that both (*An. latens* and *An. cracens*) bite humans and macaques demonstrates that these species could facilitate transmission of simian parasites from macaques to humans. It is not inconceivable that in future the parasites may be transmitted from human to human by these mosquitoes as shown in Fig. 3.

4.4 Vectorial capacity and life expectancy of knowlesi simian malaria vectors

Vectorial capacity (VC) is a measure of transmission potential of a vector-parasite system and according to Garret-Jones and Shidrawi (1969), it takes into consideration the man biting rate of the vector, its daily survival rate and the sporogonic cycle. The daily survival rate is dependent on the proportion of it being parous (Davidson, 1954) and life expectancy can be determined using these parameters (Garrett-Jones and Grab, 1964). Examination of the ovaries of wild mosquito vectors can help determine their vectorial capacity and life expectancy. However, only few studies have determined these biological characteristics (Vythilingam et al., 2018).

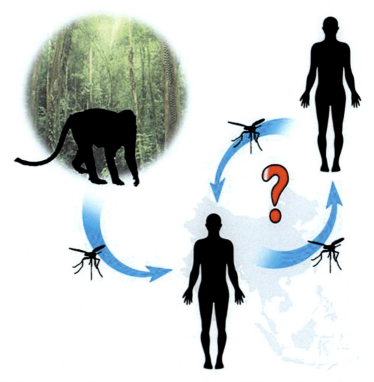

Fig. 3 Diagram depicting the current transmission of *P. knowlesi* from macaques to humans by vector mosquitoes in Southeast Asia. Whether human to human transmission is occurring is not conclusive yet.

In brief, the higher the parous rate, the higher the estimated daily survival rate and the parous rates of several simian malaria vectors, *An. latens, An. cracens* and *An. balabacensis* have been estimated to be greater than 50% in different habitats (Jiram et al., 2012; Tan et al., 2008; Wong et al., 2015). These values are high, translating to a mean daily survival rates of up to 0.9 and indicating that current control activities have only limited, if any, impact on vector survival. Besides the percentage of population of the vectors that could live long enough to become infective (10 days for *P. knowlesi* extrisnic incubation period) ranged from 13% to 31% for different vectors and habitats (Vythilingam et al., 2018). The vectorial capacity ranged from 0.6 in forest habitat in Sarawak to 3.85 in the forest habitat of Kudat, Sabah (Vythilingam et al., 2018), suggesting that people in Sabah may be at greater risk of infection compared to those in Sarawak when proximal to disease vectors.

5. Suspected vectors of knowlesi malaria in other *Anopheles* Groups

In a study that was conducted in Kapit, Sarawak (Tan, 2008) *Plasmodium* oocysts were found in *An. watsonii* and *An. donaldi* but the parasite species could not be determined with the available human and simian malaria primers. Further tests on the salivary glands, head, and thorax samples of these species with nested PCR also yielded negative results (Tan, 2008). However, only *An. latens* was positive for the simian malaria parasites. The salivary glands of other *Anopheles* species were negative on dissection (e.g. *An. vanus, An. kokhani, An. maculatus* sl, *An. tesselatus*) and a few oocyst-negative *An. latens* were also subjected to nested PCR, but all were tested negative (Tan, 2008). In Pahang where the confirmed vector *An. cracens* was present, *An. kochi* was found in high numbers in the monkey baited traps. However, none of the *An. kochi* samples were positive for oocysts or sporozoites on dissection (Jiram et al., 2012) suggesting this species is unlikely to be a vector. Studies in the 1960s indicated *An. maculatus* caught in MBTs which were positive for sporozoites failed to infect rhesus macaques (Wharton et al., 1964).

Recent studies using only molecular techniques to identify vectors of *P. knowlesi* demonstrated the presence of the parasites in vectors not incriminated previously via dissection, i.e., *An. donaldi* (Ang et al., 2020; Hawkes et al., 2019) and *An. sundaicus* (Vidhya et al., 2019). Hawkes et al. demonstrated the presence of *P. knowlesi* and *P. cynomolgi* DNA in *An. donaldi* in Keningau, Sabah (Hawkes et al., 2019). However, as whole mosquitoes were used for the investigation, it is uncertain whether the positive results came from sporozoites or oocysts. Similarly, in the Andaman Islands and Nicobar Islands, 18 pools of *An. sundaicus* were tested of which one was found to be *P. knowlesi*-positive (Vidhya et al., 2019). However, the blood for people in the area was positive only for *P. falciparum* and *P. vivax;* with further testing failing to detect *P. knowlesi*. In both studies, it is not known if the parasite DNA originated from oocysts or sporozoite stages, with the latter needed to confirm potential for onward transmission. Since *An. baimai* belonging to the Leucosphyrus Group is also found in the Andaman Islands (Dev and Sharma, 2013), more extensive studies are needed to fully characterize the range of potential vector species on these islands.

Research in Singapore also raises the possibility that non-Leucosphyrus mosquitoes may be involved in *P. knowlesi* transmission. Here, cases of

P. knowlesi were reported in humans especially from the forested areas (Jeslyn et al., 2011) but entomological sampling in these areas did not yield any Leucosphyrus Group mosquitoes, suggesting alternative *Anopheles* sp. are responsible for transmission (Jeslyn et al., 2011). Further studies should be conducted to confirm whether non Leucosphyrus *Anopheles* in this and other settings in SEA are capable of simian malaria transmission. Additionally, given the difficulty of sampling infected vectors, especially from low density populations in the fields, experimental infection studies provide a useful approach to establish vector competence.

6. Experimental transmissions of *Plasmodium knowlesi* and other simian malaria parasites in mosquitoes

Experimental infection of mosquitoes under laboratory conditions studies have provided important fundamental understanding into the life cycle and transmission of these parasites. These studies have been used to investigate a range of topics related to simian malaria transmission, pathogenicity, and drug treatment (Table 2).

Such studies on simian malarias often involve the use of monkeys, mostly rhesus monkeys (*Macaca mulatta*) as the laboratory model. Though the rhesus macaque is not a natural host of *P. knowlesi*, its susceptibility to *P. knowlesi* infection and resulting fulminating infection pattern, makes it an ideal

Table 2 Studies that involve experimental infection of mosquitoes.

Topic	Examples
Hypnozoites and malaria relapses	Joyner et al. (2016), Joyner et al. (2019)
Transmission-blocking compounds/drugs	Terzian (1970)
Sporontocidal activity of compounds	Coleman et al. (2001)
Prophylactic or curative effects of antimalarials to the liver stages including hypnozoites	Zeeman et al. (2014), Zeeman et al. (2016)
In vitro cultivation of the liver stages	Millet et al. (1994), Dembele et al. (2011)
Immunization/vaccination using attenuated/live sporozoites	Collins and Contacos (1972), Gysin et al. (1984), Wijayalath et al. (2012), Sissoko et al. (2017), Shears et al. (2020),
Mosquito bite immunization	Hickey et al. (2016)

laboratory model. However, eventual advances in *in-vitro* cultivation of simian malaria parasites including *P. knowlesi* (Armistead et al., 2018) and *P. inui* (Nguyen-Dinh et al., 1980) will enable these studies to be conducted without direct feeding of vectors on infected monkeys.

6.1 Experimental studies on *Plasmodium knowlesi* in mosquitoes

In the mammalian host, *P. knowlesi* gametocytes may take 33–36 h to mature from merozoites (Hawking et al., 1968). Early work showed that mosquitoes can be successfully infected from feeding on monkeys with 200–15,000 *P. knowlesi* gametocytes/µL blood (Singh et al., 1950). The period between 5 and 6 days after inoculation of infected blood into rhesus monkeys appeared to be optimum for generating mosquito infections (Garnham et al., 1957). Further studies found oocyst numbers are highest in *An. stephensi* fed on *P. knowlesi*-infected monkeys during the period from evening until after midnight (Hawking et al., 1968). Thus, experimental transmission of *P. knowlesi* from monkeys to mosquitoes is best performed during this time, when numbers of mature and exflagellating gametocytes are high. This peak transmission period coincides with the biting times of *Anopheles* mosquito vectors in nature (Hawking et al., 1968). For example, the peak biting time of *Anopheles latens* and *An. cracens* on monkeys is at midnight (Jiram et al., 2012; Tan et al., 2008).

In experimentally infected vectors kept at 26–28 °C, oocysts of *P. knowlesi* are observable between 5 and 6 days after an infectious blood meal, while sporozoites can be present in the salivary glands as early as 9–11 days (Garnham et al., 1957, Collins et al., 1971). *Anopheles* species from the Americas (e.g. *An. aztecus*) and Europe (*An. atroparvus*) can develop *P. knowlesi* sporozoites under laboratory conditions (Table 3). However, vector species from South Asia (e.g. *An. annularis*, *An. stephensi*) which are found close to the geographical range of *P. knowles* supported the development of these parasites more efficiently, although some vectors only developed a very small number of sporozoites in the salivary glands (Garnham et al., 1957; Hawking et al., 1957). For example, in early studies oocysts and sporozoites of *P. knowlesi* in *An. stephensi* appeared to degrade or be destroyed within days after an infectious blood meal (Hawking et al., 1957; Singh et al., 1950). Additionally, *An. freeborni* could support the growth of oocysts, but sporozoite-infected salivary glands were rare. In this case, the *P. knowlesi* sporozoites apparently failed to invade the salivary glands of *An. freeborni* (Rosenberg, 1985). Therefore, non-compatible mosquitoes

Table 3 *Anopheles* species used in experimental infection in the laboratory to check for presence of sporozoites of simian malaria parasites in their salivary glands.

Plasmodium strain/ subspecies	Mosquito species	Transmission status of sporozoites to monkeys[a]	References
Plasmodium knowlesi			
Sinton and Mulligan	*An. annularis*	Successful via inoculation of infected salivary glands or by bites.	Singh et al., 1950
	An. stephensi	Successful via inoculation of infected salivary glands	Singh et al. (1949)
	Armigeres obturbans		
	Aedes reginae	Unknown	
H	*An. cracens*	Experimentally unknown but is a natural vector	Murphy et al. (2014), Vythilingam et al. (2008)
	An. dirus (*An. balabacensis balabacensis*)	Successful by bites	Collins et al. (1967), Collins et al. (1971)
	An. dirus X		Murphy et al. (2014)
	An. freeborni	Unknown	Collins et al. (1967), Collins et al. (1971)
	An. gambiae (susceptible strain)		Collins et al. (1986)
	An. maculatus		Collins et al. (1967), Collins et al. (1971)
	An. stephensi		Collins et al. (1971)
Hackeri	*An. dirus* (*An. balabacensis balabacensis*)	Successful by bites	Collins et al. (1967), Collins et al. (1971)
	An. freeborni	Unknown	Collins et al. (1967), Collins et al. (1971)
	An. maculatus		
	An. quadrimaculatus		Collins et al. (1971)
	An. stephensi		

Continued

Table 3 *Anopheles* species used in experimental infection in the laboratory to check for presence of sporozoites of simian malaria parasites in their salivary glands.—cont'd

Plasmodium strain/ subspecies	Mosquito species	Transmission status of sporozoites to monkeys[a]	References
Nuri	*An. atroparvus (An. maculipennis atroparvus)*	Successful via inoculation of infected glands and stomachs	Hawking et al. (1957)
	An. stephensi		
Isolated in 1956 by Dr. JFB Edeson	*An. aztecus*	Successful via inoculation of infected glands and guts	Garnham et al. (1957)
	An. stephensi	Successful via inoculation of infected glands and stomachs	Hawking et al. (1957)
Plasmodium cynomolgi			
B / bastianelli	*An. freeborni*	Successful by bites or inoculation of infected salivary glands to monkeys and humans	Eyles, 1960a, Eyles et al. (1960)
	An. quadrimaculatus	Successful by bites to monkeys and humans	Beye et al. (1961)
	An. dirus (An. balabacensis balabacensis)	Successful by bites	Collins et al. (1972)
	An. stephensi		
	An. albimanus	Successful	Eyles (1960b)
	An. aztecus		Garnham (1959)
	An. kochi		Bennett et al. (1966)
	An. lesteri		
	An. maculatus		Warren and Wharton (1963)
	An. philippinensis		
	An. sundaicus		Bennett et al. (1966)

Table 3 *Anopheles* species used in experimental infection in the laboratory to check for presence of sporozoites of simian malaria parasites in their salivary glands.—cont'd

Plasmodium strain/ subspecies	Mosquito species	Transmission status of sporozoites to monkeys[a]	References
	Mansonia uniformis	Failed	Bennett et al. (1966)
	An. atroparvus (*An. maculipennis atroparvus*)	Unknown	Garnham (1959)
	An. cracens (*An. dirus B*)		Klein et al. (1991)
	An. gambiae		Collins et al. (1986)
	An. nivipes		Klein et al. (1991)
	An. takasagoensis		
Berok	*An. peditaeniatus*	Successful by bites	Collins et al. (1999)
	An. culicifacies	Successful via inoculation of sporozoites	Collins et al. (1999)
	An. dirus		
	An. quadrimaculatus		
	An. kochi	Successful	Bennett et al. (1966)
	An. maculatus		
	An. lesteri	Unknown	Bennett et al. (1966)
	An. letifer		Collins et al. (1999)
	An. sinensis		Bennett et al. (1966)
	An. sundaicus		
Cambodian	*An. maculatus*	Successful by bites to humans	Bennett and Warren (1965)
	An. kochi	Successful	Bennett et al. (1966)
	An. letifer		
	An. peditaeniatus		

Continued

Table 3 *Anopheles* species used in experimental infection in the laboratory to check for presence of sporozoites of simian malaria parasites in their salivary glands.—cont'd

Plasmodium strain/ subspecies	Mosquito species	Transmission status of sporozoites to monkeys[a]	References
	An. separatus		
	An. sinensis		
	An. sundaicus		
	An. vagus		
	An. aconitus	Failed	Bennett et al. (1966)
	An. argyropus		
	An. barbirostris		
	An. subpictus		
	Mansonia uniformis		
	An. lesteri	Unknown	Bennett et al. (1966)
	An. philippinensis		
Ceylonensis	*An. atroparvus* (*An. maculipennis atroparvus*)	Failed by bites to humans	Dissanaike et al. (1965)
	An. aztecus	Unknown	Dissanaike et al. (1965)
	An. gambiae		Collins et al. (1986)
	An. stephensi		Dissanaike et al. (1965)
Gombak	*An. farauti*	Successful by bites	Collins et al. (2005)
	An. maculatus	Successful via inoculation	Eyles (1963)
	An. dirus	Successful	Coatney et al. (1971)
	An. freeborni		Coatney et al. (1971)
	An. introlatus		Bennett et al. (1966)

Table 3 *Anopheles* species used in experimental infection in the laboratory to check for presence of sporozoites of simian malaria parasites in their salivary glands.—cont'd

Plasmodium strain/ subspecies	Mosquito species	Transmission status of sporozoites to monkeys[a]	References
	An. kochi		Bennett et al. (1966)
	An. letifer		Warren and Wharton (1963)
	An. quadrimaculatus		Coatney et al. (1971)
	An. stephensi		Coatney et al. (1971)
	An. sundaicus		Bennett et al. (1966), Collins et al. (2005)
	An. umbrosus	Failed	Warren and Wharton (1963)
	An. vagus	Unknown	Bennett et al. (1966)
M / TC / Rockefeller	*An. freeborni*	Successful by bites or inoculation of infected salivary glands	Eyles (1960a)
	An. atroparvus (*An. maculipennis atroparvus*)	Failed via inoculation of sporozoites or by bites to humans Successful by bites and inoculation of whole mosquitoes / infected salivary glands to monkeys	Sinton et al. (1938), Shortt and Garnham (1948)
	An. quadrimaculatus	Successful by bites to rhesus monkeys; Failed by bites to humans	Coggeshall (1941)
	An. kochi	Successful	Bennett et al. (1966)
	An. maculatus		
	An. sundaicus		

Continued

Table 3 *Anopheles* species used in experimental infection in the laboratory to check for presence of sporozoites of simian malaria parasites in their salivary glands.—cont'd

Plasmodium strain/ subspecies	Mosquito species	Transmission status of sporozoites to monkeys[a]	References
Smithsonian	*An. farauti*	Successful via inoculation of sporozoites	Collins et al. (2005)
	An. gambiae		
	An. stephensi		
Unknown	*An. annularis*	Successful by bites	Choudhury et al. (1963)
	An. splendidus		
	An. hyrcanus	Successful	Warren and Wharton (1963)
	An. barbirostris s.l.	Unknown	Warren and Wharton (1963)
Plasmodium inui			
Neotype/ inui/ Mulligan	*An. atroparvus (An. maculipennis atroparvus)*	Successful via inoculation of infected salivary glands and by bites	Garnham (1951)
	An. dirus	Successful via inoculation of sporozoites	Collins et al. (2007)
	An. maculatus		
	An. stephensi		
	An. quadrimaculatus	Successful via inoculation of infected salivary glands	Eyles (1960a)
	An. culicifacies	Unknown	Collins et al. (2007)
CDC	*An. freeborni*	Successful via inoculation of sporozoites	Collins et al. (2007)
	An. maculatus		
Cebu, the Philippines 1949	*An. freeborni*	Successful via inoculation of ground thoraces	Schmidt et al. (1980)
Celebes I	*An. dirus*	Successful via inoculation of sporozoites	Collins et al. (2007)
CINUI	*An. dirus*	Successful via inoculation of sporozoites	Collins et al. (2007)
	An. maculatus		

Vectors of simian malaria

Table 3 *Anopheles* species used in experimental infection in the laboratory to check for presence of sporozoites of simian malaria parasites in their salivary glands.—cont'd

Plasmodium strain/ subspecies	Mosquito species	Transmission status of sporozoites to monkeys[a]	References
Hackeri	*An. maculatus*	Successful via inoculation of sporozoites	Collins et al. (2007)
L	*An. maculatus*	Successful by bites	Collins et al. (1966)
	An. stephensi		
	An. quadrimaculatus	Unknown	Collins et al. (1966)
N-34	*An. freeborni*	Successful via inoculation	Collins et al. (2007)
	An. quadrimaculatus	Successful via inoculation of oocysts/bodies	Collins et al. (2007)
	An. gambiae (susceptible line)	Unknown	Collins et al. (2007)
OS / osmaniae / shortii	*An. maculatus*	Successful by bites to humans and monkeys	Coatney et al. (1966), Collins et al. (1966)
	An. dirus	Successful by bites	Collins et al. (1988)
	An. stephensi	Failed by bites Successful by inoculation of infected salivary glands Successful by bites	Sinha and Gajanana (1984) Shortt et al. (1963) Collins et al. (1966)
	An. aztecus	Successful via inoculation of infected salivary glands	Shortt et al. (1963)
	An. freeborni		Collins et al. (1988)
	An. quadrimaculatus	Unknown	Collins et al. (1966)
Perak	*An. dirus*	Successful via inoculation of sporozoites	Collins et al. (2007)

Continued

Table 3 *Anopheles* species used in experimental infection in the laboratory to check for presence of sporozoites of simian malaria parasites in their salivary glands.—cont'd

Plasmodium strain/ subspecies	Mosquito species	Transmission status of sporozoites to monkeys[a]	References
Taiwan I	*An. dirus*	Unknown	Collins and Warren (1998)
	An. kochi		
	An. maculatus		
Taiwan II	*An. dirus*	Unknown	Collins and Warren (1998)
	An. freeborni		
	An. maculatus		
	An. stephensi		
Walter Reed	*An. dirus*	Successful via inoculation of sporozoites	Collins et al. (2007)
	An. stephensi		
Plasmodium cynomolgi and *P. inui*			
Nilgiris, India	*An. fluviatilis*	Successful by bites	Choudhury et al. (1963)
	An. stephensi		
	An. tessellatus		
	An. mirans (An. elegans)	Unknown	Choudhury et al. (1963)
Plasmodium fieldi			
N-3	*An. dirus (An. balabacensis balabacensis)*	Successful by bites	Collins et al. (1968)
	An. maculatus		
	An. stephensi		
	An. freeborni	Successful via inoculation of sporozoites	Collins et al. (1984)
Plasmodium coatneyi			
	An. dirus (An. balabacensis balabacensis)	Successful by bites	Held and Contacos (1967), Collins et al. (2001),

Table 3 *Anopheles* species used in experimental infection in the laboratory to check for presence of sporozoites of simian malaria parasites in their salivary glands.—cont'd

Plasmodium strain/ subspecies	Mosquito species	Transmission status of sporozoites to monkeys[a]	References
	An. farauti		Collins et al. (2002)
	An. aztecus	Successful	Warren and Wharton (1963)
	An. freeborni		
	An. quadrimaculatus		
	An. maculatus	Unknown	Collins et al. (2001)
	An. stephensi		

[a]Successful: infection in monkey was observed after transmission of sporozoites, but the mechanism of transmission was not described. Failed: infection in monkey was not observed after transmission of sporozoites and the mechanism of transmission was not described. Unknown: studies did not assess or report the transmissibility of the sporozoites.

with many developing *P. knowlesi* oocysts may not necessarily have sporozoites in their salivary glands (Singh et al., 1949) or even viable sporozoites (Hawking et al., 1968). Sporogonic efficiency may vary between *P. knowlesi* strains. For example, studies using a newly isolated *P. knowlesi* strain generated higher oocyst infection rates and intensities in *An. stephensi*, and the development of infective sporozoites (Singh et al., 1950). It is possible that the absence of sporozoite infections in other studies was due to the use of a highly passaged *P. knowlesi* strain that had lost some of its transmission ability (Hawking et al., 1957).

We note that most of the experiments listed in Table 3 did not use natural vectors of *P. knowlesi* nor intact (non-splenectomised), natural monkey hosts (viz long-tailed or pig-tailed monkeys). Unnatural vector/host-parasite combinations can lead to erroneous or biased conclusions of vector competence in the wild (Ferguson and Read, 2002). In experiments using natural vectors, *An. dirus* (incorrectly identified as *An. balabacensis balabacensis*) fed on an infected monkey on the 4th and 16th day of patency developed mean oocyst burdens of 4.7 and 108 oocysts, respectively. Despite this variation in oocyst load, similar numbers of sporozoites were found in mosquito salivary glands from infections initiated on different days (Collins et al., 1967). Human-to-human, monkey-human, and human-monkey transmission of

P. *knowlesi* was experimentally demonstrated using *An. dirus* (Chin et al., 1968). In vaccine trials where mosquitoes fed on *P. knowlesi*-infected monkeys, high oocyst and sporozoite intensities were generated in *An. dirus, An. cracens* and *An. dirus X* (a cross between *An. dirus* and *An. cracens*) (Murphy et al., 2014).

Although *An. donaldi* (of the *An. barbirostris* group) can transmit *P. vivax* and *P. falciparum* to humans (Hardin et al., 1973), it is thought to be a poor vector for *P. cynomolgi*. Experimental studies showed *P. cynomolgi* rarely produced oocysts in *An. donaldi* (Bennett et al., 1966; Warren et al., 1963). Similarly, *An. donaldi* did not support the development of *P. inui* under experimental conditions (Collins and Warren, 1998). *Anopheles barbirostris s.l.* (e.g. *An. campestris*) is also unlikely to transmit *P. cynomolgi* (Collins et al., 2005; Wharton et al., 1964), although there was a report from India of *P. cynomolgi* M strain sporozoites found in *An. barbirostris* s.l. (although the exact vector species is unconfirmed (Warren and Wharton, 1963)). In contrast *An. sundaicus* has been demonstrated as an efficient vector of human malaria (*P. falciparum* and *P. vivax*) (Adak et al., 2005; Sinka et al., 2011) as well as all strains of *P. cynomolgi* (Bennett et al., 1966; Collins et al., 1999, 2005, 2009; Wharton et al., 1964) under experimental conditions.

Information on the sporogonic cycle of *P. knowlesi* and other simian malaria parasites in their natural vector hosts is incomplete. Most knowledge comes from experimental infection studies conducted with *An. dirus* and other secondary or unlikley vectors in studies between the 1950 and 1980. Nevertheless, the overall evidence suggests there is substantial variation within and between *P. knowlesi* strains in their development in different *Anopheles* species, as will be further discussed below.

6.2 Implication of experimental studies using vectors on the transmission of *P. knowlesi* and other simian malarias in nature

While *P. knowlesi* infections have become increasingly prevalent in recent years, the emergence of *P. cynomolgi* and potentially *P. inui*, warrants further investigation as zoonotic malarias of public health importance in Southeast Asia (Jeyaprakasam et al., 2020; Liew et al., 2021; Yap et al., 2021). As supporting evidence, experimental transfer of *P. cynomolgi* from human-to-human via mosquito bites was easily accomplished (Beye et al., 1961; Contacos et al., 1962; Eyles et al., 1960), and natural infection of this zoonosis in humans has been reported recently (Jeyaprakasam et al., 2020). In addition, *P. inui* could also be transmitted to humans via mosquito bites under experimental conditions (Coatney et al., 1966).

Experimental infection studies on the sporogonic cycle of a range of simian malarias have revealed differences in the length of the extrinsic incubation period between parasites (e.g. Table 4). The reason for this variation in sporogonic cycle length is unclear and may be a factor of both innate biological properties of the parasite, the vector used, and other experimental conditions.

While experimental infection studies are invaluable for demonstrating the basis of vector competence, they may not reflect natural patterns of transmission. Here we have summarized the list of vector species that have been found to be competent for simian malaria transmission under laboratory conditions (e.g. developed sporozoites in their salivary glands after experimental infection, Table 3); however more work is needed to corroborate the role of these vectors in natural settings. More extensive information on these experimental infection studies, including on vectors that did not support the parasite development can be found in Coatney et al. (1971), Warren and Wharton (1963), Bray and Garnham (1964), Bennett et al. (1966), Bray (1963), and other references therein and in Table 3.

Table 4 Extrinsic incubation period in days of the simian malaria parasites.

Parasite	Temperature conditions	Oocyst	Sporozoites	References
Plasmodium knowlesi	26–28 °C	5–6 days	9–10 days	Garnham et al. (1957), Collins et al. (1971)
Plasmodium cynomolgi	25–28 °C	At least 3 days[a]	At least 7.5 days[a]	Green (1932), Shortt and Garnham (1948), Bennett and Warren (1965), Dissanaike et al. (1965)
Plasmodium inui	25–28 °C	6 days	At least 11 days	Garnham (1951), Collins et al. (1966), Sinha and Gajanana (1984)
Plasmodium fieldi	25 ± 1 °C	At least 5 days	12 days	Coatney et al. (1971), Millet et al. (1994),
Plasmodium coatneyi	25 ± 1 °C	At least 6 days	11 days	Coatney et al. (1971)

[a]Depending on the parasite strain.

6.2.1 Mosquito:Plasmodium compatibility

Under laboratory conditions, there is considerable variation in infection outcome between different simian malaria parasites, strains, and vector species. For example, *P. cynomolgi* B strain developed completely in *An. maculatus*, but sporozoites of a different strain of *P. cynomolgi* failed to develop in this vector. On the other hand, *Anopheles introlatus*, which is a natural vector of *P. cynomolgi*, did not support the development of *P. cynomolgi* B strain under laboratory conditions (Eyles, 1963). More examples can be found in Warren and Wharton (1963). In some mosquitoes such as *An. barbirostris s.l.*, oocysts could develop from some parasite strains but quickly degenerate. However, when infected with other strains, sporozoites developed but could not invade the salivary glands (Bennett et al., 1966). Some less competent vectors can harbour high oocyst counts but do not develop sporozoites in salivary glands (Collins et al., 1984; Collins and Warren, 1998). Conversely, high sporozoite numbers can be found in the salivary glands of highly competent vectors, even though their oocyst counts may be low (Collins et al., 1984). Thus, successful development of numerous sporozoites in a mosquito vector appears to depend on the compatibility of the parasite strain and the mosquito species; and may vary considerably between experimental and natural settings.

The variability in susceptibility of vectors to malaria infection could be due to genetic makeup of the mosquitoes (Riehle et al., 2017; Zheng et al., 1997) and/or the parasite genotype. More recently, the microbiota (Gendrin and Christophides, 2013; Romoli and Gendrin, 2018) and immunity (Clayton et al., 2014; Simões et al., 2017) of the *Anopheles* mosquito have been shown to influence their vectorial capacity and ability to transmit *Plasmodium* parasites. As an example of mosquito genetic effects, the same mosquito species from different geographical areas can have differential susceptibility to the same parasite strain (Klein et al., 1991). Thus, failure to infect a particular vector species with a specific simian malaria parasite in the laboratory should not be interpreted as conclusive evidence of a general incompatibility between the vector and the parasite (Medley et al., 1993). Similarly, this also implies that failure to detect the parasites in a particular mosquito species in a given area does not mean it is not a vector also in another area. The best evidence for vector incrimination comes from field studies.

Laboratory infection studies also suggest that between–parasite strain variation in infectiousness occurs in natural vector populations. It has been hypothesized that malaria vector-parasite interactions may be shaped by local adaptation (Lambrechts and Koella, 2013; Lefevre et al., 2018), with parasite strains being more infectious in allopatric and sympatric vector populations (Harris et al., 2012; Joy et al., 2008). These local parasite strains may then be further selected for increased infectiousness in indigenous monkeys or human populations; with optimal ability to produce gametocytes in these hosts (Coatney et al., 1961; Schmidt et al., 1961; Singh et al., 1949). This might explain the variable *P. knowlesi* endemicity from one area to another, even though the same mosquito species can be found throughout. This co-adaptation may also partly explain why infection in human is usually associated with only one *P. knowlesi* genotype, while primate-derived infections are typically polyclonal, and the level of multiplicity of infection differs from one geographical area to another (Divis et al., 2017; Saleh Huddin et al., 2019). Thus, unless thorough investigations have been conducted in different localities, the dynamics of simian malaria transmission should not be assumed to be similar across wider regions.

6.2.2 Gametocytaemia and timing of simian malaria transmission to the mosquitoes

Transmission studies of simian malarias showed that infectivity to mosquitoes is not governed by gametocytaemia alone, nor is it correlated to the ratio of male: female gametocytes or exflagellation events (Collins et al., 1972; Schmidt et al., 1982). Recent studies suggest that gametocyte sex ratio in *P. falciparum* is important in mosquito transmission (Bradley et al., 2018; Tadesse et al., 2019). Whether this applies similarly to simian malaria parasites in the wild is unknown. Submicroscopic gametocyte densities can still produce infections in mosquito vectors, and there can be substantial variation in infection rate between batches of mosquitoes fed on blood of similar gametocyte density on different days (Collins et al., 1968, 2001; Contacos et al., 1962; de Arruda-Mayr et al., 1979; Green, 1932). Furthermore, increases in gametocyte number may have little effect on mosquito infection rates or oocyst counts (Collins et al., 1972; Green, 1932; Puri et al., 1989). In contrast, high gametocyte (and/or asexual parasite) counts may negatively affect simian malaria infection in the mosquitoes mediated through immune reactions in the host and/or mosquito mortality (Collins et al., 1972, 1988; Garnham et al., 1957; Murphy et al., 2014).

Another factor that may impact mosquito infection rates is the timing during vertebrate infection. Although infection to the mosquitoes can occur throughout the course of an infection in the vertebrate, there are certain windows of time when the vertebrate hosts are most infectious to the mosquitoes (Collins et al., 1971, 1984). In acute infection of *P. knowlesi*, the period between fifth and seventh day of patency in monkeys and humans is optimal for infecting the mosquitoes. This coincides with the maximum gametocyte numbers (Garnham et al., 1957) and high asexual parasite counts (Chin et al., 1968). Mosquito feedings on earlier or later days did not result in any infection. In contrast, gametocytaemia in chronic infections of *P. knowlesi* and *P. cynomolgi* may rise and fall in waves (Coatney et al., 1971; Green, 1932; Puri et al., 1989). Although infection to the mosquitoes can occur throughout the duration of such infection, mosquitoes were more likely to be infected during the peaks of the waves or during a particular wave (Collins et al., 1971; Puri et al., 1989). The pattern of infectiousness in *P. knowlesi* diverged somewhat from trends in gametocytaemia; as gametocytaemia can be higher in the first than second and subsequent waves, or at the beginning rather than end of the second wave (Collins et al., 1971). Therefore, when gametocytes are observable, a host can be most infectious to the mosquitoes during the earlier (not right at the beginning) to mid phases of the infection (not later than 27 days after mosquito bite), especially during the second wave or when gametocytaemia is rising (Collins et al., 1972, 1984, 2001; Contacos et al., 1962; Schmidt et al., 1982). General infectiousness may decrease with infection length in chronic cases, with observatiosn showing that parasites that had been in the host for some time failing to produce good infections in mosquitoes despite high gametocyte counts (Collins et al., 1984).

Simian malaria infection rates in mosquito vectors may also be influenced by their time of feeding. Under experimental conditions, infections in mosquitoes were most optimum when feedings occurred between the late afternoon and middle of the night (1700–0400 h), synchronizing both with the peak appearance of mature gametocytes (*P. knowlesi* and *P. cynomolgi*) in host blood just after midnight, and the biting time of the mosquitoes (on macaques) in nature (Anderios et al., 2010; Hawking et al., 1968). This circadian pattern of periodicity in gametocytes has also been observed in *P. inui* and *P. coatneyi* (Collins et al., 2001; Garnham and Kendall, 1974). In contrast, another report showed that mosquitoes that fed on *P. cynomolgi*-infected monkeys at 9 am and 9 pm generated similar oocyst infection rates and intensities

(Schmidt et al., 1982), similar to a study using rodent malaria which indicated that blood-feeding time does not influence transmission success to mosquitoes (O'Donnell et al., 2019). Good *P. cynomolgi* infection rates in vectors were also associated with the phase when late ring asexual stage parasites predominated or at least constituted 30% of all asexual parasites (Schmidt et al., 1982). It is possible that a combination of mature gametocytes and late ring stages in the blood from evening to midnight is optimal for transmission to vectors. Other factors that influence infectivity of malaria parasites to mosquito vectors (Hawking, 1975) include concurrent asexual density, host age, haematological factors, etc. (de Jong et al., 2020).

Given what is known from these experimental studies, some speculation could be made as to the lack of evidence of human-to-human *P. knowlesi* transmission and the general (but by no means certain) belief that it is rare compared to primate-to-primate or primate-to-human infection. This is because gametocytes are either absent or exist at very low density in most human knowlesi malaria cases (Goh et al., 2013; Grigg et al., 2016; Lee et al., 2009; Maeno et al., 2017) and even in *P. cynomolgi* infections (Contacos et al., 1962; Ta et al., 2014). Furthermore, *P. knowlesi* and *P. cynomolgi* infections in humans are typically so mild (Barber et al., 2013; Daneshvar et al., 2009; Grigg et al., 2016; Hartmeyer et al., 2019; Raja et al., 2020; Singh et al., 2004; Ta et al., 2014) that asexual and gametocyte densities may be very low. In contrast, parasite and gametocyte densities are often higher in macaque infections that transmission from monkey to mosquitoes is much more likely than that of human to mosquito (and subsequently to human) (Contacos and Coatney, 1963). Data do suggest that, monkeys and humans with low density infections (i.e. microscopically negative) can still infect mosquitoes, although there is no evidence yet to show such infections result in transmission of *P. knowlesi* or *P. cynomolgi* in nature. Nonetheless, it is important to highlight that most experimental transmission had a prerequisite for the presence of gametocytes as proxy for infection to mosquitoes.

Infected humans may also play a negligible role in transmitting simian malaria to mosquitoes because of the timing of the clinical presentation. Most knowlesi malaria patients report seeking treatment 4–6 days after disease onset (Barber et al., 2013; Daneshvar et al., 2009; Grigg et al., 2016; Ngernna et al., 2019), which precedes the optimum infectious period to mosquitoes, implying a reduced likelihood of mosquitoes becoming infected from feeding on such patients (Chin et al., 1968; Garnham et al., 1957).

Even when parasitemia is high, suggesting high gametocyte counts (Lee et al., 2009), mosquito infections may be rare, and mosquitoes that become infected may have reduced survival (Klein et al., 1986; Murphy et al., 2014). However, more evidence for this is required as reduced mosquito fitness following malaria infection may be an artefact of laboratory conditions (Ferguson and Read, 2002).

The above conjectures were surmised based on our limited understanding of simian malaria epidemiology and their natural transmission dynamics. The fact that most known *P. knowlesi* vectors do not bite inside houses may reduce the chance of human-to-human transmission (Contacos and Coatney, 1963); however this is not impossible as vectors do bite during hours when people are outside (Chua et al., 2017; Hawkes et al., 2017; Manin et al., 2016; Tan et al., 2008; Wong et al., 2015). Furthermore, the finding of human knowlesi malaria clusters and the involvement of young children in them raise a red flag of possible human-to-human transmissions (Barber et al., 2012; Herdiana et al., 2018).

6.2.3 Can some experimental vectors transmit the parasites in the wild?

Two non-Leucosphyrus Anophelines have recently been implicated in the transmission of *P. knowlesi*: *An. sundaicus* (Vidhya et al., 2019) and *An. donaldi* (Ang et al., 2020). Further investigations may reveal a wider range of Anopheline vector species than currently assumed. Experimental infection studies could provide some clues on which *Anopheles* species occurring within endemic areas are potential vectors.

It has been shown that *P. cynomolgi* can easily infect a wide range of *Anopheles* under laboratory conditions (Table 3), including those beyond its current geographical range. Similarly, *Anopheles* mosquitoes from subgenus *Cellia* (to which the Leucosphyrus Group belongs) are more susceptible to simian malaria parasites (i.e. *P. cynomolgi*) than those of subgenus *Anopheles* (Bennett et al., 1966; Warren et al., 1963); indicating that members of subgenus *Cellia* could have higher potential as carriers of simian malaria parasites. Additionally, some non-Asian vector species (e.g., the major African malaria vectors *An. gambiae*) can be infected by *P. knowlesi*, *P. cynomolgi* and *P. inui*, under laboratory conditions (Collins et al., 1986). Many of these non-native vector species also developed numerous infectious sporozoites in the laboratory. Thus, infected travellers returning to their homeland may infect local competent vector species, but further studies need to be conducted to confirm this.

One non-Leucosphyrus Anopheline that might have the capacity to transmit simian malaria in Southeast Asia is *An. maculatus*. No simian malaria parasites have so far been reported in *An. maculatus* in the wild, although almost all simian malaria parasite species and strains can infect this mosquito in the laboratory (Table 3). In Malaysia, *An. maculatus* had been historically identified as the principal human malaria vector (Reid and Weitz, 1961). This vector is mostly anthropophilic but can also be attracted to monkeys (1381 to human bait vs 345 to monkey bait) (Wharton et al., 1964). Furthermore *An. maculatus* is found in jungle, villages, plantations, and other *peri* domestic areas where there is potential to transmit malaria from monkeys to humans (Warren et al., 1970). However more recent studies showed that *An. maculatus* was not attracted to monkeys (61 to HBT and 3 to MBT) (Jiram et al., 2012); thus, the potential for *An. maculatus* to act as a bridge vector is unclear. *Anopheles sundaicus* has similar traits in that it is anthropophilic but also occasionally bites monkeys (Warren et al., 1963). This species has now been postulated to be a vector for *P. knowlesi* in Andaman Islands (Vidhya et al., 2019). It will become a major concern if anthropophilic vectors such as *An. maculatus* or *An. sundaicus* become natural vectors for simian malaria. As it is, the simio-anthropophilic mosquitoes viz. *An. latens* (Tan et al., 2008) and *An. balabacensis* (Wong et al., 2015) are both already incriminated vectors for *P. knowlesi*. Increased adaptation of simian malaria parasites to other anthropophilic vectors and vice versa, would lead to a greater possibility for human-to-human transmission of these parasites (Bray, 1963; Contacos and Coatney, 1963).

Finally, the possibility of other genera such as *Mansonia*, *Aedes*, *Armigeres* and *Culex* being competent for simian malarias has been investigated. In a few such studies, oocysts were observed in these non-Anopheline species, but very few developed sporozoites in their salivary glands (Bennett et al., 1966; Warren et al., 1962), or became infectious. Many culicine mosquitoes are also attracted to the monkey (Warren and Wharton, 1963) and humans, but there is no evidence to show that they can be efficinet vectors for simian malaria parasites.

7. Control of vectors of *P. knowlesi* and other simian malarias

7.1 Tools for control of simian malaria

The primary focus of malaria eradication agenda (malERA) has been on *Plasmodium falciparum* (Alonso et al., 2011), given this parasite accounts for most of the global mortality and morbidity (WHO, 2020). So far there has been minimal consideration of control or elimination strategies for zoonotic malaria. The growing public health burden of *P. knowlesi* in Malaysia demands attention and there is an urgent need to identify strategies for control as well as eventual elimination.

In contrast to standard human malaria parasite species, control of zoonotic malaria will require a much more diverse range of strategies. One Health approaches integrating control in the wildlife reservoir in addition to human and vector populations will be needed to reduce spillover infections (Scott, 2020). Here we briefly review the prospects for vector control using existing and novel approaches.

7.2 Vector control for simian malaria in Southeast Asia

Control of mosquito vectors is an integral component of malaria control. At present, Insecticide Treated Nets and Indoor Residual Spraying are the only core interventions recommended by the World Health Organization (WHO, 2019). Both these interventions target mosquitoes inside houses, where most of the human exposure occurs in Africa. However, as reviewed above, *P. knowlesi* vectors are typically highly exophagic, exophilic and early feeders thus unlikely to be targeted by indoor-based interventions. This is particularly true in the epicentre of human cases in Malaysian Borneo where the primary vectors almost never enter houses (Jiram et al., 2012; Manin et al., 2016; Tan et al., 2008).

Additionally, it was originally hypothesized that most human exposure occurs away from the home when people are working in forest or plantation environments (Moyes et al., 2014). For example, it has been estimated that ~50% of *P. knowlesi cases* occurring in Sabah, Malaysia in 2018 were in people working in agriculture or plantations; with the remainder in those doing forest related work (Chin et al., 2020). However, recent evidence from case-control in Sabah, Malaysian Borneo (Manin et al., 2016) and human mobility studies (Fornace et al., 2019) suggest that exposure may also occur in peridomestic and forest edge environments. Given the limitations of existing vector control methods, a broader range of approaches may be required that are better suited to the distinct ecology and behaviour of *P. knowlesi* vectors. There is a need to identify methods that could protect high risk groups who are exposed to vectors when outside of the home. Effective vector control for simian malaria must cover all key habitats where humans are exposed.

7.2.1 Insecticidal nets and indoor residual spraying

Malaria control programmes within the epicentre of *P. knowlesi* transmission in Malaysian Borneo currently rely on ITNs and IRS (Manin et al., 2016).

So far there is limited evidence that these methods are effective for *P. knowlesi*. A case-control study in Sabah found no significant association between bednet use and *P. knowlesi* risk (Grigg et al., 2017); in line with current understanding that *P. knowlesi* vectors do not bite indoors. Insecticide treated nets could offer personal protection if used by people during overnight trips for forest work. However, a study of forest workers in Central Vietnam indicated that people rarely take ITNs into forests for overnight work (Bannister-Tyrrell et al., 2018). Thus, there may be a need to find delivery formats that are easier or more appealing for use.

In contrast to ITNs, there is some evidence that IRS may reduce *P. knowlesi* risk. In a case -control study carried out in Sabah; IRS was associated with reduced risk of clinical *P. knowlesi* (Grigg et al., 2017). This may be due to the excito-repellancy of chemicals used in IRS, which could be sufficient to repel mosquitoes from both the inside and peridomestic areas of houses. In addition to IRS, there has been recent investigation of a new pyrethroid (PolyZone) formulation for use in Outdoor Residual Spraying (ORS, spraying outer walls of houses, and nearby vegetation) against *P. knowlesi* vectors in Sabah (Rohani et al., 2020). The impact of this formulation on mosquito survival was compared when applied indoors and outdoors, and at different concentrations (Rohani et al., 2020). Initial results indicate PolyZone can kill up to 90% of the primary *P. knowlesi* vector *An. balabacensis* after landing on treated surface; although the killing effect varied substantially between wall types and was lower when applied outdoors than inside walls (Rohani et al., 2020). Additionally, the impact of ORS on non-target insects in the outdoor environment is poorly understood. Further investigation of long-term outdoor and indoor residual spraying is warranted for *P. knowlesi* vector control.

7.2.2 Larvicides

As the exophilic behaviour of most *P. knowlesi* vectors limits the impact of indoor-based interventions, an alternative approach could be to target larvae in their aquatic habitats. Use of chemical or microbial larvicides has been shown to reduce malaria vector populations and malaria incidence in some settings in Africa (Choi et al., 2019); but may be considerably more challenging with *P. knowlesi vectors* due to the wider diversity and cryptic nature of their aquatic habitats. For example, vectors such as *An. balabacensis* and *An. maculatus* use a range of larval habitats including temporary ground pools, tire tracks, and slow flowing streams; with habitats distributed across oil palm, coconut and rubber plantations, and forest fringe habitats

(Ahmad et al., 2018; Rohani et al., 2010). Implementation of a larviciding programme that could achieve sufficient coverage across this diversity of habitats, in all environments, may be unfeasible. For this reason, larviciding is not being considered for control of *P. knowlesi* at present.

7.2.3 Insecticide-treated hammocks

Insecticide-treated hammocks (ITHs) have been evaluated for protection against other malaria parasites species in forest settings. Their use has been shown to reduce exposure to malaria vectors in small scale studies e.g. (Sochantha et al., 2010) and malaria incidence in randomized control studies carried out in forested-dwelling communities in Vietnam and Venezuela (Duc et al., 2009; Magris et al., 2007). However, even within the context of a randomized control study where hammocks were provided for free, their use was relatively low during evening and night-time periods (Grietens et al., 2012). Low usage rates may be due to perceived impracticality of carrying hammock nets into the forest by workers or insufficient durability (Bannister-Tyrrell et al., 2018). Another limitation of ITHs is that they still only provide protection during sleeping hours, which may be later than the typical host seeking period of *P. knowlesi* vectors. However, given the demonstrated protection gained from ITHs in other forest malaria contexts, their further investigation for control of *P. knowlesi* is warranted.

7.2.4 Topical repellents

Topical repellents could be considered for provision of personal protection for high-risk groups who have greatest exposure to infection (e.g., those involved in forest or plantation work). Topical repellents can be effective in reducing outdoor biting rates by Asian vector species e.g. (Tangena et al., 2018), however a systematic review on the uptake of malaria interventions by forest-goers indicated that repellents were not commonly used; with the high cost cited as main reason (Nofal et al., 2019). Even when repellents are used, it is unclear whether associated reductions in mosquito biting are of sufficient magnitude to reduce infection risk. Results from a recent cluster randomized trial showed no protective effect of a topical repellent on malaria risk in Myanmar (Agius et al., 2020). Similarly, a recent Cochrane review concluded there is no clear evidence that topical repellents are protective against malaria infection at present, although insecticide treated clothing was shown to be effective in some settings in the absence of ITN use (Maia et al., 2018). To our knowledge, neither topical repellents, insecticide treated clothing or insecticide-treated hammocks have been specifically evaluated for protection against *P. knowlesi*. While questions remain about the acceptability and uptake of these interventions in forest habitats, they hold potential for personal protection against simian malaria in high transmission areas.

7.2.5 Spatial repellents

In contrast to topical repellents which provide personal protection just to the individual user, there is growing interest in the use of spatial repellents for household or community-level protection against mosquito-borne diseases (Achee et al., 2012). Unlike topical repellents, another advantage of spatial repellents is that they do not need daily application or maintenance (Achee et al., 2012). Spatial repellents can be disseminated through emanators or treated materials (e.g. (Achee et al., 2012, Govella et al., 2015, Norris and Coats, 2017, Ogoma et al., 2017)). Small-scale field trials in Cambodia found spatial repellents could reduce mosquito landing rates on people by 50% or more (Charlwood et al., 2016) and have relatively good acceptability to users (Liverani et al., 2017). At present, only one cluster-randomized trial of spatial repellents for malaria control been conducted, with no clear evidence of a protective effect found (Syafruddin et al., 2020). However further investigation of this intervention for *P. knowlesi* could be beneficial.

7.2.6 Endectocides

Over the last decade, endectocides have been increasingly investigated as a novel strategy for malaria vector control (Chaccour, 2021). Here the principle is that the presence of endectocides such as ivermectin in host blood will kill mosquito vectors that feed upon them. Laboratory and semi-field studies indicate that ivermectin in blood meals can substantially impair malaria vector fitness and suppress their populations (Lyimo et al., 2017; Ng'habi et al., 2018). This killing effect has been demonstrated in a range of mosquito species including the *P. knowlesi* vector *An. dirus* (Kobylinski et al., 2020). These entomological effects may be sufficient to generate epidemiological impact. In a recent study, mass drug administration of ivermectin in humans reduced malaria incidence in children in west Africa (Foy et al., 2019). An additional advantage of ivermectin for simian malaria control is that it has been shown to inhibit the development of the primate malaria *P. cynomologi* in vitro (Mendes et al., 2017). However, this effect was not repeatable in in vivo studies with rhesus macaques (Vanachayangkul et al., 2020).

To be effective against *P. knowlesi*, endectocides would need to be administered to the macaque reservoir population. The application of endectocides in wildlife populations has been investigated in several other zoonotic disease systems; including gerbil and prairie dog hosts of plague (Poche et al., 2018; Poché et al., 2020a), mice hosts of Lyme disease (Poché et al., 2020b), and avian hosts of West Nile Virus (Nguyen et al., 2019). The estimated impact of endectocides in wildlife varies between ectoparasite vectors, but there is clear evidence of reduced exposure rates in some scenarios. Further investigation of its potential use in wild primate populations would be required to assess feasibility for *P. knowlesi* control.

8. Challenges

Major knowledge gaps remain on the ecology, behaviour and larval habitats of simian malaria vectors. In the early 1920s, although drugs were available to treat malaria cases, attempts were focused on destroying and/or modifying breeding sites to reduce density of the vectors. This environmental modification was successfully achieved by subsoil drainage and bunding (Watson, 1921). It is clear that better understanding of vector ecology (Ferguson et al., 2010; Godfray, 2013) is vital for progress with disease control. Without knowing where the vectors are resting and breeding; targeted control measures are not possible. Studies carried out in villages and forested areas where *P. knowlesi* transmission is high in Sabah failed to capture any known vectors using resting buckets, sticky resting buckets and CDC Backpack aspirators (Brown et al., 2018). Thus, the resting behaviour of *P. knowlesi* vectors and their host choice remains a major knowledge gap.

The inability to capture resting mosquitoes is only one of several limitations for the surveillance of simian malaria vectors. Despite attempts to find alternatives (Hawkes et al., 2017), presently human landing collection is the most efficient way to sample host seeking vectors of simian malaria. HLC also requires one to carry out sampling in forested areas which may lead to encounters with wildlife, and also raises ethical concern through potentially exposing participants to malaria or other mosquito-borne infections. A recent report has shown that the Mosquito Magnet traps (MM) can be used as an alternative sampling tool for the Leucosphyrus Group of *Anopheles* mosquitoes (Jeyaprakasam et al., 2021). However, the MM is relatively expensive, and ways to use them efficiently should be investigated further.

Another challenge for controlling simian malaria vectors is the uncertainty about their distribution and abundance. For example, the landscape in peninsular Malaysia is not homogenous, and considerably less is known about vectors of *P. knowlesi* here than in Sabah and Sarawak. A detailed distribution of *Anopheles* in Malaya was published by Reid in 1960's (Reid, 1968), which is probably outdated as there have been changes to the landscape, urbanization, and deforestation. Thus, it is important to determine the finer-scale distribution of vectors throughout the country, and investigate the association between local heterogeneity in macaque, vectors and human cases. Such spatial analysis will help elucidate the geographic risk factors related to *P. knowlesi* infection.

Describing ecological associations must also take account of the rapid rate of deforestation occurring in areas where parasites and the macaque reservoir are present, and lack of effective control strategies for simian malaria vectors. The rapid deforestation taking place in Southeast Asia is driving the zoonotic transmission of *P. knowlesi* (Davidson et al., 2019; Hawkes et al., 2019). However, we do not have the tool sets to eliminate or even control simian malaria vectors. Currently the natural transmission of simian malaria to humans cannot be ignored if we want to succeed with malaria elimination in Southeast Asia.

A further challenge to understanding the epidemiology and ultimately controlling simian malaria is the their potential interactions with human parasite species. There is a possibility that people can be exposed to both human and simian malaria infections from the same vector population. In the specimens of *An. dirus* from Southern Vietnam both human and simian (knowlesi) parasites were detected (Maeno et al., 2015; Chinh et al., 2019). The question arises whether these mosquitoes were infected by *P. knowlesi* (from a macaque) and *P. falciparum* (from a human) on separate feeding events, or whether both parasite species were picked up from a co-infected person. Furthermore, it was observed some patients who had *P. knowlesi* were also co-infected with *P. falciparum* or *P. vivax* (Maeno et al., 2017).

Additionally, the same allelic types of *pfg* 377, *pvs* 25 and *pks* 25 were found in both human and mosquito infections in Vietnam, which may suggest *An. dirus* was transmitting *P. knowlesi* from humans to humans (Maeno et al., 2017). Some support for this view is the detection of *P. knowlesi* gametocytes in human blood by microscopy (Lee et al., 2009; Ta et al., 2014) and molecular tools (Grigg et al., 2016), indicating transmission stage parasites can develop in humans to infect mosquitoes.

9. Conclusions and the way forward

The Asia Pacific Region has been slated for human malaria elimination by 2030 (Baird, 2015; WHO, 2020). Currently it is known that *P. knowlesi* is the predominant malaria parasite species occurring in Malaysia (Chin et al., 2020); although other simian malarias like *P. cynomolgi* and *P. inui* are also being reported (Liew et al., 2021; Yap et al., 2021). While the elimination of human malarias in SEA would be a major achievement, progress could be reversed if *P. knowlesi* and other simian malarias parasites become increasingly adapted to humans with direct human-to-human transmission occurring rather than via spillover from the macaque reservoir. Such cross-species host switching is common in the evolution of the malaria parasites (Hayakawa et al., 2008; Martinsen et al., 2008). Thus, surveillance and control of simian malarias must be pursued alongside the elimination of human malaria.

Currently, most control programmes are singularly focussed on human malaria elimination targets, which is justifiable considering they constitute the majority of cases at the global level. However, the original hypothesis that spillover of simian malaria was likely to be rare and of negligible importance made in the 1960s (Warren et al., 1970) is clearly no longer valid. Since this time, the situation has radically changed in recent years to a point where zoonotic malaria is now a major public health problem in at least some areas of SEA. It would be timely now to reconsider simian malaria as a priority for surveillance and control, before malaria elimination status can be declared (Anstey and Grigg, 2019; Baird, 2015; Ekawati et al., 2020; Verhulst et al., 2012). Thus, distribution of simian malaria vectors throughout Southeast Asia should be mapped to enable vector surveillance and control measures to be instituted to achieve malaria elimination.

Acknowledgement

The first author was funded by the Ministry of Higher Education of Malaysia Long Term Research Grant Scheme (LRGS), grant no. LRGS 1/2018/UM/01/1/3.

References

Achee, N.L., Bangs, M.J., Farlow, R., Killeen, G.F., Lindsay, S., Logan, J.G., Moore, S.J., Rowland, M., Sweeney, K., Torr, S.J., 2012. Spatial repellents: from discovery and development to evidence-based validation. Malar. J. 11, 1–9.

Adak, T., Singh, O., Das, M., Wattal, S., Nanda, N., 2005. Comparative susceptibility of three important malaria vectors *Anopheles stephensi, Anopheles fluviatilis*, and *Anopheles sundaicus* to *Plasmodium vivax*. J. Parasitol. 91, 79–82.

Agius, P.A., Cutts, J.C., Han Oo, W., Thi, A., O'Flaherty, K., Zayar Aung, K., Kyaw Thu, H., Poe Aung, P., Mon Thein, M., Nyi Zaw, N., 2020. Evaluation of the effectiveness of topical repellent distributed by village health volunteer networks against *Plasmodium* spp. infection in Myanmar: a stepped-wedge cluster randomised trial. PLoS Med. 17, e1003177.

Ahmad, R., Ali, W.N.W.M., Omar, M.H., Abd Rahman, A.A., Majid, M.A., Nor, Z.M., Xin, Y.K., Jelip, J., Husin, T., Lim, L.H., 2018. Characterization of the larval breeding sites of *Anopheles balabacensis* (Baisas), in Kudat, Sabah, Malaysia. Southeast Asian J. Trop. Med. Public Health 49, 566–579.

Ahmed, M.A., Fauzi, M., Han, E.-T., 2018. Genetic diversity and natural selection of *Plasmodium knowlesi* merozoite surface protein 1 paralog gene in Malaysia. Malar. J. 17, 1–11.

Alonso, P.L., Brown, G., Arevalo-Herrera, M., Binka, F., Chitnis, C., Collins, F., Doumbo, O.K., Greenwood, B., Hall, B.F., Levine, M.M., 2011. A research agenda to underpin malaria eradication. PLoS Med. 8, e1000406.

Anderios, F., NoorRain, A., Vythilingam, I., 2010. In vivo study of human *Plasmodium knowlesi* in *Macaca fascicularis*. Exp. Parasitol. 124, 181–189.

Ang, J.X.D., Kadir, K.A., Mohamad, D.S.A., Matusop, A., Divis, P.C.S., Yaman, K., Singh, B., 2020. New vectors in northern Sarawak, Malaysian Borneo, for the zoonotic malaria parasite, *Plasmodium knowlesi*. Parasit. Vectors 13, 1–13.

Anstey, N.M., Grigg, M.J., 2019. Zoonotic Malaria: The Better You Look, the More You Find. Oxford University Press US.

Arisue, N., Hashimoto, T., Kawai, S., Honma, H., Kume, K., Horii, T., 2019. Apicoplast phylogeny reveals the position of *Plasmodium vivax* basal to the Asian primate malaria parasite clade. Sci. Rep. 9, 1–9.

Arisue, N., Hashimoto, T., Mitsui, H., Palacpac, N.M., Kaneko, A., Kawai, S., Hasegawa, M., Tanabe, K., Horii, T., 2012. The *Plasmodium* apicoplast genome: conserved structure and close relationship of *P. ovale* to rodent malaria parasites. Mol. Biol. Evol. 29, 2095–2099.

Armistead, J.S., Barros, R.R.M., Gibson, T.J., Kite, W.A., Mershon, J.P., Lambert, L.E., Orr-Gonzalez, S.E., Sá, J.M., Adams, J.H., Wellems, T.E., 2018. Infection of mosquitoes from in vitro cultivated *Plasmodium knowlesi* H strain. Int. J. Parasitol. 48, 601–610.

Baird, J.K., 2015. Malaria in the Asia-Pacific Region. Asia-Pacific J. Japan Focus 13, 1–9.

Bannister-Tyrrell, M., Xa, N.X., Kattenberg, J.H., Van Van, N., Dung, V.K.A., Hieu, T.M., Van Hong, N., Rovira-Vallbona, E., Thao, N.T., Duong, T.T., Rosanas-Urgell, A., 2018. Micro-epidemiology of malaria in an elimination setting in Central Vietnam. Malar. J. 17, 1–15.

Barber, B.E., Rajahram, G.S., Grigg, M.J., William, T., Anstey, N.M., 2017. World malaria report: time to acknowledge *Plasmodium knowlesi* malaria. Malar. J. 16, 1–3.

Barber, B.E., William, T., Dhararaj, P., Anderios, F., Grigg, M.J., Yeo, T.W., Anstey, N.M., 2012. Epidemiology of *Plasmodium knowlesi* malaria in north-east Sabah, Malaysia: family clusters and wide age distribution. Malar. J. 11 (1), 1–8.

Barber, B.E., William, T., Grigg, M.J., Menon, J., Auburn, S., Marfurt, J., Anstey, N.M., Yeo, T.W., 2013. A prospective comparative study of knowlesi, falciparum, and vivax malaria in Sabah, Malaysia: high proportion with severe disease from *Plasmodium knowlesi* and *Plasmodium vivax* but no mortality with early referral and artesunate therapy. Clin. Infect. Dis. 56, 383–397.

Benavente, E.D., Gomes, A.R., De Silva, J.R., Grigg, M., Walker, H., Barber, B.E., William, T., Yeo, T.W., de Sessions, P.F., Ramaprasad, A., 2019. Whole genome sequencing of amplified *Plasmodium knowlesi* DNA from unprocessed blood reveals genetic exchange events between Malaysian Peninsular and Borneo subpopulations. Sci. Rep. 9, 1–11.

Bennett, G.F., Warren, M., 1965. Transmission of a new strain of *Plasmodium cynomolgi* to man. J. Parasitol. 51, 79–80.

Bennett, G.F., Warren, M., Cheong, W., 1966. Biology of the simian malarias of southeast Asia. II. The susceptibility of some Malaysian mosquitoes to infection with five strains of *Plasmodium cynomolgi*. J. Parasitol. 52, 625–631.

Beye, H.K., Getz, M.E., Coatney, G.R., Elder, H.A., Eyles, D.E., 1961. Simian malaria in man. Am. J. Trop. Med. Hyg. 10, 311–316.

Boundenga, L., Ollomo, B., Rougeron, V., Mouele, L.Y., Mve-Ondo, B., Delicat-Loembet, L.M., Moukodoum, N.D., Okouga, A.P., Arnathau, C., Elguero, E., 2015. Diversity of malaria parasites in great apes in Gabon. Malar. J. 14, 1–8.

Bradley, J., Stone, W., Da, D.F., Morlais, I., Dicko, A., Cohuet, A., Guelbeogo, W.M., Mahamar, A., Nsango, S., Soumaré, H.M., Diawara, H., 2018. Predicting the likelihood and intensity of mosquito infection from sex specific *Plasmodium falciparum* gametocyte density. elife 7, e34463.

Brant, H.L., Ewers, R.M., Vythilingam, I., Drakeley, C., Benedick, S., Mumford, J.D., 2016. Vertical stratification of adult mosquitoes (Diptera: Culicidae) within a tropical rainforest in Sabah, Malaysia. Malar. J. 15, 370.

Brasil, P., Zalis, M.G., de Pina-Costa, A., Siqueira, A.M., Júnior, C.B., Silva, S., Areas, A.L.L., Pelajo-Machado, M., de Alvarenga, D.A.M., da Silva Santelli, A.C.F., 2017. Outbreak of human malaria caused by *Plasmodium simium* in the Atlantic Forest in Rio de Janeiro: a molecular epidemiological investigation. Lancet Glob. Health 5, e1038–e1046.

Bray, R.S., 1963. Malaria Infections in Primates and their Importance to Man. In: Ergebnisse der Mikrobiologie, Immunitatsforschung und experimentellen Therapie. vol. 36. Springer Vetlag, Berlin, Heidelberg city, pp. 168–213.

Bray, R.S., Garnham, P.C.C., 1964. *Anopheles* as vectors of animal malaria parasites. Bull. World Health Organ. 31, 143–147.

Brown, R., Chua, T.H., Fornace, K., Drakeley, C., Vythilingam, I., Ferguson, H.M., 2020. Human exposure to zoonotic malaria vectors in village, farm and forest habitats in Sabah, Malaysian Borneo. PLOS Negl. Trop. Dis. 14, e0008617.

Brown, R., Hing, C.T., Fornace, K., Ferguson, H.M., 2018. Evaluation of resting traps to examine the behaviour and ecology of mosquito vectors in an area of rapidly changing land use in Sabah, Malaysian Borneo. Parasit. Vectors 11, 346.

Byrne, I., Aure, W., Manin, B.O., Vythilingam, I., Ferguson, H.M., Drakeley, C.J., Chua, T.H., Fornace, K.M., 2021. Environmental and spatial risk factors for the larval habitats of *Plasmodium knowlesi* vectors in Sabah, Malaysian Borneo. Sci. Rep. 11, 1–11.

Carlton, J.M., Adams, J.H., Silva, J.C., Bidwell, S.L., Lorenzi, H., Caler, E., Crabtree, J., Angiuoli, S.V., Merino, E.F., Amedeo, P., 2008. Comparative genomics of the neglected human malaria parasite *Plasmodium vivax*. Nature 455, 757–763.

Chaccour, C., 2021. Veterinary endectocides for malaria control and elimination: prospects and challenges. Philos. Trans. R. Soc. B 376, 20190810.

Charlwood, J., Nenhep, S., Protopopoff, N., Sovannaroth, S., Morgan, J., Hemingway, J., 2016. Effects of the spatial repellent metofluthrin on landing rates of outdoor biting anophelines in Cambodia, Southeast Asia. Med. Vet. Entomol. 30, 229–234.

Chin, A.Z., Maluda, M.C.M., Jelip, J., Jeffree, M.S.B., Culleton, R., Ahmed, K., 2020. Malaria elimination in Malaysia and the rising threat of *Plasmodium knowlesi*. J. Physiol. Anthropol. 39, 1–9.

Chin, W., Contacos, P.G., Coatney, G.R., Kimball, H.R., 1965. A naturally acquired quotidian-type malaria in man transferable to monkeys. Science 149, 865.

Chin, W., Contacos, P.G., Collins, W.E., Jeter, M.H., Alpert, E., 1968. Experimental mosquito-transmission of *Plasmodium knowlesi* to man and monkey. Am. J. Trop. Med. Hyg. 17, 355–358.

Chinh, V.D., Masuda, G., Hung, V.V., Takagi, H., Kawai, S., Annoura, T., Maeno, Y., 2019. Prevalence of human and non-human primate *Plasmodium* parasites in anopheline mosquitoes: a cross-sectional epidemiological study in Southern Vietnam. Trop. Med. Health 47, 1–6.

Choi, L., Majambere, S., Wilson, A.L., 2019. Larviciding to prevent malaria transmission. Cochrane Database Syst. Rev. 2019, CD012736.

Chong, E.T.J., Neoh, J.W.F., Lau, T.Y., Lim, Y.A.-L., Chai, H.C., Chua, K.H., Lee, P.-C., 2020. Genetic diversity of circumsporozoite protein in *Plasmodium knowlesi* isolates from Malaysian Borneo and Peninsular Malaysia. Malar. J. 19, 1–7.

Choudhury, D., Mohan, B., Prakash, S., Ramakrishnan, S., 1963. Experimental susceptibility of Anopheline mosquitoes to simian malaria in the Nilgiris, Madras State, South India. Indian J. Malariol. 17, 237–242.

Chua, T.H., Manin, B.O., Daim, S., Vythilingam, I., Drakeley, C., 2017. Phylogenetic analysis of simian Plasmodium spp. infecting *Anopheles balabacensis* Baisas in Sabah, Malaysia. PLoS Negl. Trop. Dis. 11, e0005991.

Chua, T.H., Manin, B.O., Vythilingam, I., Fornace, K., Drakeley, C.J., 2019. Effect of different habitat types on abundance and biting times of *Anopheles balabacensis* Baisas (Diptera: Culicidae) in Kudat district of Sabah, Malaysia. Parasit. Vectors 12, 1–13.

Clayton, A.M., Dong, Y., Dimopoulos, G., 2014. The *Anopheles* innate immune system in the defense against malaria infection. J. Innate Immun. 6, 169–181.

Coatney, G., Collins, W., Warren, M., Contacos, P., 1971. The Primate Malarias. US Government Printing Office, Washington DC, p. 366.

Coatney, G.R., 1963. Simian malaria: its importance to world-wide eradication of malaria. J. Am. Med. Assoc. 184, 876–877.

Coatney, G.R., Chin, W., Contacos, P.G., King, H.K., 1966. *Plasmodium inui*, a quartan-type malaria parasite of old world monkeys transmissible to man. J. Parasitol. 52, 660–663.

Coatney, G.R., Elder, H.A., Contacos, P.G., Getz, M.E., Greenland, R., Rossan, R.N., Schmidt, L., 1961. Transmission of the M strain of *Plasmodium cynomolgi* to man. Am. J. Trop. Med. Hyg. 10, 673–678.

Coggeshall, L., 1941. Infection of *Anopheles quadrimaculatus* with *Plasmodium cynomolgi*, a monkey malaria parasite, and with *Plasmodium lophurae*, an avian malaria parasite. Am. J. Trop. Med. Hyg. 1, 525–530.

Coleman, R.E., Polsa, N., Eikarat, N., Kollars Jr., T.M., Sattabongkot, J., 2001. Prevention of sporogony of *Plasmodium vivax* in *Anopheles dirus* mosquitoes by transmission-blocking antimalarials. Am. J. Trop. Med. Hyg. 65, 214–218.

Colless, D., 1956. The *Anopheles leucosphyrus* group. Trans. R. Entomol. Soc. Lond. 108, 37–116.

Collins, F.H., Sakai, R.K., Vernick, K.D., Paskewitz, S., Seeley, D.C., Miller, L.H., Collins, W.E., Campbell, C.C., Gwadz, R.W., 1986. Genetic selection of a Plasmodium-refractory strain of the malaria vector *Anopheles gambiae*. Science 234, 607–610.

Collins, W.E., Contacos, P.G., 1972. Transmission of *Plasmodium falciparum* from monkey to monkey by the bite of infected *Anopheles freeborni* mosquitoes. Trans. R. Soc. Trop. Med. Hyg. 66, 371–372.

Collins, W.E., Contacos, P.G., Guinn, E.G., 1967. Studies on the transmission of simian malarias II. Transmission of the H strain of *Plasmodium knowlesi* by *Anopheles balabacensis balabacensis*. J. Parasitol. 53, 841–844.

Collins, W.E., Contacos, P.G., Guinn, E.G., Held, J.R., 1966. Studies on the transmission of simian malarias, I. Transmission of two strains of *Plasmodium inui* by *Anopheles maculatus* and *A. stephensi*. J. Parasitol. 52, 664–668.

Collins, W.E., Contacos, P.G., Guinn, E.G., Held, J.R., 1968. Transmission of *Plasmodium fieldi* by *Anopheles maculatus*, *A. stephensi*, and *A. balabacensis balabacensis*. J. Parasitol. 54, 376.

Collins, W.E., Contacos, P.G., Skinner, J.C., Guinn, E.G., 1971. Studies on the transmission of simian malaria. IV. Further studies on the transmission of *Plasmodium knowlesi* by *Anopheles balabacensis balabacensis* mosquitoes. J. Parasitol. 57, 961–966.

Collins, W.E., Contacos, P.G., Skinner, J.C., Guinn, E.G., 1972. Studies on the transmission of simian malaria V. Infection and transmission of the B strain of *Plasmodium cynomolgi*. J. Parasotol. 58, 653–659.

Collins, W.E., Jeffery, G.M., Sullivan, J.S., Nace, D., Williams, T., Gall, G.G., Williams, A., Barnwell, J.W., 2009. Infection of mosquitoes with *Plasmodium falciparum* by feeding on humans and on Aotus monkeys. Am. J. Trop. Med. Hyg. 81, 529–533.

Collins, W.E., Skinner, J.C., Filipski, V., Wilson, C., Broderson, J.R., Stanfill, P.S., 1988. Transmission of the OS strain of *Plasmodium inui* to *Saimiri sciureus boliviensis* and *Aotus azarae boliviensis* monkeys by *Anopheles dirus* mosquitoes. J. Parasitol. 74, 502–503.

Collins, W.E., Skinner, J.C., Stanfill, P.S., Sutton, B.B., Huong, A.Y., 1984. Infection and transmission studies with the N-3 strain of *Plasmodium fieldi* in the *Macaca mulatta* monkey. J. Parasitol. 70, 422–427.

Collins, W.E., Sullivan, J.S., Galland, G.G., Nace, D., Williams, A., Williams, T., Barnwell, J.W., 2007. Isolates of *Plasmodium inui* adapted to *Macaca mulatta* monkeys and laboratory-reared Anopheline mosquitoes for experimental study. J. Parasitol. 93, 1061–1069.

Collins, W.E., Sullivan, J.S., Nace, D., Williams, T., Sullivan, J.J., Galland, G.G., Grady, K.K., Bounngaseng, A., 2002. Experimental infection of *Anopheles farauti* with different species of *Plasmodium*. J. Parasitol. 88, 295–298.

Collins, W.E., Warren, M., 1998. Studies on infections with two strains of *Plasmodium inui* from Taiwan in rhesus monkeys and different anopheline mosquitoes. J. Parasitol. 84, 547–551.

Collins, W.E., Warren, M., Galland, G.G., 1999. Studies on infections with the Berok strain of *Plasmodium cynomolgi* in monkeys and mosquitoes. J. Parasitol. 85, 268–272.

Collins, W.E., Warren, M., Sullivan, J.S., Galland, G.G., 2001. *Plasmodium coatneyi*: observations on periodicity, mosquito infection, and transmission to *Macaca mulatta* monkeys. Am. J. Trop. Med. Hyg. 64, 101–110.

Collins, W.E., Warren, M., Sullivan, J.S., Galland, G.G., Nace, D., Williams, A., Williams, T., Barnwell, J.W., 2005. Studies on two strains of *Plasmodium cynomolgi* in New World and Old World monkeys and mosquitoes. J. Parasitol. 91, 280–283.

Contacos, P.G., Coatney, G.R., 1963. Experimental adaptation of simian malarias to abnormal hosts. J. Parasitol. 49, 912–918.

Contacos, P.G., Elder, H.A., Coatney, G.R., Genther, C., 1962. Man to man transfer of two strains of *Plasmodium cynomolgi* by mosquito bite. Am. J. Trop. Med. Hyg. 11, 186–193.

Daneshvar, C., Davis, T.M., Cox-Singh, J., Rafa'ee, M.Z., Zakaria, S.K., Divis, P.C., Singh, B., 2009. Clinical and laboratory features of human *Plasmodium knowlesi* infection. Clin. Infect. Dis. 49, 852–860.

Davidson, G., 1954. Estimation of survival rate of anopheline mosquitoes in nature. Nature 174, 792–793.

Davidson, G., Chua, T.H., Cook, A., Speldewinde, P., Weinstein, P., 2019. The role of ecological linkage mechanisms in *Plasmodium knowlesi* transmission and spread. EcoHealth 1, 1–7.

de Arruda-Mayr, M., Cochrane, A.H., Nussenzweig, R.S., 1979. Enhancement of a simian malarial infection (*Plasmodium cynomolgi*) in mosquitoes fed on rhesus (*Macaca mulatta*) previously infected with an unrelated malaria (*Plasmodium knowlesi*). Am. J. Trop. Med. Hyg. 28, 627–633.

de Jong, R.M., Tebeje, S.K., Meerstein-Kessel, L., Tadesse, F.G., Jore, M.M., Stone, W., Bousema, T., 2020. Immunity against sexual stage *Plasmodium falciparum* and *Plasmodium vivax* parasites. Immunol. Rev. 293, 190–215.

Dembele, L., Gego, A., Zeeman, A.-M., Franetich, J.-F., Silvie, O., Rametti, A., Le Grand, R., Dereuddre-Bosquet, N., Sauerwein, R., van Gemert, G.-J., 2011. Towards an in vitro model of *Plasmodium* hypnozoites suitable for drug discovery. PLoS One 6, e18162.

Dev, V., Sharma, V.P., 2013. The dominant mosquito vectors of human malaria in India. *Anopheles* mosquitoes. In: Manguin, S. (Ed.), *Anopheles* Mosquitoes -New Insights Into Malaria Vectors. IntechOpen, Rijeka, Croatia, pp. 239–272.

Dissanaike, A., Nelson, P., Garnham, P., 1965. Two new malaria parasites, *Plasmodium cynomolgi ceylonensis* subup. nov. and *Plasmodium fragile* sp. Nov., from Monkeys in Ceylon. Ceylon J. Med. Sci. 14, 1–9.

Divis, P.C., Lin, L.C., Rovie-Ryan, J.J., Kadir, K.A., Anderios, F., Hisam, S., Sharma, R.S., Singh, B., Conway, D.J., 2017. Three divergent subpopulations of the malaria parasite *Plasmodium knowlesi*. Emerg. Infect. Dis. 23, 616.

Duc, T.N., Erhart, A., Speybroeck, N., Xuan, X.N., Ngoc, T.N., Van, K.P., Le Xuan, H., Le Khanh, T., Coosemans, M., D'Alessandro, U., 2009. Long-lasting insecticidal hammocks for controlling forest malaria: a community-based trial in a rural area of Central Vietnam. PLoS One 4, e7369.

Ekawati, L.L., Johnson, K.C., Jacobson, J.O., Cueto, C.A., Zarlinda, I., Elyazar, I.R., Fatah, A., Sumiwi, M.E., Noviyanti, R., Cotter, C., 2020. Defining malaria risks among forest workers in Aceh, Indonesia: a formative assessment. Malar. J. 19, 1–14.

Escalante, A.A., Ayala, F.J., 1994. Phylogeny of the malarial genus *Plasmodium*, derived from rRNA gene sequences. Proc. Natl. Acad. Sci. 91, 11373–11377.

Escalante, A.A., Cornejo, O.E., Freeland, D.E., Poe, A.C., Durrego, E., Collins, W.E., Lal, A.A., 2005. A monkey's tale: the origin of *Plasmodium vivax* as a human malaria parasite. Proc. Natl. Acad. Sci. 102, 1980–1985.

Eyles, D., 1960a. Susceptibility of *Anopheles albimanus* to primate and avian malarias. Mosq. News 20, 368–371.

Eyles, D.E., 1960b. *Anopheles freeborni* and *A. quadrimaculatus* as experimental vectors of *Plasmodium cynomolgi* and *P. inui*. J. Parasitol. 46, 540.

Eyles, D.E., 1963. The species of simian malaria: taxonomy, morphology, life cycle, and geographical distribution of the monkey species. J. Parasitol. 49, 866–887.

Eyles, D.E., Coatney, G.R., Getz, M.E., 1960. *Vivax*-type malaria parasite of macaques transmissible to man. Science 131, 1812–1813.

Ferguson, H.M., Dornhaus, A., Beeche, A., Borgemeister, C., Gottlieb, M., Mulla, M.S., Gimnig, J.E., Fish, D., Killeen, G.F., 2010. Ecology: a prerequisite for malaria elimination and eradication. PLoS Med. 7, e1000303.

Ferguson, H.M., Read, A.F., 2002. Why is the effect of malaria parasites on mosquito survival still unresolved? Trends Parasitol. 18, 256–261.

Fong, M.Y., Ahmed, M.A., Wong, S.S., Lau, Y.L., Sitam, F., 2015. Genetic diversity and natural selection of the *Plasmodium knowlesi* circumsporozoite protein nonrepeat regions. PLoS One 10, e0137734.

Fornace, K.M., Alexander, N., Abidin, T.R., Brock, P.M., Chua, T.H., Vythilingam, I., Ferguson, H.M., Manin, B.O., Wong, M.L., Ng, S.H., 2019. Local human movement patterns and land use impact exposure to zoonotic malaria in Malaysian Borneo. elife 8, e47602.

Fornace, K.M., Nuin, N.A., Betson, M., Grigg, M.J., William, T., Anstey, N.M., Yeo, T.W., Cox, J., Ying, L.T., Drakeley, C.J., 2016. Asymptomatic and submicroscopic carriage of *Plasmodium knowlesi* malaria in household and community members of clinical cases in Sabah, Malaysia. J. Infect. Dis. 213, 784–787.

Foy, B.D., Alout, H., Seaman, J.A., Rao, S., Magalhaes, T., Wade, M., Parikh, S., Soma, D.D., Sagna, A.B., Fournet, F., Slater, H.C., 2019. Efficacy and risk of harms of repeat ivermectin mass drug administrations for control of malaria (RIMDAMAL): a cluster-randomised trial. Lancet 393, 1517–1526.

Galen, S.C., Borner, J., Martinsen, E.S., Schaer, J., Austin, C.C., West, C.J., Perkins, S.L., 2018. The polyphyly of *Plasmodium*: comprehensive phylogenetic analyses of the malaria parasites (order Haemosporida) reveal widespread taxonomic conflict. R. Soc. Open Sci. 5, 171780.

Garnham, P., 1951. The mosquito transmission of *Plasmodium inui* Halberstaedter and Prowazek, and its pre-erythrocytic development in the liver of the rhesus monkey. Trans. R. Soc. Trop. Med. Hyg. 45, 45–52.

Garnham, P., 1959. A new sub-species of *Plasmodium cynomolgi*. Riv. Parassitol. 20, 273–278.

Garnham, P.C.C., 1966. Malaria Parasites and Other Haemosporidia. Blackwell Scientific, Oxford, UK.

Garnham, P., Lainson, R., Cooper, W., 1957. The tissue stages and sporogony of *Plasmodium knowlesi*. Trans. R. Soc. Trop. Med. Hyg. 51, 384–396.

Garnham, P.C.C., Kendall, G.P., 1974. Periodicity of infectivity of plasmodial gametocytes: the "Hawking phenomenon". Int. J. Parasitol. 4, 103–106.

Garrett-Jones, C., Grab, B., 1964. The assessment of insecticidal impact on the malaria mosquito's vectorial capacity, from data on the proportion of parous females. Bull. World Health Organ. 31, 71–86.

Garret-Jones, C., Shidrawi, G.R., 1969. Malaria vectorial capacity of a population of *Anopheles gambiae*, an exercise in epidemiological entomology. Bull. World Health Organ. 40, 531–545.

Gendrin, M., Christophides, G.K., 2013. The *Anopheles* mosquito microbiota and their impact on pathogen transmission. In: Manguin, S. (Ed.), *Anopheles* Mosquitoes -New Insights Into Malaria Vectors. IntechOpen, Rijeka, Croatia, pp. 525–548.

Godfray, H.C.J., 2013. Mosquito ecology and control of malaria. J. Anim. Ecol. 82, 15–25.

Goh, X.T., Lim, Y.A., Vythilingam, I., Chew, C.H., Lee, P.C., Ngui, R., Tan, T.C., Yap, N.J., Nissapatorn, V., Chua, K.H., 2013. Increased detection of *Plasmodium knowlesi* in Sandakan division, Sabah as revealed by PlasmoNex™. Malar. J. 12, 1–14.

Govella, N.J., Ogoma, S.B., Paliga, J., Chaki, P.P., Killeen, G., 2015. Impregnating hessian strips with the volatile pyrethroid transfluthrin prevents outdoor exposure to vectors of malaria and lymphatic filariasis in urban Dar es Salaam, Tanzania. Parasit. Vectors 8, 1–9.

Green, R., 1932. A malarial parasite of Malayan monkeys and its development in anopheline mosquitoes. Trans. R. Soc. Trop. Med. Hyg. 25, 455–477.

Grietens, K.P., Xuan, X.N., Ribera, J.M., Duc, T.N., van Bortel, W., Ba, N.T., Van, K.P., Le Xuan, H., D'Alessandro, U., Erhart, A., 2012. Social determinants of long lasting insecticidal hammock-use among the Ra-Glai ethnic minority in Vietnam: implications for forest malaria control. PLoS One 7, e29991.

Grigg, M.J., Cox, J., William, T., Jelip, J., Fornace, K.M., Brock, P.M., von Seidlein, L., Barber, B.E., Anstey, N.M., Yeo, T.W., 2017. Individual-level factors associated with the risk of acquiring human *Plasmodium knowlesi* malaria in Malaysia: a case-control study. Lancet Planet. Health 1, e97–e104.

Grigg, M.J., William, T., Menon, J., Dhanaraj, P., Barber, B.E., Wilkes, C.S., Von Seidlein, L., Rajahram, G.S., Pasay, C., McCarthy, J.S., 2016. Artesunate–mefloquine versus chloroquine for treatment of uncomplicated *Plasmodium knowlesi* malaria in Malaysia (ACT KNOW): an open-label, randomised controlled trial. Lancet Infect. Dis. 16, 180–188.

Grignard, L., Shah, S., Chua, T.H., William, T., Drakeley, C.J., Fornace, K.M., 2019. Natural human infections with *Plasmodium cynomolgi* and other malaria species in an elimination setting in Sabah, Malaysia. J. Infect. Dis. 220, 1946–1949.

Gysin, J., Barnwell, J., Schlesinger, D., Nussenzweig, V., Nussenzweig, R., 1984. Neutralization of the infectivity of sporozoites of *Plasmodium knowlesi* by antibodies to a synthetic peptide. J. Exp. Med. 160, 935–940.

Hardin, S., Santa Maria, M., Liaw, C., World Health Organization, 1973. Experimental Infection of *Anopheles donaldi* Reid With *Plasmodium falciparum* and *Plasmodium vivax*. World Health Organization.

Harris, A.F., McKemey, A.R., Nimmo, D., Curtis, Z., Black, I., Morgan, S.A., Oviedo, M.N., Lacroix, R., Naish, N., Morrison, N.I., 2012. Successful suppression of a field mosquito population by sustained release of engineered male mosquitoes. Nat. Biotechnol. 30, 828–830.

Harrison, T., Krigbaum, J., Manser, J., 2006. Primate Biogeography and Ecology on the Sunda Shelf Islands: A Paleontological and Zooarchaeological Perspective. Springer, Boston, MA, pp. 331–372. 2006.

Hartmeyer, G.N., Stensvold, C.R., Fabricius, T., Marmolin, E.S., Hoegh, S.V., Nielsen, H.V., Kemp, M., Vestergaard, L.S., 2019. *Plasmodium cynomolgi* as cause of malaria in tourist to Southeast Asia, 2018. Emerg. Infect. Dis. 25, 1936.

Hawkes, F., Manin, B.O., Ng, S.H., Torr, S.J., Drakeley, C., Chua, T.H., Ferguson, H.M., 2017. Evaluation of electric nets as means to sample mosquito vectors host-seeking on humans and primates. Parasit. Vectors 10, 1–13.

Hawkes, F.M., Manin, B.O., Cooper, A., Daim, S., Homathevi, R., Jelip, J., Husin, T., Chua, T.H., 2019. Vector compositions change across forested to deforested ecotones in emerging areas of zoonotic malaria transmission in Malaysia. Sci. Rep. 9, 1–12.

Hawking, F., 1975. Circadian and other rhythms of parasites. In: Advances Parasitol. Elsevier, pp. 123–182.

Hawking, F., Mellanby, H., Terry, E., Webber, W.A., 1957. Transmission of *Plasmodium knowlesi* by *Anopheles stephensi*. Trans. R. Soc. Trop. Med. Hyg. 51, 397–402.

Hawking, F., Worms, M.J., Gammage, K., 1968. 24-and 48-hour cycles of malaria parasites in the blood; their purpose, production and control. Trans. R. Soc. Trop. Med. Hyg. 62, 731–760.

Hayakawa, T., Culleton, R., Otani, H., Horii, T., Tanabe, K., 2008. Big bang in the evolution of extant malaria parasites. Mol. Biol. Evol. 25, 2233–2239.

Held, J.R., Contacos, P.G., 1967. Studies of the exoerythrocytic stages of simian malaria. II. *Plasmodium coatneyi*. J. Parasitol. 53, 910–918.

Herdiana, H., Irnawati, I., Coutrier, F.N., Munthe, A., Mardiati, M., Yuniarti, T., Sariwati, E., Sumiwi, M.E., Noviyanti, R., Pronyk, P., Hawley, W.A., 2018. Two clusters of *Plasmodium knowlesi* cases in a malaria elimination area, Sabang Municipality, Aceh, Indonesia. Malar. J. 17, 1–10.

Hickey, B.W., Lumsden, J.M., Reyes, S., Sedegah, M., Hollingdale, M.R., Freilich, D.A., Luke, T.C., Charoenvit, Y., Goh, L.M., Berzins, M.P., 2016. Mosquito bite immunization with radiation-attenuated *Plasmodium falciparum* sporozoites: safety, tolerability, protective efficacy and humoral immunogenicity. Malar. J. 15, 1–18.

Hii, J., Vythilingam, I., Roca-Feltrer, A., 2018. Human and simian malaria in the Greater Mekong Subregion and challenges for elimination. In: Manguin, S. (Ed.), Towards Malaria Elimination—A Leap Forward. IntechOpen, Rijeka, Croatia, pp. 95–127.

Imwong, M., Madmanee, W., Suwannasin, K., Kunasol, C., Peto, T.J., Tripura, R., von Seidlein, L., Nguon, C., Davoeung, C., Day, N.P., 2019. Asymptomatic natural human infections with the simian malaria parasites *Plasmodium cynomolgi* and *Plasmodium knowlesi*. J. Infect. Dis. 219, 695–702.

Jaswant, S., Ray, A., Nair, C., 1949. Transmission experiments with *P. knowlesi*. Indian J. Malariol. 3, 145–150.

Jeslyn, W.P.S., Huat, T.C., Vernon, L., Irene, L.M.Z., Sung, L.K., Jarrod, L.P., Singh, B., Ching, N.L., 2011. Molecular epidemiological investigation of *Plasmodium knowlesi* in humans and macaques in Singapore. Vector Borne Zoonotic Dis. 11, 131–135.

Jeyaprakasam, N.K., Liew, J.W.K., Low, V.L., Wan-Sulaiman, W.-Y., Vythilingam, I., 2020. *Plasmodium knowlesi* infecting humans in Southeast Asia: what's next? PLoS Negl. Trop. Dis. 14, e0008900.

Jeyaprakasam, N.K., Pramasivan, S., Liew, J.W.K., Low, V.L., Wan-Sulaiman, W.Y., Ngui, R., Jelip, J., Vythilingam, I., 2021. Evaluation of Mosquito Magnet and other collection tools for *Anopheles* mosquito vectors of simian malaria. Parasit. Vectors 14, 1–13.

Jiram, A.I., Ooi, C.H., Rubio, J.M., Hisam, S., Karnan, G., Sukor, N.M., Artic, M.M., Ismail, N.P., Alias, N.W., 2019. Evidence of asymptomatic submicroscopic malaria in low transmission areas in Belaga district, Kapit division, Sarawak, Malaysia. Malar. J. 18, 1–12.

Jiram, A.I., Vythilingam, I., NoorAzian, Y.M., Yusof, Y.M., Azahari, A.H., Fong, M.Y., 2012. Entomologic investigation of *Plasmodium knowlesi* vectors in Kuala Lipis, Pahang, Malaysia. Malar. J. 11, 213.

Joy, D.A., Feng, X., Mu, J., Furuya, T., Chotivanich, K., Krettli, A.U., Ho, M., Wang, A., White, N.J., Suh, E., 2003. Early origin and recent expansion of *Plasmodium falciparum*. Science 300, 318–321.

Joy, D.A., Gonzalez-Ceron, L., Carlton, J.M., Gueye, A., Fay, M., McCutchan, T.F., Su, X.Z., 2008. Local adaptation and vector-mediated population structure in *Plasmodium vivax* malaria. Mol. Biol. Evol. 25, 1245–1252.

Joyner, C., Moreno, A., Meyer, E.V., Cabrera-Mora, M., Ma, H.C., Kissinger, J.C., Barnwell, J.W., Galinski, M.R., 2016. *Plasmodium cynomolgi* infections in rhesus macaques display clinical and parasitological features pertinent to modelling vivax malaria pathology and relapse infections. Malar. J. 15, 451.

Joyner, C.J., Brito, C.F., Saney, C.L., Joice Cordy, R., Smith, M.L., Lapp, S.A., Cabrera-Mora, M., Kyu, S., Lackman, N., Nural, M.V., DeBarry, J.D., 2019. Humoral immunity prevents clinical malaria during *Plasmodium* relapses without eliminating gametocytes. PLoS Pathog. 15, e1007974.

Klein, T., Harrison, B., Dixon, S., Burge, J., 1991. Comparative susceptibility of Southeast Asian *Anopheles* mosquitoes to the simian malaria parasite *Plasmodium cynomolgi*. J. Am. Mosq. Control Assoc. 7, 481–487.

Klein, T., Harrison, B., Grove, J., Dixon, S., Andre, R., 1986. Correlation of survival rates of *Anopheles dirus* A (Diptera: Culicidae) with different infection densities of *Plasmodium cynomolgi*. Bull. World Health Organ. 64, 901.

Knowles, R., Gupta, D., 1933. BM (1932) A study of monkey-malaria, and its experimental transmission to man. Ind. Med. Gaz. 67, 301–320.

Kobylinski, K.C., Jittamala, P., Hanboonkunupakarn, B., Pukrittayakamee, S., Pantuwatana, K., Phasomkusolsil, S., Davidson, S.A., Winterberg, M., Hoglund, R.M., Mukaka, M., van der Pluijm, R.W., 2020. Safety, pharmacokinetics, and mosquito-lethal effects of ivermectin in combination with dihydroartemisinin-piperaquine and primaquine in healthy adult thai subjects. Clin. Pharmacol. Ther. 107 (5), 1221–1230.

Krief, S., Escalante, A.A., Pacheco, M.A., Mugisha, L., André, C., Halbwax, M., Fischer, A., Krief, J.-M., Kasenene, J.M., Crandfield, M., 2010. On the diversity of malaria parasites in African apes and the origin of *Plasmodium falciparum* from Bonobos. PLoS Pathog. 6, e1000765.

Lalremruata, A., Magris, M., Vivas-Martínez, S., Koehler, M., Esen, M., Kempaiah, P., Jeyaraj, S., Perkins, D.J., Mordmüller, B., Metzger, W.G., 2015. Natural infection of *Plasmodium brasilianum* in humans: man and monkey share quartan malaria parasites in the Venezuelan Amazon. EBioMedicine 2, 1186–1192.

Lambrechts, L., Koella, J.C., 2013. Evolutionary Aspects of *Anopheles-Plasmodium* Interactions. Wageningen Academic Publishers, Wageningen.

Lee, K.-S., Cox-Singh, J., Singh, B., 2009. Morphological features and differential counts of *Plasmodium knowles* parasites in naturally acquired human infections. Malar. J. 8, 1–10.

Lee, K.-S., Divis, P.C., Zakaria, S.K., Matusop, A., Julin, R.A., Conway, D.J., Cox-Singh, J., Singh, B., 2011. *Plasmodium knowlesi*: reservoir hosts and tracking the emergence in humans and macaques. PLoS Pathog. 7, e1002015.

Lefevre, T., Ohm, J., Dabiré, K.R., Cohuet, A., Choisy, M., Thomas, M.B., Cator, L., 2018. Transmission traits of malaria parasites within the mosquito: genetic variation, phenotypic plasticity, and consequences for control. Evol. Appl. 11, 456–469.

Liew, J.W.K., MohdBukhari, F.D., Jeyaprakasam, N.K., Phang, W.K., Vythilingam, I., Lau, Y.L., 2021. Natural *Plasmodium inui* infections in humans and *Anopheles cracens* mosquito, Malaysia. Emerg. Infect. Dis. 27 (10), (in press) October issue. https://doi.org/10.3201/eid2710.210412.

Liu, W., Li, Y., Learn, G.H., Rudicell, R.S., Robertson, J.D., Keele, B.F., Ndjango, J.-B.N., Sanz, C.M., Morgan, D.B., Locatelli, S., 2010. Origin of the human malaria parasite *Plasmodium falciparum* in gorillas. Nature 467, 420–425.

Liu, W., Li, Y., Shaw, K.S., Learn, G.H., Plenderleith, L.J., Malenke, J.A., Sundararaman, S.A., Ramirez, M.A., Crystal, P.A., Smith, A.G., 2014. African origin of the malaria parasite *Plasmodium vivax*. Nat. Commun. 5, 1–10.

Liverani, M., Charlwood, J.D., Lawford, H., Yeung, S., 2017. Field assessment of a novel spatial repellent for malaria control: a feasibility and acceptability study in Mondulkiri, Cambodia. Malar. J. 16, 1–12.

Loy, D.E., Plenderleith, L.J., Sundararaman, S.A., Liu, W., Gruszczyk, J., Chen, Y.-J., Trimboli, S., Learn, G.H., MacLean, O.A., Morgan, A.L., 2018. Evolutionary history of human *Plasmodium vivax* revealed by genome-wide analyses of related ape parasites. Proc. Natl. Acad. Sci. 115, E8450–E8459.

Lutz, H.L., Patterson, B.D., Peterhans, J.C.K., Stanley, W.T., Webala, P.W., Gnoske, T.P., Hackett, S.J., Stanhope, M.J., 2016. Diverse sampling of East African haemosporidians reveals chiropteran origin of malaria parasites in primates and rodents. Mol. Phylogenet. Evol. 99, 7–15.

Lyimo, I.N., Kessy, S.T., Mbina, K.F., Daraja, A.A., Mnyone, L.L., 2017. Ivermectin-treated cattle reduces blood digestion, egg production and survival of a free-living population of Anopheles arabiensis under semi-field condition in southeastern Tanzania. Malar. J. 16, 1–12.

Maeno, Y., Culleton, R., Quang, N., Kawai, S., Marchand, R., Nakazawa, S., 2017. *Plasmodium knowlesi* and human malaria parasites in Khan Phu, Vietnam: gametocyte production in humans and frequent co-infection of mosquitoes. Parasitology 144, 527.

Maeno, Y., Quang, N.T., Culleton, R., Kawai, S., Masuda, G., Nakazawa, S., Marchand, R.P., 2015. Humans frequently exposed to a range of non-human primate malaria parasite species through the bites of *Anopheles dirus* mosquitoes in South-central Vietnam. Parasit. Vectors 8, 376.

Magris, M., Rubio-Palis, Y., Alexander, N., Ruiz, B., Galván, N., Frias, D., Blanco, M., Lines, J., 2007. Community-randomized trial of lambdacyhalothrin-treated hammock nets for malaria control in Yanomami communities in the Amazon region of Venezuela. Tropical Med. Int. Health 12, 392–403.

Maia, M.F., Kliner, M., Richardson, M., Lengeler, C., Moore, S.J., 2018. Mosquito repellents for malaria prevention. Cochrane Database Syst. Rev. 2.

Manin, B.O., Ferguson, H.M., Vythilingam, I., Fornace, K., William, T., Torr, S.J., Drakeley, C., Chua, T.H., 2016. Investigating the contribution of peri-domestic transmission to risk of zoonotic malaria infection in humans. PLoS Negl. Trop. Dis. 10, e0005064.

Marchand, R.P., Culleton, R., Maeno, Y., Quang, N.T., Nakazawa, S., 2011. Co-infections of *Plasmodium knowlesi, P. falciparum, and P. vivax* among humans and *Anopheles dirus* mosquitoes, southern Vietnam. Emerg. Infect. Dis. 17, 1232–1239.

Martinsen, E.S., Perkins, S.L., Schall, J.J., 2008. A three-genome phylogeny of malaria parasites (Plasmodium and closely related genera): evolution of life-history traits and host switches. Mol. Phylogenet. Evol. 47, 261–273.

Medley, G., Sinden, R., Fleck, S., Billingsley, P., Tirawanchap, N., Rodriguez, M., 1993. Heterogeneity in patterns of malarial oocyst infections in the mosquito vector. Parasitology 106, 441–449.

Mendes, A.M., Albuquerque, I.S., Machado, M., Pissarra, J., Meireles, P., Prudêncio, M., 2017. Inhibition of *Plasmodium* liver infection by ivermectin. Antimicrob. Agents Chemother. 61, e02005-16.

Millet, P., Anderson, P., Collins, W.E., 1994. In vitro cultivation of exoerythrocytic stages of the simian malaria parasites *Plasmodium fieldi* and *Plasmodium simiovale* in rhesus monkey hepatocytes. J. Parasitol., 384–388.

Moyes, C.L., Henry, A.J., Golding, N., Huang, Z., Singh, B., Baird, J.K., Newton, P.N., Huffman, M., Duda, K.A., Drakeley, C.J., 2014. Defining the geographical range of the *Plasmodium knowlesi* reservoir. PLoS Negl. Trop. Dis. 8, e2780.

Mu, J., Joy, D.A., Duan, J., Huang, Y., Carlton, J., Walker, J., Barnwell, J., Beerli, P., Charleston, M.A., Pybus, O.G., Su, X.Z., 2005. Host switch leads to emergence of *Plasmodium vivax* malaria in humans. Mol. Biol. Evol. 22, 1686–1693.

Mueller, A.-K., Kohlhepp, F., Hammerschmidt, C., Michel, K., 2010. Invasion of mosquito salivary glands by malaria parasites: prerequisites and defense strategies. Int. J. Parasitol. 40, 1229–1235.

Murphy, J.R., Weiss, W.R., Fryauff, D., Dowler, M., Savransky, T., Stoyanov, C., Muratova, O., Lambert, L., Orr-Gonzalez, S., Zeleski, K.L., 2014. Using infective mosquitoes to challenge monkeys with *Plasmodium knowlesi* in malaria vaccine studies. Malar. J. 13, 215.

Nakazawa, S., Marchand, R.P., Quang, N.T., Culleton, R., Manh, N.D., Maeno, Y., 2009. *Anopheles dirus* co-infection with human and monkey malaria parasites in Vietnam. Int. J. Parasitol. 39, 1533–1537.

Nelson, P., Jayasuriya, J., 1971. The establishment of *Anopheles elegans* as the natural vector of simian malaria in Ceylon. Ceylon J. Med. Sci. 20, 46–51.

Ng'habi, K., Viana, M., Matthiopoulos, J., Lyimo, I., Killeen, G., Ferguson, H.M., 2018. Mesocosm experiments reveal the impact of mosquito control measures on malaria vector life history and population dynamics. Sci. Rep. 8, 1–12.

Ngernna, S., Rachaphaew, N., Thammapalo, S., Prikchoo, P., Kaewnah, O., Manopwisedjaroen, K., Phumchuea, K., Suansomjit, C., Roobsoong, W., Sattabongkot, J., 2019. Case report: case series of human *Plasmodium knowlesi* infection on the Southern border of Thailand. Am. J. Trop. Med. Hyg. 101, 1397–1401.

Nguyen-Dinh, P., Campbell, C.C., Collins, W.E., 1980. Cultivation in vitro of the quartan malaria parasite *Plasmodium inui*. Science 209, 1249–1251.

Nguyen, C., Gray, M., Burton, T.A., Foy, S.L., Foster, J.R., Gendernalik, A.L., Rückert, C., Alout, H., Young, M.C., Boze, B., 2019. Evaluation of a novel West Nile virus transmission control strategy that targets *Culex tarsalis* with endectocide-containing blood meals. PLoS Negl. Trop. Dis. 13, e0007210.

Nishimoto, Y., Arisue, N., Kawai, S., Escalante, A.A., Horii, T., Tanabe, K., Hashimoto, T., 2008. Evolution and phylogeny of the heterogeneous cytosolic SSU rRNA genes in the genus *Plasmodium*. Mol. Phylogenet. Evol. 47, 45–53.

Nofal, S.D., Peto, T.J., Adhikari, B., Tripura, R., Callery, J., Bui, T.M., von Seidlein, L., Pell, C., 2019. How can interventions that target forest-goers be tailored to accelerate malaria elimination in the Greater Mekong Subregion? A systematic review of the qualitative literature. Malar. J. 18, 1–10.

Norris, E.J., Coats, J.R., 2017. Current and future repellent technologies: the potential of spatial repellents and their place in mosquito-borne disease control. Int. J. Environ. Res. Public Health 14, 1–15.

O'Connell, J.F., Allen, J., Williams, M.A., Williams, A.N., Turney, C.S., Spooner, N.A., Kamminga, J., Brown, G., Cooper, A., 2018. When did Homo sapiens first reach Southeast Asia and Sahul? Proc. Natl. Acad. Sci. 115, 8482–8490.

O'Donnell, A.J., Rund, S.S., Reece, S.E., 2019. Time-of-day of blood-feeding: effects on mosquito life history and malaria transmission. Parasit. Vectors 12, 1–16.

Ogoma, S.B., Mmando, A.S., Swai, J.K., Horstmann, S., Malone, D., Killeen, G.F., 2017. A low technology emanator treated with the volatile pyrethroid transfluthrin confers long term protection against outdoor biting vectors of lymphatic filariasis, arboviruses and malaria. PLoS Negl. Trop. Dis. 11, e0005455.

Pacheco, M.A., Matta, N.E., Valkiūnas, G., Parker, P.G., Mello, B., Stanley Jr., C.E., Lentino, M., Garcia-Amado, M.A., Cranfield, M., Kosakovsky Pond, S.L., Escalante, A.A., 2018. Mode and rate of evolution of haemosporidian mitochondrial genomes: timing the radiation of avian parasites. Mol. Biol. Evol. 35, 383–403.

Pain, A., Böhme, U., Berry, A.E., Mungall, K., Finn, R.D., Jackson, A.P., Mourier, T., Mistry, J., Pasini, E.M., Aslett, M.A., Balasubrammaniam, S., 2008. The genome of the simian and human malaria parasite *Plasmodium knowlesi*. Nature 455, 799–803.

Perkins, S.L., Schall, J., 2002. A molecular phylogeny of malarial parasites recovered from cytochrome b gene sequences. J. Parasitol. 88, 972–978.

Poché, D., Clarke, T., Tseveenjav, B., Torres-Poché, Z., 2020a. Evaluating the use of a low dose fipronil bait in reducing black-tailed prairie dog (*Cynomys ludovicianus*) fleas at reduced application rates. Int. J. Parasitol. 13, 292–298.

Poché, D.M., Franckowiak, G., Clarke, T., Tseveenjav, B., Polyakova, L., Poché, R.M., 2020b. Efficacy of a low dose fipronil bait against blacklegged tick (*Ixodes scapularis*) larvae feeding on white-footed mice (*Peromyscus leucopus*) under laboratory conditions. Parasit. Vectors 13, 1–15.

Poche, D.M., Torres-Poche, Z., Yeszhanov, A., Poche, R.M., Belyaev, A., Dvořák, V., Sayakova, Z., Polyakova, L., Aimakhanov, B., 2018. Field evaluation of a 0.005% fipronil bait, orally administered to Rhombomys opimus, for control of fleas (Siphonaptera: Pulicidae) and phlebotomine sand flies (Diptera: Psychodidae) in the Central Asian Republic of Kazakhstan. PLoS Negl. Trop. Dis. 12, e0006630.

Prugnolle, F., Durand, P., Neel, C., Ollomo, B., Ayala, F.J., Arnathau, C., Etienne, L., Mpoudi-Ngole, E., Nkoghe, D., Leroy, E., Delaporte, E., 2010. African great apes are natural hosts of multiple related malaria species, including *Plasmodium falciparum*. Proc. Natl. Acad. Sci. 107, 1458–1463.

Prugnolle, F., Rougeron, V., Becquart, P., Berry, A., Makanga, B., Rahola, N., Arnathau, C., Ngoubangoye, B., Menard, S., Willaume, E., Ayala, F.J., 2013. Diversity, host switching and evolution of *Plasmodium vivax* infecting African great apes. Proc. Natl. Acad. Sci. 110, 8123–8128.

Puri, S., Kamboj, K., Dutta, G., 1989. Infectivity studies on *Anopheles stephensi* using *Plasmodium cynomolgi* B infection in rhesus monkeys. Trop. Med. Parasitol. 40, 409–411.

Qari, S.H., Shi, Y.P., Pieniazek, N.J., Collins, W.E., Lal, A.A., 1996. Phylogenetic relationship among the malaria parasites based on small subunit rRNA gene sequences: monophyletic nature of the human malaria parasite, *Plasmodium falciparum*. Mol. Phylogenet. Evol. 6, 157–165.

Raja, T.N., Hu, T.H., Kadir, K.A., Mohamad, D.S.A., Rosli, N., Wong, L.L., Hii, K.C., Divis, P.C.S., Singh, B., 2020. Naturally acquired human *Plasmodium cynomolgi* and *P. knowlesi* infections, Malaysian Borneo. Emerg. Infect. Dis. 26, 1801–1809.

Rattanarithkul, R., Harrison, B.A., Harbach, R.E., Panthusiri, P., Coleman, R.E., 2006. Illustrated keys to the mosquitoes of Thailand. IV. *Anopheles*. Southeast Asian J. Trop. Med. Public Health 37, 1–128.

Reid, J., Weitz, B., 1961. Anopheline mosquitoes as vectors of animal malaria in Malaya. Ann. Trop. Med. Parasitol. 55, 180–186.

Reid, J.A., 1968. Anopheline Mosquitoes of Malaya and Borneo. Institute of Medical Research Malaysia.

Riehle, M.M., Bukhari, T., Gneme, A., Guelbeogo, W.M., Coulibaly, B., Fofana, A., Pain, A., Bischoff, E., Renaud, F., Beavogui, A.H., Traore, S.F., 2017.

The *Anopheles gambiae* 2La chromosome inversion is associated with susceptibility to *Plasmodium falciparum* in Africa. elife 6, e25813.

Rohani, A., Fakhriy, H.A., Suzilah, I., Zurainee, M., Najdah, W.W., Ariffin, M.M., Shakirudin, N.M., Afiq, M.M., Jenarun, J., Tanrang, Y., 2020. Indoor and outdoor residual spraying of a novel formulation of deltamethrin K-Othrine[®](Polyzone) for the control of simian malaria in Sabah, Malaysia. PLoS One 15, e0230860.

Rohani, A., Wan Najdah, W., Zamree, I., Azahari, A., Mohd Noor, I., Rahimi, H., Lee, H., 2010. Habitat characterization and mapping of *Anopheles maculatus* (Theobald) mosquito larvae in malaria endemic areas in Kuala Lipis, Pahang, Malaysia. Southeast Asian J. Trop. Med. Public Health 41, 821–830.

Romoli, O., Gendrin, M., 2018. The tripartite interactions between the mosquito, its microbiota and *Plasmodium*. Parasit. Vectors 11, 1–8.

Rosenberg, R., 1985. Inability of *Plasmodium knowlesi* sporozoites to invade *Anopheles freeborni* salivary glands. Am. J. Trop. Med. Hyg. 34, 687–691.

Roy, S.W., Irimia, M., 2008. Origins of human malaria: rare genomic changes and full mitochondrial genomes confirm the relationship of *Plasmodium falciparum* to other mammalian parasites but complicate the origins of *Plasmodium vivax*. Mol. Biol. Evol. 25, 1192–1198.

Russell, T.L., Farlow, R., Min, M., Espino, E., Mnzava, A., Burkot, T.R., 2020. Capacity of national malaria control programmes to implement vector surveillance: a global analysis. Malar. J. 19, 1–9.

Rutledge, G.G., Böhme, U., Sanders, M., Reid, A.J., Cotton, J.A., Maiga-Ascofare, O., Djimdé, A.A., Apinjoh, T.O., Amenga-Etego, L., Manske, M., Barnwell, J.W., 2017. *Plasmodium malariae* and *P. ovale* genomes provide insights into malaria parasite evolution. Nature 542, 101–104.

Saleh Huddin, A., Md Yusuf, N., Razak, M., Ogu Salim, N., Hisam, S., 2019. Genetic diversity of Plasmodium knowlesi among human and long-tailed macaque populations in Peninsular Malaysia: the utility of microsatellite markers. Infect. Genet. Evol. 75, 103952.

Sallum, M.A.M., Foster, P.G., Li, C., Sithiprasasna, R., Wilkerson, R.C., 2007. Phylogeny of the Leucosphyrus Group of *Anopheles* (Cellia)(Diptera: Culicidae) based on mitochondrial gene sequences. Ann. Entomol. Soc. Am. 100, 27–35.

Sallum, M.A.M., Peyton, E.L., Harrison, B.A., Wilkerson, R.C., 2005a. Revision of the Leucosphyrus group of *Anopheles* (Cellia)(Diptera, Culicidae). Rev. Bras. Entomol. 49, 01–152.

Sallum, M.A.M., Peyton, E.L., Wilkerson, R.C., 2005b. Six new species of the *Anopheles leucosphyrus* group, reinterpretation of *An. elegans* and vector implications. Med. Vet. Entomol. 19, 158–199.

Schmidt, L., Fradkin, R., Harrison, J., Rossan, R.N., Squires, W., 1980. The course of untreated *Plasmodium inui* infections in the rhesus monkey (*Macaca mulatta*). Am. J. Trop. Med. Hyg. 29, 158–169.

Schmidt, L., Genther, C.S., Rossan, R.N., 1982. IV. Acquisition of Anopheles quadrimaculatus infected with the M strain and Anopheles freeborni infected with the M, B, or Ro strain. Am. J. Trop. Med. Hyg. 31, 681–698.

Schmidt, L., Greenland, R., Genther, C.S., 1961. The transmission of *Plasmodium cynomolgi* to man. Am. J. Trop. Med. Hyg. 10, 679–688.

Scott, J., 2020. Proposed integrated control of zoonotic *Plasmodium knowlesi* in Southeast Asia using themes of one health. Trop. Med. Infect. Dis. 5, 175.

Shears, M.J., Seilie, A.M., Sim, B.K.L., Hoffman, S.L., Murphy, S.C., 2020. Quantification of *Plasmodium knowlesi* versus *Plasmodium falciparum* in the rhesus liver: implications for malaria vaccine studies in rhesus models. Malar. J. 19, 1–9.

Shortt, H., Baker, J., Nesbitt, P., 1963. The pre-erythrocytic stage of *Plasmodium osmaniae*. J. Trop. Med. Hyg. 66, 127–129.

Shortt, H., Garnham, P., 1948. The pre-erythrocytic development of *Plasmodium cynomolgi* and *Plasmodium vivax*. Trans. R. Soc. Trop. Med. Hyg. 41, 785–795.

Simões, M.L., Mlambo, G., Tripathi, A., Dong, Y., Dimopoulos, G., 2017. Immune regulation of *Plasmodium* is *Anopheles* species specific and infection intensity dependent. MBio 8, 5. e01631-17.

Singh, B., Kadir, K., Hu, T., Raja, T., Mohamad, D., Lin, L., Hii, K., 2018. Naturally acquired human infections with the simian malaria parasite, *Plasmodium cynomolgi*, in Sarawak, Malaysian Borneo. Int. J. Infect. Dis. 73, 68.

Singh, B., Sung, L.K., Matusop, A., Radhakrishnan, A., Shamsul, S.S.G., Cox-Singh, J., Thomas, A., Conway, D.J., 2004. A large focus of naturally acquired *Plasmodium knowlesi* infections in human beings. Lancet 363, 1017–1024.

Singh, J., Ray, A.P., Nair, C.P., 1949. Preliminary investigations on the chemotherapeutic activity of atebrin, paludrine, resochin, camoquin, metachloridine and aphacrine on simian malaria. Indian J. Malariol. 3, 387–403.

Singh, J., Ray, A.P., Nair, G.P., 1950. Transmission experiments with *P. knowlesi*. Indian J. Malariol. 3, 145–150.

Sinha, S., Gajanana, A., 1984. First report of natural infection with quartan malaria parasite *Plasmodium shortti* in *Macaca fascicularis umbrosa* (= *irus*) of Nicobar Islands. Trans. R. Soc. Trop. Med. Hyg. 78, 567.

Sinka, M.E., Bangs, M.J., Manguin, S., Chareonviriyaphap, T., Patil, A.P., Temperley, W.H., Gething, P.W., Elyazar, I.R.F., Kabaria, C.W., Harbach, R.E., 2011. The dominant *Anopheles* vectors of human malaria in the Asia-Pacific region: occurrence data, distribution maps and bionomic précis. Parasit. Vectors 4, 1–46.

Sinton, J., Hutton, E., Shute, P., 1938. Failure to transmit an Infection of *Plasmodium cynomolgi* to man by blood inoculation and by mosquitobBites. J. Trop. Med. Hyg. 41, 245–246.

Sissoko, M.S., Healy, S.A., Katile, A., Omaswa, F., Zaidi, I., Gabriel, E.E., Kamate, B., Samake, Y., Guindo, M.A., Dolo, A., 2017. Safety and efficacy of PfSPZ Vaccine against *Plasmodium falciparum* via direct venous inoculation in healthy malaria-exposed adults in Mali: a randomised, double-blind phase 1 trial. Lancet Infect. Dis. 17, 498–509.

Sochantha, T., Van Bortel, W., Savonnaroth, S., Marcotty, T., Speybroeck, N., Coosemans, M., 2010. Personal protection by long-lasting insecticidal hammocks against the bites of forest malaria vectors. Tropical Med. Int. Health 15, 336–341.

Syafruddin, D., Asih, P.B., Rozi, I.E., Permana, D.H., Hidayati, A.P.N., Syahrani, L., Zubaidah, S., Sidik, D., Bangs, M.J., Bøgh, C., 2020. Efficacy of a spatial repellent for control of malaria in Indonesia: a cluster-randomized controlled trial. Am. J. Trop. Med. Hyg. 103, 344–358.

Ta, T.H., Hisam, S., Lanza, M., Jiram, A.I., Ismail, N., Rubio, J.M., 2014. First case of a naturally acquired human infection with *Plasmodium cynomolgi*. Malar. J. 13, 68.

Tachibana, S.I., Sullivan, S.A., Kawai, S., Nakamura, S., Kim, H.R., Goto, N., Arisue, N., Palacpac, N.M., Honma, H., Yagi, M., Tougan, T., 2012. *Plasmodium cynomolgi* genome sequences provide insight into *Plasmodium vivax* and the monkey malaria clade. Nat. Genet. 44, 1051–1055.

Tadesse, F.G., Meerstein-Kessel, L., Gonçalves, B.P., Drakeley, C., Ranford-Cartwright, L., Bousema, T., 2019. Gametocyte sex ratio: the key to understanding *Plasmodium falciparum* transmission? Trends Parasitol. 35, 226–238.

Tan, C.H., 2008. Identification of Vectors of *Plasmodium knowlesi* and Other Malaria Parasites, and Studies on Their Bionomics in Kapit, Sarawak, Malaysia. MSc Thesis, University Malaysia, Sarawak (UNIMAS).

Tan, C.H., Vythilingam, I., Matusop, A., Chan, S.T., Singh, B., 2008. Bionomics of *Anopheles latens* in Kapit, Sarawak, Malaysian Borneo in relation to the transmission of zoonotic simian malaria parasite *Plasmodium knowlesi*. Malar. J. 7, 52.

Tangena, J.-A.A., Thammavong, P., Chonephetsarath, S., Logan, J.G., Brey, P.T., Lindsay, S.W., 2018. Field evaluation of personal protection methods against outdoor-biting mosquitoes in Lao PDR. Parasit. Vectors 11, 1–13.

Terzian, L.A., 1970. A note on the effects of antimalarial drugs on the sporogonous cycle of *Plasmodium cynomolgi* in *Anopheles stephensi*. Parasitology 61, 191–194.

Tsukamoto, M., Miyata, A., Miyagi, I., 1978. Surveys on simian malaria parasites and their vector in Palawan Island, the Philippines. Trop. Med. 20, 39–50.

Vanachayangkul, P., Im-Erbsin, R., Tungtaeng, A., Kodchakorn, C., Roth, A., Adams, J.H., Chaisatit, C., Saingam, P., Sciotti, R.J., Reichard, G.A., Nolan, C.K., 2020. Safety, pharmacokinetics, and liver-stage *Plasmodium cynomolgi* effect of high-dose ivermectin and chloroquine against the liver stage of Plasmodium cynomolgi infection in rhesus macaques. Antimicrob. Agents Chemother. 64, e00741-20.

Verhulst, N.O., Smallegange, R.C., Takken, W., 2012. Mosquitoes as potential bridge vectors of malaria parasites from non-human primates to humans. Front. Physiol. 3, 197.

Vidhya, P.T., Sunish, I.P., Maile, A., Zahid, A.K., 2019. *Anopheles sundaicus* mosquitoes as vector for *Plasmodium knowlesi*, Andaman and Nicobar Islands, India. Emerg. Infect. Dis. 25, 817–820.

Vythilingam, I., Hii, J., 2013. Simian malaria parasites: special emphasis on *Plasmodium knowlesi* and their *Anopheles* vectors in Southeast Asia. In: Manguin, S. (Ed.), *Anopheles* Mosquitoes—New Insights Into Malaria Vectors. In Tech, Rijeka, Croatia, pp. 487–510.

Vythilingam, I., Lim, Y.A., Venugopalan, B., Ngui, R., Leong, C.S., Wong, M.L., Khaw, L., Goh, X., Yap, N., Sulaiman, W.Y.W., 2014. *Plasmodium knowlesi* malaria an emerging public health problem in Hulu Selangor, Selangor, Malaysia (2009-2013): epidemiologic and entomologic analysis. Parasit. Vectors 7, 436.

Vythilingam, I., NoorAzian, Y.M., Huat, T.C., Jiram, A.I., Yusri, Y.M., Azahari, A.H., NorParina, I., NoorRain, A., LokmanHakim, S., 2008. *Plasmodium knowlesi* in humans, macaques and mosquitoes in peninsular Malaysia. Parasit. Vectors 1, 1–10.

Vythilingam, I., Tan, C.H., Asmad, M., Chan, S.T., Lee, K.S., Singh, B., 2006. Natural transmission of *Plasmodium knowlesi* to humans by *Anopheles latens* in Sarawak, Malaysia. Trans. R. Soc. Trop. Med. Hyg. 100, 1087–1088.

Vythilingam, I., Wong, M., Wan-Yussof, W., 2018. Current status of *Plasmodium knowlesi* vectors: a public health concern? Parasitology 145, 32–40.

Warren, M., Eyles, D., Wharton, R., 1962. Primate malaria infections in *Mansonia uniformis*. Mosq. News 22, 303–304.

Warren, M., Eyles, D., Wharton, R., Ow Yang, C., 1963. The susceptibility of malayan anophelines to *Plasmodium cynomolgi bastianellii*. Indian J. Malariol. 17, 85–105.

Warren, M.W., Cheong, W.H., Fredericks, H.K., Coatney, G.R., 1970. Cycles of jungle malaria in West Malaysia. Am. J. Trop. Med. Hyg. 19, 383–393.

Warren, M.W., Wharton, R.H., 1963. The vectors of simian malaria: identity, biology, and geographical distribution. J. Parasitol. 49, 892–904.

Watson, M., 1921. The Prevention of Malaria in the Federated Malay States: A Record of Twenty Years' Progress. EP Dutton & Company.

Wharton, R.H., Eyles, D.E., 1961. *Anopheles hackeri*, a vector of *Plasmodium knowlesi* in Malaya. Science 134, 279–280.

Wharton, R.H., Eyles, D.E., Warren, M., Cheong, W.H., 1964. Studies to determine the vectors of monkey malaria in Malaya. Ann. Trop. Med. Parasitol. 58, 56–77.

WHO, 2016. Eliminating Malaria. World Health Organization, Geneva.

WHO, 2018. Malaria Surveillance, Monitoring & Evaluation: A Reference Manual. World Health Organization, Geneva, p. 206.

WHO, 2019. Guidelines for Malaria Vector Control. World Health Organization, Geneva.

WHO, 2020. World Malaria Report: 20 Years of Global Progress and Challenges. World Health Organisation, Geneva.

Widiarti, T., Garjito, A., Widyastuti, U., 2016. Genetic diversity of *Anopheles balabacensis*, Baisas base on the second internal transcribed spacer (Its2) ribosomal gene sequence at several areas in Indonesia. Bul. Penel. Kes. 44, 1–12.

Wijayalath, W., Cheesman, S., Tanabe, K., Handunnetti, S., Carter, R., Pathirana, S., 2012. Strain-specific protective effect of the immunity induced by live malarial sporozoites under chloroquine cover. PLoS One 7, e45861.

Wong, M.L., Ahmed, M.A., Sulaiman, W.Y.W., Manin, B.O., Leong, C.S., Quan, F.S., Chua, T.H., Drakeley, C., Snounou, G., Vythilingam, I., 2019. Genetic diversity of zoonotic malaria parasites from mosquito vector and vertebrate hosts. Infect. Genet. Evol. 73, 26–32.

Wong, M.L., Chua, T.H., Leong, C.S., Khaw, L.T., Fornace, K., Wan-Sulaiman, W.-Y., William, T., Drakeley, C., Ferguson, H.M., Vythilingam, I., 2015. Seasonal and spatial dynamics of the primary vector of *Plasmodium knowlesi* within a major transmission focus in Sabah, Malaysia. PLoS. Negl. Trop. Dis. 9, e0004135.

Yap, N.J., Goh, X.T., Koehler, A.V., William, T., Yeo, T.W., Vythilingam, I., Gasser, R.B., Lim, Y.A., 2017. Genetic diversity in the C-terminus of merozoite surface protein among *Plasmodium knowlesi* isolates from Selangor and Sabah Borneo, Malaysia. Infect. Genet. Evol. 54, 39–46.

Yap, N.J., Hossain, H., Raja, T.N., Ngui, R., Muslim, A., Hoh, B.P., Khaw, L.T., Abdul Kadir, K., Divis, P.C.S., Vythilingam, I., Singh, B., Lim, Y.A.L., 2021. Natural human infections with *Plasmodium cynomolgi, Plasmodium inui*, and 4 other simian malaria parasites, Malaysia. Emerg. Infect. Dis. 27, 2187–2191.

Yusof, R., Ahmed, M.A., Jelip, J., Ngian, H.U., Mustakim, S., Hussin, H.M., Fong, M.Y., Mahmud, R., Sitam, F.T., Japning, J.R.-R., Snounou, G., Escalante, A.A., Lau, Y.L., 2016. Phylogeographic evidence for 2 genetically distinct zoonotic *Plasmodium knowlesi* parasites, Malaysia. Emerg. Infect. Dis. 22, 1371–1380.

Zeeman, A.M., Lakshminarayana, S.B., van der Werff, N., Klooster, E.J., Voorberg-van der Wel, A., Kondreddi, R.R., Bodenreider, C., Simon, O., Sauerwein, R., Yeung, B.K., Diagana, T.T., 2016. PI4 kinase is a prophylactic but not radical curative target in *Plasmodium vivax*-type malaria parasites. Antimicrob. Agents Chemother. 60, 2858–2863.

Zeeman, A.M., Van Amsterdam, S.M., McNamara, C.W., Voorberg-Van Der Wel, A., Klooster, E.J., Van Den Berg, A., Remarque, E.J., Plouffe, D.M., Van Gemert, G.J., Luty, A., Sauerwein, R., 2014. KAI407, a potent non-8-aminoquinoline compound that kills *Plasmodium cynomolgi* early dormant liver stage parasites in vitro. Antimicrob. Agents Chemother. 58, 1586–1595.

Zheng, L., Cornel, A.J., Wang, R., Erfle, H., Voss, H., Ansorge, W., Kafatos, F.C., Collins, F.H., 1997. Quantitative trait loci for refractoriness of *Anopheles gambiae* to *Plasmodium cynomolgi* B. Science 276, 425–428.

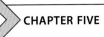

CHAPTER FIVE

Molecular epidemiology and population genomics of *Plasmodium knowlesi*

Paul C.S. Divis[a], Balbir Singh[a], and David J. Conway[a,b,*]
[a]Malaria Research Centre, Universiti Malaysia Sarawak, Kota Samarahan, Sarawak, Malaysia
[b]Department of Infection Biology, London School of Hygiene and Tropical Medicine, London, United Kingdom
[*]Corresponding author: e-mail address: david.conway@lshtm.ac.uk

Contents

1. Molecular detection in discovery of *Plasmodium knowlesi* as a significant zoonosis — 192
2. Molecular surveys of the distribution of *P. knowlesi* infections in humans — 193
   2.1 *P. knowlesi* in humans — 193
   2.2 *P. knowlesi* in primate reservoir hosts — 195
   2.3 *P. knowlesi* in mosquito vectors — 195
3. Early utility of a few genetic loci for analysis of *P. knowlesi* polymorphism — 198
   3.1 Initial informative studies involving sequencing of individual genes — 198
   3.2 Mitochondrial genome sequencing and haplotype relationships — 203
4. Multi-locus microsatellite analyses of *P. knowlesi* uncovers population structure — 205
5. Whole-genome sequence analysis of *P. knowlesi* subpopulation divergence — 208
6. Loci under positive natural selection in the *P. knowlesi* genome — 211
7. Assays for efficient surveillance of different *P. knowlesi* subpopulations — 213
8. Adaptation and the future of *P. knowlesi* emerging from local zoonoses — 215
References — 217

Abstract

Molecular epidemiology has been central to uncovering *P. knowlesi* as an important cause of human malaria in Southeast Asia, and to understanding the complex nature of this zoonosis. Species-specific parasite detection and characterization of sequences were vital to show that *P. knowlesi* was distinct from the human parasite species that had been presumed to cause all malaria. With established sensitive and specific molecular detection tools, surveys subsequently indicated the distribution of *P. knowlesi* infections in humans, wild primate reservoir host species, and mosquito vector species. The importance of studying *P. knowlesi* genetic polymorphism was indicated initially by analysing a few nuclear gene loci as well as the mitochondrial genome, and subsequently by multi-locus microsatellite analyses and whole-genome sequencing. Different human infections generally have unrelated *P. knowlesi* genotypes, acquired from the diverse local parasite reservoirs in macaques. However, individual human infections are usually less genetically complex than those of wild macaques which experience more frequent superinfection with different *P. knowlesi* genotypes. Multi-locus analyses have revealed deep population subdivisions within *P. knowlesi*, which are structured both geographically and in relation to different macaque reservoir host species. Simplified genotypic discrimination assays now enable efficient large-scale surveillance of the sympatric *P. knowlesi* subpopulations within Malaysian Borneo. The whole-genome sequence analyses have also identified loci under recent positive natural selection in the *P. knowlesi* genome, with evidence that different loci are affected in different populations. These provide a foundation to understand recent adaptation of the zoonotic parasite populations, and to track and interpret future changes as they emerge.

1. Molecular detection in discovery of *Plasmodium knowlesi* as a significant zoonosis

Molecular tools have been central to the identification and subsequent understanding of *P. knowlesi* as an important zoonotic parasite. This was initiated by a study on the epidemiology of malaria two decades ago in Malaysian Borneo which led to the discovery of *Plasmodium knowlesi* as a significant cause of human malaria (Singh et al., 2004). At that time, the main cause of malaria in Sarawak state of Malaysian Borneo was *P. vivax*, followed by *P. falciparum* and infections diagnosed by microscopy as '*P. malariae*', although the epidemiology of these '*P. malariae*' infections appeared unusual. While *P. vivax* infections were widely distributed across all the administrative divisions of the state and affected both adults and children, almost half of the '*P. malariae*' cases were reported in the Kapit Division and were mostly in adults. Elsewhere, *P. malariae* infections have usually had relatively low parasitaemia (Garnham, 1966), whereas many of the supposed '*P. malariae*' infections in Kapit required hospitalization and had parasitaemia above 5000 parasites per μL blood. Initial analysis by nested PCR assays based on the small subunit ribosomal (SSUr) RNA genes (Singh et al., 1999) of DNA from 5 blood samples of patients at Kapit Hospital infected with '*P. malariae*' revealed that they contained *Plasmodium* DNA but were negative for *P. malariae* and the other 3 human malaria parasite species.

This initial observation suggested that these patients were either infected with a newly emergent *Plasmodium* species or with a variant of *P. malariae* that had been described elsewhere in Asia (Liu et al., 1998). The first phylogenetic analysis of the partial sequence of the SSU rRNA gene of one of these '*P. malariae*' isolates indicated it was genetically identical with the macaque malaria parasite species *P. knowlesi* and clearly very different from actual *P. malariae*. Subsequent analysis of larger portions of the SSU rRNA genes derived from eight of the supposed '*P. malariae*' patients produced similar results, showing that parasites had a high level of sequence identity with the H strain of *P. knowlesi* that had been isolated from a long-tailed macaque in Peninsular Malaysia decades previously (Chin et al., 1965; Coatney et al., 1971). PCR primers for *P. knowlesi* were developed and together with primers for the human malarias were used to examine blood samples from 208 malaria patients admitted at Kapit Hospital between 2000 and 2002, 141 (68%) of whom were diagnosed by microscopy as having '*P. malariae*' infections. The nested PCR assays revealed that none of the patients was actually infected with *P. malariae*, and that 120 (58%) had either single *P. knowlesi* infections or *P. knowlesi* infections mixed with one of the other human malaria parasite species. The reason for the misdiagnosis by microscopy was that asexual forms of *P. knowlesi* look morphologically similar to those of *P. malariae* on stained slides (Lee et al., 2009), indicating that it is essential to utilize molecular detection methods for correct identification of *P. knowlesi*.

2. Molecular surveys of the distribution of *P. knowlesi* infections in humans

2.1 *P. knowlesi* in humans

The findings of a large focus of human infections with *P. knowlesi* in the Kapit Division of Sarawak led to subsequent reports of human cases of knowlesi malaria at other locations, all of which required the use of molecular methods for identification. The first of these was of a man who had acquired his infection in 2000 in southern Thailand (Jongwutiwes et al., 2004), followed by an extensive study showing the widespread distribution of knowlesi malaria in the states of Sarawak and Sabah in Malaysian Borneo and in Pahang State in Peninsular Malaysia (Cox-Singh et al., 2008) (Table 1). By the end of 2009, knowlesi malaria had been described in Myanmar (Zhu et al., 2006), Singapore (Ng et al., 2008), the Philippines (Luchavez et al., 2008) and Vietnam (Van Den Eede et al., 2009), and reports over the following years indicated that the range extended to Kalimantan (Figtree et al., 2010) and Sumatra (Lubis et al., 2017) in Indonesia, Brunei (UK Health Protection Agency, 2011), Laos (Iwagami et al., 2018), and the Andaman and Nicobar Islands of India (Tyagi et al., 2013).

Many of the initial reports from individual countries were of a single or a relatively small number of knowlesi malaria cases, based mainly on malaria patients at hospitals (Table 1). However, as more extensive studies using molecular detection methods were undertaken in communities as well as hospitals, it became clear that human infections with *P. knowlesi* were more prevalent and widespread than previously thought in Thailand

Table 1 Initial reports of human *P. knowlesi* malaria cases at various locations in Asia using molecular methods of detection.

Location	Detection methods used	No of cases	Dates of infections	Reference
Sarawak, Malaysian Borneo	Nested PCR and sequencing	120	2000–2002	Singh et al. (2004)
Thailand	Nested PCR and sequencing	1	2000	Jongwutiwes et al. (2004)
Myanmar	Nested PCR	1	1998	Zhu et al. (2006)
Pahang, Peninsular Malaysia	Nested PCR	5	2004–2005	Cox-Singh et al. (2008)
Sabah, Malaysian Borneo	Nested PCR	41	2003–2005	Cox-Singh et al. (2008)
Palawan, Philippines	Nested PCR	5	2006	Luchavez et al. (2008)
Singapore	Nested PCR and sequencing	1	2007	Ng et al. (2008)
South Kalimantan, Indonesia	Nested PCR and sequencing	1	2010	Figtree et al. (2010)
Cambodia	Nested PCR and sequencing	2	2007–2010	Khim et al. (2011)
Vietnam	Nested PCR and sequencing	3	2004	Van Den Eede et al. (2009)
Brunei	Not stated	1	2006	UK Health Protection Agency (2011)
Andaman and Nicobar Islands, India	Nested PCR and sequencing	53	2004–2010	Tyagi et al. (2013)
North Sumatra, Indonesia	Nested PCR	377	2015	Lubis et al. (2017)
Laos	Real-time PCR and sequencing	1	2016	Iwagami et al. (2018)

(Jongwutiwes et al., 2011; Putaporntip et al., 2009), Myanmar (Jiang et al., 2010), Malaysia (Cooper et al., 2020; Cox-Singh et al., 2008; Joveen-Neoh et al., 2011; Naing et al., 2011; Siner et al., 2017; Vythilingam et al., 2008; Yusof et al., 2014), Laos (Pongvongsa et al., 2018), Vietnam (Marchand et al., 2011; Pongvongsa et al., 2018) and Indonesia (Herdiana et al., 2018).

Furthermore, asymptomatic infections of *P. knowlesi* were described in Vietnam (Pongvongsa et al., 2018; Van Den Eede et al., 2009), Cambodia (Imwong et al., 2019), Malaysian Borneo (Fornace et al., 2016b; Siner et al., 2017) and Peninsular Malaysia (Jiram et al., 2016), indicating the importance of community-based sampling to more fully understand the epidemiology of knowlesi malaria.

2.2 *P. knowlesi* in primate reservoir hosts

Long-tailed macaques (*Macaca fascicularis*) were first implicated as natural hosts for *P. knowlesi* by early studies at the Calcutta School of Tropical Medicine in India in the 1930s on macaques imported from Singapore (Knowles and Das Gupta, 1932). Over the following decades, *P. knowlesi* was detected by slide examination of blood from long-tailed macaques sampled elsewhere in Southeast Asia, as well as from pig-tailed macaques (*M. nemestrina*), and occasionally from leaf monkeys (Coatney et al., 1971). More recently, using molecular detection methods, the presence of *P. knowlesi* has been confirmed in wild long-tailed macaques in Peninsular Malaysia (Akter et al., 2015; Vythilingam et al., 2008), Malaysian Borneo (Lee et al., 2011), Thailand (Putaporntip et al., 2010), Singapore (Jeslyn et al., 2011; Li et al., 2021), the Philippines (Gamalo et al., 2019) and Laos (Zhang et al., 2016) (Table 2). Molecular methods have also detected *P. knowlesi* in pig-tailed macaques in Thailand (Putaporntip et al., 2010) and Malaysian Borneo (Lee et al., 2011), in dusky leaf monkeys (*Trachypithecus obscurus*) in Thailand (Putaporntip et al., 2010), and in a stump-tailed macaque (*Macaca arctoides*) in Thailand (Fungfuang et al., 2020) (Table 2).

2.3 *P. knowlesi* in mosquito vectors

Anopheles hackeri was the first vector described for *P. knowlesi*, shown by inoculating sporozoites from a wild-caught mosquito into a laboratory-bred rhesus macaque (*M. mulatta*) (Coatney et al., 1971). More recently, molecular detection assays for malaria parasites have improved the means to correctly identify sporozoites within mosquitoes, thereby making it simpler to identify vectors of particular malaria parasite species. Molecular approaches were first employed in entomological studies to identify vectors of knowlesi malaria in the Kapit Division of Sarawak, and *An. latens* was incriminated as the vector (Tan et al., 2008; Vythilingam et al., 2006). Similar approaches were utilized in other parts of Malaysian Borneo (Ang et al., 2020, 2021; Brown et al., 2020; Hawkes et al., 2019; Wong et al., 2015), Peninsular Malaysia (Jiram et al., 2012; Vythilingam et al., 2008), and Vietnam (Nakazawa et al., 2009), showing that the main vector species for knowlesi

Table 2 Prevalence of *Plasmodium knowlesi* infections in non-human primate host species using molecular methods of detection in surveys of different areas in Southeast Asia.

Locality	Non-human primate	Total no. examined	*P.k.* positive	% *P.k.* positive	Dates of samples	Reference
Sarawak, Malaysian Borneo	*Macaca fascicularis*	82	71	86.6	2004–2008	Lee et al. (2011)
Sarawak, Malaysian Borneo	*M. nemestrina*	26	13	50	2004–2008	Lee et al. (2011)
Pahang, Peninsular Malaysia	*M. fascicularis*	75	10	6.9	2007	Vythilingam et al. (2008)
Hulu Selangor, Peninsular Malaysia	*M. fascicularis*	70	21	30	2014	Akter et al. (2015)
Western Catchment, Singapore	*M. fascicularis*	3	3	100	2007 and 2009	Jeslyn et al. (2011)
Western Catchment, Singapore	*M. fascicularis*	379	142	37.5	2009–2017	Li et al. (2021)
Narathiwat, Thailand	*M. fascicularis*	186	1	0.5	2008–2009	Putaporntip et al. (2010)
Narathiwat, Thailand	*M. nemestrina*	373	5	1.3	2008–2009	Putaporntip et al. (2010)
Narathiwat, Thailand	*Trachypithecus obscurus*	7	1	14.3	2008–2009	Putaporntip et al. (2010)
Prachuap Kiri Khan, Thailand	*M. arctoides*	32	1	3.1	2017–2019	Fungfuang et al. (2020)
Laos	*M. fascicularis*	44	1	2.3	2013	Zhang et al. (2016)
Palawan, Philippines	*M. fascicularis*	95	18	18.9	2017	Gamalo et al. (2019)

Table 3 Surveys identifying *P. knowlesi* infections in mosquito vector species using molecular methods of detection.

Locality	Vector identified	Detection method	Period of study	Reference
Kapit district, Sarawak, Malaysian Borneo	*An. latens*	Nested PCR	2005–2006	Vythilingam et al. (2006), Tan et al. (2008)
Lawas district, Sarawak, Malaysian Borneo	*An. latens, An. donaldi*	Nested PCR and sequencing of SSU rRNA gene	2014–2015	Ang et al. (2020)
Betong district, Sarawak, Malaysian Borneo	*An. latens, An. introlatus, An. roperi, An. collessi*	Nested PCR and sequencing of SSU rRNA gene	2015–2016	Ang et al. (2021)
Kuala Lipis district, Pahang, Peninsular Malaysia	*An. cracens*	Nested PCR	2007–2008	Vythilingam et al. (2008), Jiram et al. (2012)
Banggi Island and Kudat district, Sabah, Malaysian Borneo	*An. balabacensis*	Nested PCR	2013–2015	Wong et al. (2015)
Ranau district, Sabah, Malaysian Borneo	*An. balabacensis*	Nested PCR	2015–2016	Hawkes et al. (2019)
Keningau district, Sabah, Malaysian Borneo	*An. donaldi*	Nested PCR	2015–2016	Hawkes et al. (2019)
Pitas district, Sabah, Malaysian Borneo	*An. balabacensis*	Nested PCR	2016	Brown et al. (2020)
Khanh Vinh district, Khanh Hoa, Vietnam	*An. dirus*	Nested PCR, PCR and sequencing of *csp* gene	2008	Nakazawa et al. (2009)
Khanh Phu, Khanh Hoa, Vietnam	*An. dirus*	Nested PCR and PCR of *csp* gene	2009–2010	Marchand et al. (2011)

malaria varied at different locations (Table 3). Furthermore, in addition to members of the Leucosphyrus Group which were initially thought to be the only vectors capable of transmitting *P. knowlesi* in nature, members of the Umbrosus Group were also found to be capable of transmitting *P. knowlesi* in the Betong district of Sarawak, Malaysian Borneo (Ang et al., 2021).

3. Early utility of a few genetic loci for analysis of *P. knowlesi* polymorphism

3.1 Initial informative studies involving sequencing of individual genes

A common purpose of sequencing an individual parasite gene is to confirm the identification of the parasite species within a sample from a vertebrate host or mosquito. Although such analysis is limited in scope, it is preferable to merely counting a sample as positive by detecting a PCR product using species-specific primers. A main reason is that natural nucleotide polymorphisms normally commonly occur among parasite samples of any species, and identification of nucleotide differences among different samples can help confirm that PCR-positivity is not a result of laboratory PCR-contamination. Indeed, such natural sequence polymorphisms within-species often exist in loci that are widely used for discriminating different species, such as the small subunit ribosomal RNA (SSUrRNA) gene, or single-copy essential protein-coding genes.

Extending this, analysis of a second or third gene for species confirmation gives added confidence that contamination or misidentification has not occurred. This was done in the initial characterization of *P. knowlesi* as a major zoonosis in Malaysian Borneo (Singh et al., 2004), which is illustrated here by showing sequence variation in the circumsporozoite (*csp*) gene in the first clinical isolates of *P. knowlesi* that were analysed when the existence of the zoonosis was not already known (Fig. 1). This was done at the time for further confirmation, as the sequences of the SSUrRNA gene in the samples had also been analysed in parallel, showing nucleotide polymorphism that clearly indicated that the samples were from a natural *P. knowlesi* population that was unexpected in humans (Singh et al., 2004).

Following this first molecular description of the zoonosis, characterization of *P. knowlesi* clinical infections in Thailand included analysis of SSUrRNA gene sequences, which showed polymorphism as would be

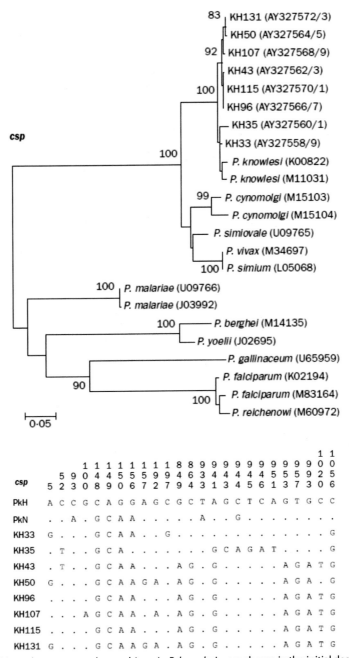

Fig. 1 Natural sequence polymorphisms in *P. knowlesi* were shown in the initial description of zoonotic cases in Malaysian Borneo. This figure shows data for the circumsporozoite protein (*csp*) gene in the first eight clinical isolates analysed (labelled 'KH' for Kapit Hospital). The top panel indicates that the clinical isolates clustered closely with the two previously available *P. knowlesi* sequences from parasites maintained in laboratory macaques, confirming the species identification, and that the sequences of the individual samples were not identical. The bottom panel shows an alignment of the polymorphic nucleotide sites for these samples together with the two previous *P. knowlesi* sequences. *Figure incorporating reproduction with permission.* Singh, B., Kim Sung, L., Matusop, A., Radhakrishnan, A., Shamsul, S. S., Cox-Singh, J., Thomas, A., Conway, D.J., 2004. A large focus of naturally acquired Plasmodium knowlesi infections in human beings. Lancet 363, 1017–1024.

expected from a natural zoonotic infection (Jongwutiwes et al., 2004; Putaporntip et al., 2009). Although only a few local samples from macaques positive for *P. knowlesi* were available at the time, they showed sequences similar to those in the human infections, consistent with the local human infections being zoonotic (Putaporntip et al., 2009). Subsequent analysis in Thailand included a few more samples of *P. knowlesi* from macaques along with human cases, and analysed sequences of the merozoite surface protein 1 (*msp1*) gene which gave consistent results, showing that the diversity of sequences among different patients was similar to the diversity of sequences from local macaques (Jongwutiwes et al., 2011).

There are ongoing examples of local identification of zoonoses, where description of natural sequence variation is a part of the initial description, and this is now being done in analyses of *P. cynomolgi* in humans alongside *P. knowlesi*. For example, samples of zoonotic *P. knowlesi* and *P. cynomolgi* infections in the south of Thailand show polymorphism in the mitochondrial cytochrome *b* (*cytb*) gene within each parasite species, as expected for local zoonoses (Fig. 2) (Putaporntip et al., 2021). It is known that both of these species are transmitted to humans from wild macaques, although the numbers of cases of *P. knowlesi* are much higher than those of *P. cynomolgi*.

Analysis of *P. knowlesi* in multiple samples of humans and macaques from the same area was first focused on the Kapit District of Sarawak in Malaysian Borneo, where most zoonotic cases were first described. This showed that the macaques had more *P. knowlesi* genotypes per infection, as illustrated for *csp* gene sequence data (Fig. 3), most individual human infections having an unmixed parasite allele sequence and most macaque infections containing multiple alleles, consistent with the expectation that transmission is more common among macaques which causes superinfection of different parasite genotypes. However, at the local population level the overall sequence variation was similar among infections of humans and macaques, with no evidence of only a restricted set of genotypes being seen in either (Fig. 3).

A study of sequence variation in the merozoite surface protein 1 gene (*msp1*) in a small number of *P. knowlesi* isolates from humans and macaques of Thailand suggested higher haplotype diversity in *P. knowlesi* isolated from humans than those of macaques (Putaporntip et al., 2013). However, the numbers of samples were very small, and as *msp1* is under strong natural

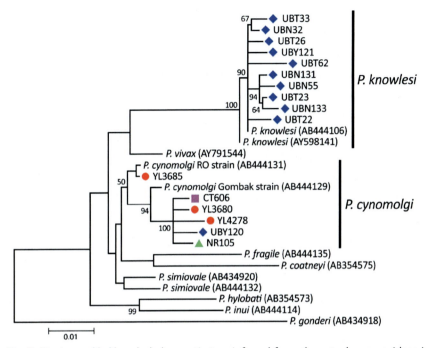

Fig. 2 Maximum-likelihood phylogenetic tree inferred from the cytochrome oxidase I (*cox1*) gene in the parasite mitochondrial genome. Isolates of *Plasmodium cynomolgi* and *P. knowlesi* from Thailand are compared with selected sequence data previously obtained from these and other species (GenBank accession numbers in parentheses). Colours and symbols indicate different provinces in Thailand from which the individual human cases were sampled. Bootstrap confidence values exceeding 50% are shown on the branches. Scale bar indicates nucleotide substitutions per site. *Figure reproduced under Creative Commons licence. Putaporntip, C., Kuamsab, N., Pattanawong, U., Yanmanee, S., Seethamchai, S., Jongwutiwes, S., 2021. Plasmodium cynomolgi co-infections among symptomatic malaria patients, Thailand. Emerg. Infect. Dis. 27, 590–593.*

selection in most parasite species its use as a single marker was not ideal. This emphasized the need to study different genetic loci, including those in which variation is largely selectively neutral.

It is clear that sequence analysis of one or a few genes is useful for confirmation of parasite species, and to give an initial assessment of whether individual samples are genetically different from each other. Beyond this, application of sequencing and genotyping for molecular epidemiological studies of malaria benefit from analysis of multiple genetic loci. The information from the sequence of each gene is very limited, and distribution of

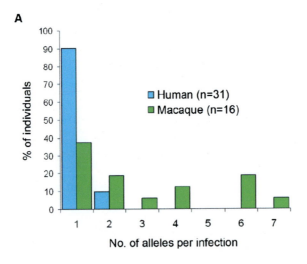

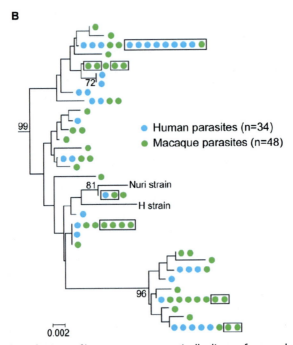

Fig. 3 *P. knowlesi* infections of humans are as genetically diverse from each other as infections of local reservoir hosts, but are less mixed genotypically. The panels show data from analyses of *P. knowlesi* circumsporozoite protein gene (*csp*) gene sequences from infections of macaques and humans in the Kapit division of Sarawak in Malaysian Borneo. (A) Histogram showing proportion of human (blue) and macaque (green) individuals with different numbers of *P. knowlesi csp* alleles detected per infection. (B) Diversity of *P. knowlesi csp* alleles as indicated by a Neighbour-Joining tree diagram based on a distance matrix of pairwise sequence differences in the non-repeat region of the gene. Figures on the branches are bootstrap confidence percentages above 70%, and scale bar indicates proportion of nucleotide differences per site. *Figure reproduced under Creative Commons licence. Lee, K.S., Divis, P.C., Zakaria, S.K., Matusop, A., Julin, R.A., Conway, D.J., Cox-Singh, J., Singh, B., 2011. Plasmodium knowlesi: reservoir hosts and tracking the emergence in humans and macaques. PLoS Pathog. 7, e1002015.*

polymorphism seen among samples for any one gene is not reliably representative of what would be seen in other genes. As frequent recombination normally occurs in malaria parasite populations, the patterns of polymorphism seen at different loci in the genome are not linked, so analysis of multiple loci is required to understand how individual samples or geographical sub-populations are related.

3.2 Mitochondrial genome sequencing and haplotype relationships

The two extrachromosomal genomes of the parasite, in the mitochondria and apicoplast organelles, are exceptional in this respect. As they are not subject to recombination, analysis of sequences of these organellar genomes allow a phylogenetic perspective on relatedness between individuals or population samples. The greatest information on the mitochondrial and apicoplast lineages is derived from analysis of the entire genomes of 6 kb and 35 kb respectively. For *P. knowlesi*, such analysis was first performed for the mitochondrial genome by comparing samples from humans and wild macaques in the area of Malaysian Borneo where most cases were initially described (Lee et al., 2011). This confirmed that there was greater within-infection sequence diversity in most macaque infections compared to each human infection, but that the sequence variants were shared among samples from humans and macaques suggesting that there is no distinct genetic subpopulation infecting humans (Fig. 4).

Further analysis of the *P. knowlesi* mitochondrial DNA SNPs and haplotype tree structure in the same study suggested that the parasite derived from an ancestral parasite population more than approximately 100,000 years ago, before human settlement in Southeast Asia. As is the case today, the local macaque species were likely the major natural hosts throughout this time. However, the shape of the mitochondrial DNA phylogeny also suggested that *P. knowlesi* may have had significant population expansion approximately 30,000–40,000 years ago, at a time when Borneo was part of mainland Southeast Asia and when the human population was growing in the region (Lee et al., 2011).

Another question arising from early gene sequencing studies is whether *P. knowlesi* had significant geographical population substructure, and initial analyses of sequence variation in individual genes indicated divergence

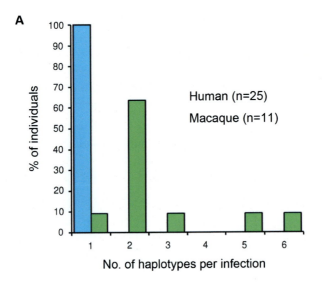

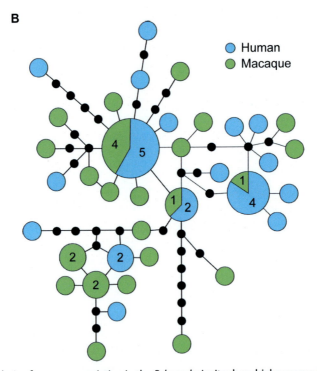

Fig. 4 Analysis of sequence variation in the *P. knowlesi* mitochondrial genome (mtDNA) in the Kapit Division of Sarawak confirms that most human infections are genotypically unmixed, but that they are as diverse from each other as infections in local reservoir hosts. (A) Histogram showing proportion of human (blue) and macaque (green) individuals containing different numbers of *P. knowlesi* mtDNA haplotypes per infection. (B) Schematic diagram showing relationship among 37 mtDNA haplotypes of *P. knowlesi*. Numbers in larger circles represent number of haplotypes and unnumbered circles represent a single haplotype. Each line connecting the circles represents a mutational step and black dots represent hypothetical missing intermediates. *Figure adapted under Creative Commons licence. Lee, K.S., Divis, P.C., Zakaria, S.K., Matusop, A., Julin, R.A., Conway, D.J., Cox-Singh, J., Singh, B., 2011. Plasmodium knowlesi: reservoir hosts and tracking the emergence in humans and macaques. PLoS Pathog. 7, e1002015.*

between parasites from Borneo and mainland Southeast Asia. Several separate studies focused on genes encoding the Duffy binding protein (DBP)-α (Fong et al., 2015), one of its paralogues DBP-γ (Fong et al., 2016), a normocyte-binding protein homologue NBPXa (Ahmed et al., 2016), mitochondrial cytochrome oxidase I (Yusof et al., 2016), as well as the SSUrRNA gene (Yusof et al., 2016), each giving concordant overall results. Each of these indicated that, as would be expected, there is significant genetic subdivision between geographical populations of the parasite that have been separated by the South China Sea since the end of the last ice age approximately 13,000 years ago. However, to gain sufficient information for a more complete understanding of population genetic structure requires simultaneous analysis of a larger number of loci.

4. Multi-locus microsatellite analyses of *P. knowlesi* uncovers population structure

As noted above, to study population genetic structure, the use of multiple genetic markers that are not under selection is recommended. Therefore a *P. knowlesi* genotyping toolkit was developed, based on 10 microsatellite loci distributed across the genome (Divis et al., 2015), chosen from a wide range of potential loci identified from examining the original *P. knowlesi* reference genome sequence (Pain et al., 2008). These assays involve targeted amplification of polymorphic simple sequence repeat loci, using a two-step heminested PCR with dye-labelled internal primer for each locus, enabling some multiplexing of loci in the process of electrophoretic analysis of allele sequence lengths.

This toolkit was initially applied to analyse *P. knowlesi* infections in humans and wild macaques from Kapit division of Sarawak state, Malaysian Borneo, and uncovered a quite unexpected population genetic substructure. Of 167 human *P. knowlesi* infections tested, a statistical Bayesian model-based analysis indicated approximately two thirds were of a genetic subpopulation (termed Cluster 1) which is also associated with long-tailed macaque hosts, while approximately one third were of another genetic subpopulation (termed Cluster 2) otherwise associated with pig-tailed macaque hosts (Divis et al., 2015) (Fig. 5).

Further surveillance using multilocus microsatellite analysis was then conducted on more human and macaque infections across Malaysia. Analysis of 583 *P. knowlesi* infections from nine localities across Malaysian

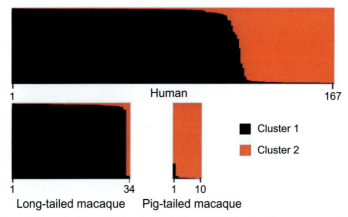

Fig. 5 Two divergent *P. knowlesi* subpopulations in Malaysian Borneo associated with different macaque host species. Multi-locus microsatellite analysis on *P. knowlesi* isolated from patients (*N* = 167) and wild macaques (*N* = 44) in Kapit division of Sarawak reveals an admixture of two divergent subpopulations in humans that are otherwise associated with long-tailed macaque (Cluster 1 in 33 out of 34) and pig-tailed macaque (Cluster 2 in all 10) hosts. Each individual infection is represented vertically in the scheme, with proportional assignment to either of the two subpopulation clusters as defined by STRUCTURE analysis. *Figure incorporating reproduction under Creative Commons licence. Divis, P.C., Singh, B., Anderios, F., Hisam, S., Matusop, A., Kocken, C.H., Assefa, S.A., Duffy, C.W., Conway, D.J., 2015. Admixture in humans of two divergent Plasmodium knowlesi populations associated with different macaque host species. PLoS Pathog. 11, e1004888.*

Borneo from the first (Divis et al., 2015) and subsequent (Divis et al., 2017) studies showed Cluster 1 and Cluster 2 subpopulations to be widely distributed in Malaysian Borneo (Fig. 6). Cluster 1 parasites were predominant in frequency at most of the sites, although Cluster 2 was more common at two of the sites (in Kanowit and Miri Districts of Sarawak). Although Cluster 2 subpopulation is associated with pig-tailed macaque reservoir hosts, it is unknown if differences in abundance of this macaque species determines the variation in the distribution, or if it is due to different mosquito vectors being responsible, as more studies are needed on the transmission.

Genetic differentiation between *P. knowlesi* infections in Malaysian Borneo and Peninsular Malaysia was expected, given the geographical separation of macaques in these different landmass areas for approximately 13,000 years since the last glacial period (Fa and Lindberg, 1996; Ziegler et al., 2007). Allopatric divergence in the parasite would be inevitably

Molecular and genomic epidemiology of *P. knowlesi*

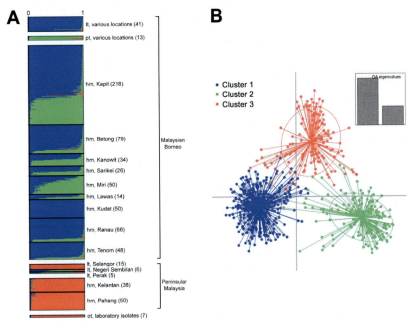

Fig. 6 Population genetic structure of *P. knowlesi* across Malaysia, as inferred by multi-locus microsatellite analysis of 751 infections in humans ('hm') and macaques ('lt' indicates long-tailed *M. fascicularis*, and 'pt' pig-tailed *M. nemestrina*). Three divergent subpopulations of *P. knowlesi* are revealed using different tests, illustrated by (A) STRUCTURE k-means cluster assignment analysis (each infection is represented horizontally on the scheme, with numbers of infections in each area being shown in brackets), and (B) discriminant analysis of principal components (DAPC) (each infection is represented by a single point on this scheme). While Cluster 1 and Cluster 2 subpopulations occur in Malaysian Borneo with each associated with different macaque hosts, the Cluster 3 subpopulation occurs in peninsular Malaysia. *Figure incorporating reproduction under Creative Commons licence. Divis, P.C., Lin, L.C., Rovie-Ryan, J.J., Kadir, K.A., Anderios, F., Hisam, S., Sharma, R.S., Singh, B., Conway, D.J., 2017. Three divergent subpopulations of the malaria parasite Plasmodium knowlesi. Emerg. Infect. Dis. 23, 616–624.*

caused by the ocean barrier between mainland Southeast Asia and Borneo which restricts the movement of the macaque hosts (Liedigk et al., 2015). With the inclusion of more *P. knowlesi* clinical infections from Peninsular Malaysia, microsatellite analysis confirmed a genetically separate subpopulation (Cluster 3) divergent from those in Malaysian Borneo (Fig. 6) (Divis et al., 2017), which had been indicated by genome sequencing of older laboratory-maintained isolates as described below (Assefa et al., 2015).

5. Whole-genome sequence analysis of *P. knowlesi* subpopulation divergence

Divergence between the genetically-distinct *P. knowlesi* subpopulation Clusters 1 and 2 in Malaysian Borneo was supported by the analysis of whole genome sequences from a subset of the clinical isolates that had been analysed by microsatellite analyses (Assefa et al., 2015) (Fig. 5), and also seen in a separate study of genome sequences from a few other clinical isolates in Malaysian Borneo (Pinheiro et al., 2015). The population substructure defined by genome sequences gave concordant classification with the microsatellite analysis, including evidence for a third genetic subpopulation (Cluster 3) which was initially represented by older laboratory isolates that had originated from Peninsular Malaysia.

Genome sequence analysis of 103 clinical isolates sampled across Malaysia shows the three subpopulation clusters (Fig. 7) (Assefa et al., 2015; Divis et al., 2018; Hocking et al., 2020). A genome-wide scan shows similar level of nucleotide diversity within both Cluster 1 and Cluster 3 subpopulations, but a lower diversity within the Cluster 2 subpopulation (Fig. 7). The reduced genetic diversity of the Cluster 2 subpopulation suggests an initial bottleneck during formation of this subpopulation in the pig-tailed macaque natural hosts (Divis et al., 2018). The timing of genetic divergence between the different *P. knowlesi* subpopulation clusters remains to be determined, but it is likely to be more recent than when the different macaque reservoir host species diverged.

Pairwise comparisons of genome-wide scans among the three *P. knowlesi* subpopulations shows substantial divergence in all of the 14 different parasite chromosomes (Fig. 8). There are some variations in the levels of divergence genome-wide which are usefully examined with each of the pairwise comparisons. For example, comparison between the sympatric Cluster 1 and Cluster 2 from Malaysian Borneo shows particularly high level of divergence in chromosomes 7, 12 and 13, which exceeds the level of divergence in the comparison between the allopatric Cluster 1 and Cluster 3 (the latter being from Peninsular Malaysia) (Hocking et al., 2020).

Genome-wide scan of fixation indices (F_{ST}) between Cluster 1 and Cluster 2 subpopulations shows heterogeneity across the genome due to the mosaic structure of diversity within Cluster 2 (Divis et al., 2018; Hocking et al., 2020). This enabled the identification of genomic islands of

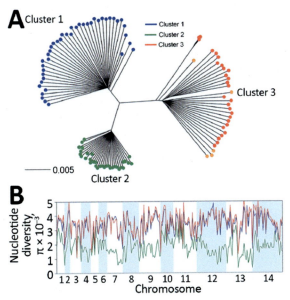

Fig. 7 Genome-wide sequence analysis of *P. knowlesi* clinical isolates sampled across Malaysia. (A) Population genomic structure of *P. knowlesi* infections as shown by a Neighbour-Joining dendrogram of the pairwise genetic distance based on single nucleotide polymorphisms. (B) Genome-wide scans on non-overlapping windows of 50 kb show similar pattern of nucleotide diversity for Cluster 1 (blue) and Cluster 3 (red) subpopulations across 14 chromosomes which are overall higher than the Cluster 2 (green) subpopulation. *Figure incorporating reproduction under Creative Commons licence. Hocking, S.E., Divis, P.C.S., Kadir, K.A., Singh, B., Conway, D.J., 2020. Population genomic structure and recent evolution of Plasmodium knowlesi, Peninsular Malaysia. Emerg. Infect. Dis. 26, 1749–1758.*

differentiation, and definition of high divergence regions (HDR) and low divergence regions (LDR) (Fig. 9). Considering the standard deviations of the mean genome-wide F_{ST} values between Cluster 1 and Cluster 2 subpopulations, contiguous windows of HDRs were mainly covering chromosomes 7, 12 and 13, while none were found in chromosome 3, 5 and 10. The Cluster 2 subpopulation showed reduced mean nucleotide diversity in the HDRs compared to Cluster 1, consistent with the possibility of a bottleneck event in the formation of the Cluster 2 subpopulation (Divis et al., 2018).

Analysis of the population genetic structure of *P. knowlesi* Cluster 3 in Peninsular Malaysia also indicates an unexpected feature. A minority of the clinical cases analysed contained highly-related *P. knowlesi* genome

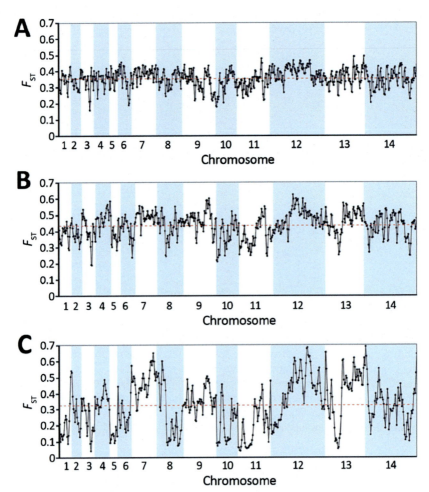

Fig. 8 Genome-wide scan of divergence between *P. knowlesi* subpopulations. The fixation index (F_{ST}) scan of divergence was performed to compare different pairs of subpopulation clusters: (A) Cluster 1 vs Cluster 3, (B) Cluster 2 vs Cluster 3, and (C) Cluster 1 vs Cluster 2. The F_{ST} scores, marked as solid dots, are mean values within windows of 500 consecutive SNPs with overlapping by 250 SNPs. *Figure incorporating reproduction under Creative Commons licence. Hocking, S.E., Divis, P.C.S., Kadir, K.A., Singh, B., Conway, D.J., 2020. Population genomic structure and recent evolution of Plasmodium knowlesi, Peninsular Malaysia. Emerg. Infect. Dis. 26, 1749–1758.*

sequences, which contrasts to the general pattern in which all other *P. knowlesi* infections have unrelated sequences (Hocking et al., 2020). Although uncommon, clinical cases with this unusual parasite type (provisionally termed Cluster 3C) were identified in different hospitals in 3

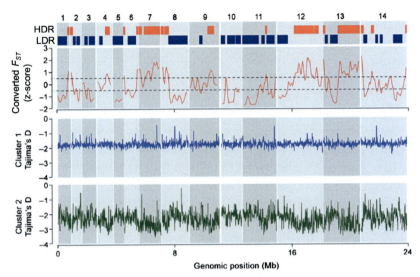

Fig. 9 Contiguous high and low divergence regions (HDR and LDR) throughout the *P. knowlesi* genome in comparison of Cluster 1 and Cluster 2 subpopulations in Malaysian Borneo. The highest divergence between Cluster 1 and Cluster 2 is observed in chromosomes 7, 12 and 13 where HDRs cover most of the respective chromosome lengths. Both subpopulations show skew towards low-frequency variants, based on scans of Tajima's *D* values in 10-kb windows genome-wide, with Cluster 1 subpopulation exhibiting less genome-wide variation of the frequency spectrum compared to Cluster 2. *Figure incorporating reproduction under Creative Commons licence. Divis, P.C.S., Duffy, C.W., Kadir, K.A., Singh, B., Conway, D.J., 2018. Genome-wide mosaicism in divergence between zoonotic malaria parasite subpopulations with separate sympatric transmission cycles. Mol. Ecol. 2, 860–870.*

different states in Peninsular Malaysia, so further sampling and analysis is needed to indicate if this is an emerging new sub-population or if it reflects an unknown and distinct zoonotic cycle (Hocking et al., 2020).

6. Loci under positive natural selection in the *P. knowlesi* genome

The genome-wide scan also showed a strong skew towards low allele frequency variants in all three *P. knowlesi* subpopulations based on the Tajima's *D* statistics, indicating long-term population size expansion (Divis et al., 2018) (Fig. 9). However, the mean genome-wide *D* values for Cluster 2 were lower than for the sympatric Cluster 1. There are also apparent differences when individual genes expected to be under balancing selection are considered. A few well-studied genes that are likely targets of immunity were indicated to be under balancing selection in a subpopulation-specific manner, including the *csp* and *trap* genes in Cluster 1, the *ama1* gene in Cluster 2, and a 6-cysteine protein gene and *msp7*-like gene in Cluster 3 (Assefa et al., 2015; Divis et al., 2018; Hocking et al., 2020). From these examples, it appears that there may be variation in the strength or targets of balancing selection in the divergent subpopulations of *P. knowlesi*.

Moreover, scans for evidence of recent positive directional selection, indicated by extended haplotype homozygosity on particular chromosomal loci, have implicated different loci in different *P. knowlesi* subpopulations. Particularly, the initial study of Cluster 1 in Malaysian Borneo indicated recent selection on several genomic loci, the strongest signature being identified on chromosome 8 (Assefa et al., 2015). This signature of positive selection on chromosome 8 was confirmed by a secondary analysis of the sequence data performed after mapping to an alternatively-generated reference genome sequence (Diez Benavente et al., 2017). In contrast, analysis of the Cluster 3 subpopulation in Peninsular Malaysia did not indicate such a strong signature of selection on chromosome 8, but indicated that there are loci on four other chromosomes (numbers 1, 7, 9 and 12) that have been under recent positive directional selection (Hocking et al., 2020) (Fig. 10).

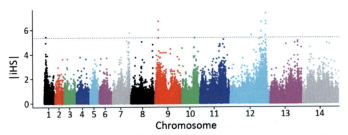

Fig. 10 Evidence of *P. knowlesi* genomic regions under recent positive directional selection in Peninsular Malaysia (Cluster 3 subpopulation) using the standardized integrated haplotype score |iHS| index. Examination of the ranges of extended haplotype homozygosity for individual SNPs identified four distinct genomic windows with high |iHS| values. Two of these regions (on chromosomes 1 and 9) spanned across members of *SICAvar* and *kir* multigene families, while the other two (on chromosomes 7 and 12) did not include *SICAvar* or *kir* genes. These genomic regions are different from those implicated to be under selection in the Cluster 1 subpopulation of *P. knowlesi* in Malaysian Borneo in a separate study (Assefa et al., 2015), indicating that signatures of recent selection are population-specific as expected. *Figure incorporating reproduction under Creative Commons licence. Hocking, S.E., Divis, P.C.S., Kadir, K.A., Singh, B., Conway, D.J., 2020. Population genomic structure and recent evolution of Plasmodium knowlesi, Peninsular Malaysia. Emerg. Infect. Dis. 26, 1749–1758.*

This confirms that adaptation and evolution of the different *P. knowlesi* subpopulations is proceeding independently, and they can be considered as distinct zoonoses, from each of which new and distinct parasite phenotypes may emerge. Understanding this is important for the molecular epidemiology of zoonotic *P. knowlesi* malaria, including tracking of the parasite populations as they adapt to environmental changes.

7. Assays for efficient surveillance of different *P. knowlesi* subpopulations

Given the occurrence of two genetically divergent *P. knowlesi* subpopulations in Malaysian Borneo (Clusters 1 and 2) associated with different macaque reservoir hosts (Assefa et al., 2015; Divis et al., 2015), which was revealed by analysing multiple loci as noted above, a simpler genotyping method has been developed to discriminate these in large scale surveys. Allele-specific PCR primers that were diagnostic for the alternative *P. knowlesi* subpopulation Clusters 1 and 2 were designed based on fixed SNP differences identified from the analysis of whole-genome sequences of clinical isolates. Each PCR assay showed a high level of sensitivity and specificity in detecting the respective subpopulation (Assefa et al., 2015; Divis et al., 2020), indicating a potentially useful method to identify the source of *P. knowlesi* infections in humans associated with different macaque host species in Borneo.

This simple PCR method of discriminating the sympatric *P. knowlesi* Clusters 1 and 2 is much less costly and time-consuming compared to multi-locus microsatellite analysis or genome sequencing. A first application of this method was performed, in analysis of samples from 1492 infections that had been previously collected in Malaysian Borneo over a 20-year period. This confirmed that overall approximately 70% of human infections were of the Cluster 1 type and approximately 30% of the Cluster 2 type, with few cases containing both (Fig. 11). The relative proportions of these vary across Malaysian Borneo, with Cluster 1 being the most common in many areas, but a few areas having Cluster 2 as the predominant subpopulation. It is most plausible that this spatial variation in the relative proportions of these types in human infections is due to differences in the local relative abundance or habitat preference of the two macaque reservoir host species, although this has yet to be confirmed through systematic sampling of reservoir hosts in different parts of Malaysian Borneo (Fig. 11).

Temporal analysis on 1204 *P. knowlesi* infections in Kapit division in Malaysian Borneo show stable relative frequencies over 20 years, with

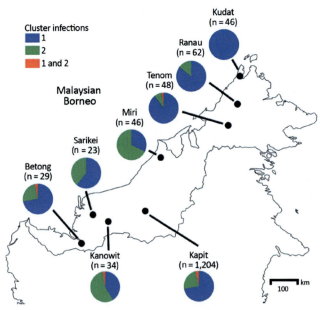

Fig. 11 Proportions of human *P. knowlesi* infections with Cluster 1 and Cluster 2 subpopulations across Malaysian Borneo. Cluster 1 subpopulations predominate in many locations compared to Cluster 2 subpopulations, which is consistent with long-tailed macaques being generally more common than pig-tailed macaques, although there may be other reasons for the variation apart from different reservoir host abundance. The genotyping of different divergent subpopulations *P. knowlesi* can be performed rapidly using simple allele-specific PCR assays. *Figure incorporating reproduction under Creative Commons licence. Divis, P.C.S., Hu, T.H., Kadir, K.A., Mohammad, D.S.A., Hii, K.C., Daneshvar, C., Conway, D.J., Singh, B., 2020. Efficient surveillance of Plasmodium knowlesi genetic subpopulations, Malaysian Borneo, 2000-2018. Emerg. Infect. Dis. 26, 1392–1398.*

approximately two thirds of infections being of the Cluster 1 type and one third of the Cluster 2 type (Fig. 12). This indicates a steady qualitative pattern of transmission of the two divergent parasite subpopulations from macaque hosts to humans, with the relative frequency also remaining similar throughout different times of year. However, the overall numbers of cases and Cluster 1 infections in particular were higher in the most recent year analysed (Fig. 12), and temporally varying numbers of overall cases may be related to environmental changes associated with deforestation, likely to alter the macaque and mosquito vector behaviour and distribution, as was observed in Sabah state of Malaysian Borneo in recent years (Cooper et al., 2020; Fornace et al., 2016a).

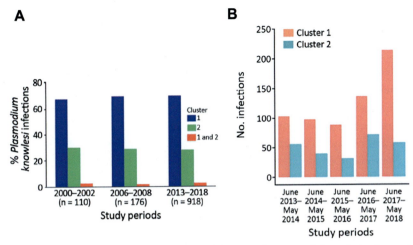

Fig. 12 Temporal analysis of frequencies of the two divergent *P. knowlesi* subpopulations in human cases in Kapit division of Sarawak. (A) The relatively high frequency of the Cluster 1 subpopulation compared to Cluster 2 remained steady since 2000, with low numbers of mixed-genotype infections being detected. (B) Analysis of the later years in more detail showed increasing numbers of Cluster 1 in the most recent year, indicating that ongoing surveillance will be needed to identify if there are changes to the previously described distribution. *Figure incorporating reproduction under Creative Commons licence. Divis, P.C.S., Hu, T.H., Kadir, K.A., Mohammad, D.S.A., Hii, K.C., Daneshvar, C., Conway, D.J., Singh, B., 2020. Efficient surveillance of Plasmodium knowlesi genetic subpopulations, Malaysian Borneo, 2000-2018. Emerg. Infect. Dis., 26, 1392–1398.*

8. Adaptation and the future of *P. knowlesi* emerging from local zoonoses

The genome sequence analyses have given clear illustration that the different *P. knowlesi* populations are responding to selection, as expected for natural parasite populations, and future adaptation will depend on environmental conditions. The potential speed of *P. knowlesi* adaptation has been well illustrated by laboratory studies, particularly those indicating adaptation of blood stage parasites to culture growth in different types of erythrocytes, a process depending on use of alternative merozoite ligands for invasion (Lim et al., 2013; Moon et al., 2013, 2016). Indeed, the parasite strain from which the reference *P. knowlesi* genome sequence was derived had been originally isolated decades ago (Chin et al., 1965), then maintained by asexual transfer in laboratory macaques for many years, and the *AP2-G2* gene that is normally involved in malaria parasite sexual stage development for mosquito transmission now has a premature stop codon in this line (Assefa et al., 2015).

Loss-of-function genomic changes selected under artificial laboratory conditions have been seen in other malaria parasite species (Claessens et al., 2017), but specific gain-of-function is generally harder to predict and detect, as there are many possible gene functional alterations and phenotype modifications that may only be potentially discerned after highly focused research efforts. Laboratory systems for analysis of *P. knowlesi* in culture, including genetic manipulation (Kocken et al., 2002; Mohring et al., 2019) and mosquito infection (Armistead et al., 2018), are potentially amenable for testing whether naturally occurring changes have effects on some candidate phenotypes. However, testing for other phenotypes would require experimental infection studies in laboratory macaques (Galinski et al., 2018), and there are technical and ethical limits to the availability of the most relevant macaque host species, as well as very few laboratory mosquito colonies of natural vector species.

In natural populations, ecological changes due to environmental modifications may alter mosquito feeding behaviour and change the habitats for mosquito breeding, resulting in changes in vector composition (Moyes et al., 2016). Local *P. knowlesi* populations are likely to adapt in response to such changes, as illustrated by data indicating that *P. falciparum* has locally-adapted to different mosquito vectors (Molina-Cruz et al., 2020; Ukegbu et al., 2020). Recent molecular entomological surveys in Sarawak show additional *Anopheles* species being incriminated as *P. knowlesi* vectors (Ang et al., 2020, 2021), so we recommend future studies of parasite genomic variation in samples from naturally-infected vectors of different species from throughout the natural range of *P. knowlesi*. Laboratory methods of selective whole genome amplification are able to increase the *P. knowlesi* genome sequence coverage obtained from samples with low amounts of parasite genomic DNA (Diez Benavente et al., 2019), which will be useful for sequencing parasites from individual mosquitoes or low-level infections in some blood samples.

It should also be noted that *P. knowlesi* population genomic analyses have focused on the core genome, as this is most easily analysed by mapping short-read sequences to a reference genome. In contrast, large multigene families such as *SICAVAR* and *KIR* have not been analysed in population studies, as these need different methods for sequence assembly and analysis (Lapp et al., 2018), and understanding their more extreme polymorphism and distinct evolutionary genetic processes would be a separate challenge.

It is important to know whether *P. knowlesi* is adapting to be transmitted more efficiently from humans to mosquitoes, and whether this will cause more cases to be acquired through a human–mosquito–human route. If so, *P. knowlesi* could eventually become endemic, as happened pre-historically for other human malaria parasite species, all of which were originally acquired from non-human primate reservoir hosts. To fully investigate these questions requires multiple disciplines, alongside molecular and genomic epidemiology, but current understanding of the parasite population structure and adaptation indicates that there is no intrinsic barrier to such potential changes. To date, the underlying population genomics of *P. knowlesi* appears to be dictated by the common reservoir hosts and the geographical structure, and against this background new patterns of emerging population structure or adaptation might be detected in future. This should encourage more prospective sampling and genome sequence analysis from throughout the range of *P. knowlesi*, at different sites and in different hosts and vectors.

References

Ahmed, M.A., Fong, M.Y., Lau, Y.L., Yusof, R., 2016. Clustering and genetic differentiation of the normocyte binding protein (nbpxa) of *Plasmodium knowlesi* clinical isolates from Peninsular Malaysia and Malaysia Borneo. Malar. J. 15, 241.

Akter, R., Vythilingam, I., Khaw, L.T., Qvist, R., Lim, Y.A., Sitam, F.T., Venugopalan, B., Sekaran, S.D., 2015. Simian malaria in wild macaques: first report from Hulu Selangor district, Selangor, Malaysia. Malar. J. 14, 386.

Ang, J.X.D., Kadir, K.A., Mohamad, D.S.A., Matusop, A., Divis, P.C.S., Yaman, K., Singh, B., 2020. New vectors in northern Sarawak, Malaysian Borneo, for the zoonotic malaria parasite, *Plasmodium knowlesi*. Parasit. Vectors 13, 472.

Ang, J.X.D., Yaman, K., Kadir, K.A., Matusop, A., Singh, B., 2021. New vectors that are early feeders for *Plasmodium knowlesi* and other simian malaria parasites in Sarawak, Malaysian Borneo. Sci. Rep. 11, 7739.

Armistead, J.S., Moraes Barros, R.R., Gibson, T.J., Kite, W.A., Mershon, J.P., Lambert, L.E., Orr-Gonzalez, S.E., Sa, J.M., Adams, J.H., Wellems, T.E., 2018. Infection of mosquitoes from *in vitro* cultivated *Plasmodium knowlesi* H strain. Int. J. Parasitol. 48, 601–610.

Assefa, S., Lim, C., Preston, M.D., Duffy, C.W., Nair, M.B., Adroub, S.A., Kadir, K.A., Goldberg, J.M., Neafsey, D.E., Divis, P., Clark, T.G., Duraisingh, M.T., Conway, D.J., Pain, A., Singh, B., 2015. Population genomic structure and adaptation in the zoonotic malaria parasite *Plasmodium knowlesi*. Proc. Natl. Acad. Sci. U. S. A. 112, 13027–13032.

Brown, R., Chua, T.H., Fornace, K., Drakeley, C., Vythilingam, I., Ferguson, H.M., 2020. Human exposure to zoonotic malaria vectors in village, farm and forest habitats in Sabah, Malaysian Borneo. PLoS Negl. Trop. Dis. 14, e0008617.

Chin, W., Contacos, P.G., Coatney, G.R., Kimball, H.R., 1965. A naturally acquired quotidian-type malaria in man transferable to monkeys. Science 149, 865.

Claessens, A., Affara, M., Assefa, S.A., Kwiatkowski, D.P., Conway, D.J., 2017. Culture adaptation of malaria parasites selects for convergent loss-of-function mutants. Sci. Rep. 7, 41303.

Coatney, G.R., Collins, W.E., Mcwilson, W., Contacos, P.G., 1971. The Primate Malarias. US Department of Health, Education and Welfare.

Cooper, D.J., Rajahram, G.S., William, T., Jelip, J., Mohammad, R., Benedict, J., Alaza, D.A., Malacova, E., Yeo, T.W., Grigg, M.J., Anstey, N.M., Barber, B.E., 2020. *Plasmodium knowlesi* malaria in Sabah, Malaysia, 2015-2017: ongoing increase in incidence despite near-elimination of the human-only *Plasmodium* species. Clin. Infect. Dis. 70, 361–367.

Cox-Singh, J., Davis, T.M., Lee, K.S., Shamsul, S.S., Matusop, A., Ratnam, S., Rahman, H.A., Conway, D.J., Singh, B., 2008. *Plasmodium knowlesi* malaria in humans is widely distributed and potentially life threatening. Clin. Infect. Dis. 46, 165–171.

Diez Benavente, E., Florez De Sessions, P., Moon, R.W., Holder, A.A., Blackman, M.J., Roper, C., Drakeley, C.J., Pain, A., Sutherland, C.J., Hibberd, M.L., Campino, S., Clark, T.G., 2017. Analysis of nuclear and organellar genomes of *Plasmodium knowlesi* in humans reveals ancient population structure and recent recombination among host-specific subpopulations. PLoS Genet. 13, e1007008.

Diez Benavente, E., Gomes, A.R., De Silva, J.R., Grigg, M., Walker, H., Barber, B.E., William, T., Yeo, T.W., De Sessions, P.F., Ramaprasad, A., Ibrahim, A., Charleston, J., Hibberd, M.L., Pain, A., Moon, R.W., Auburn, S., Ling, L.Y., Anstey, N.M., Clark, T.G., Campino, S., 2019. Whole genome sequencing of amplified *Plasmodium knowlesi* DNA from unprocessed blood reveals genetic exchange events between Malaysian peninsular and Borneo subpopulations. Sci. Rep. 9, 9873.

Divis, P.C., Singh, B., Anderios, F., Hisam, S., Matusop, A., Kocken, C.H., Assefa, S.A., Duffy, C.W., Conway, D.J., 2015. Admixture in humans of two divergent *Plasmodium knowlesi* populations associated with different macaque host species. PLoS Pathog. 11, e1004888.

Divis, P.C., Lin, L.C., Rovie-Ryan, J.J., Kadir, K.A., Anderios, F., Hisam, S., Sharma, R.S., Singh, B., Conway, D.J., 2017. Three divergent subpopulations of the malaria parasite *Plasmodium knowlesi*. Emerg. Infect. Dis. 23, 616–624.

Divis, P.C.S., Duffy, C.W., Kadir, K.A., Singh, B., Conway, D.J., 2018. Genome-wide mosaicism in divergence between zoonotic malaria parasite subpopulations with separate sympatric transmission cycles. Mol. Ecol. 2, 860–870.

Divis, P.C.S., Hu, T.H., Kadir, K.A., Mohammad, D.S.A., Hii, K.C., Daneshvar, C., Conway, D.J., Singh, B., 2020. Efficient surveillance of *Plasmodium knowlesi* genetic sub-populations, Malaysian Borneo, 2000-2018. Emerg. Infect. Dis. 26, 1392–1398.

Fa, J.E., Lindberg, D.G., 1996. Evolution and Ecology of Macaque Societies. Cambridge University Press.

Figtree, M., Lee, R., Bain, L., Kennedy, T., Mackertich, S., Urban, M., Cheng, Q., Hudson, B.J., 2010. *Plasmodium knowlesi* in human, Indonesian Borneo. Emerg. Infect. Dis. 16, 672–674.

Fong, M.Y., Rashdi, S.A., Yusof, R., Lau, Y.L., 2015. Distinct genetic difference between the Duffy binding protein (PkDBPalphaII) of *Plasmodium knowlesi* clinical isolates from North Borneo and Peninsular Malaysia. Malar. J. 14, 91.

Fong, M.Y., Rashdi, S.A., Yusof, R., Lau, Y.L., 2016. Genetic diversity, natural selection and haplotype grouping of *Plasmodium knowlesi* gamma protein region II (PkgammaRII): comparison with the Duffy binding protein (PkDBPalphaRII). PLoS One 11, e0155627.

Fornace, K.M., Abidin, T.R., Alexander, N., Brock, P., Grigg, M.J., Murphy, A., William, T., Menon, J., Drakeley, C.J., Cox, J., 2016a. Association between landscape factors and spatial patterns of *Plasmodium knowlesi* infections in Sabah, Malaysia. Emerg. Infect. Dis. 22, 201–208.

Fornace, K.M., Nuin, N.A., Betson, M., Grigg, M.J., William, T., Anstey, N.M., Yeo, T.W., Cox, J., Ying, L.T., Drakeley, C.J., 2016b. Asymptomatic and submicroscopic carriage of *Plasmodium knowlesi* malaria in household and community members of clinical cases in Sabah, Malaysia. J. Infect. Dis. 213, 784–787.

Fungfuang, W., Udom, C., Tongthainan, D., Kadir, K.A., Singh, B., 2020. Malaria parasites in macaques in Thailand: stump-tailed macaques (*Macaca arctoides*) are new natural hosts for *Plasmodium knowlesi*, *Plasmodium inui*, *Plasmodium coatneyi* and *Plasmodium fieldi*. Malar. J. 19, 350.

Galinski, M.R., Lapp, S.A., Peterson, M.S., Ay, F., Joyner, C.J., Kg, L.E.R., Fonseca, L.L., Voit, E.O., Mahpic, C., 2018. *Plasmodium knowlesi*: a superb in vivo nonhuman primate model of antigenic variation in malaria. Parasitology 145, 85–100.

Gamalo, L.E., Dimalibot, J., Kadir, K.A., Singh, B., Paller, V.G., 2019. *Plasmodium knowlesi* and other malaria parasites in long-tailed macaques from the Philippines. Malar. J. 18, 147.

Garnham, P.C.C., 1966. Malaria Parasites and Other Haemosporidia. Blackwell Scientific Publications, Oxford.

Hawkes, F.M., Manin, B.O., Cooper, A., Daim, S., Homathevi, R., Jelip, J., Husin, T., Chua, T.H., 2019. Vector compositions change across forested to deforested ecotones in emerging areas of zoonotic malaria transmission in Malaysia. Sci. Rep. 9, 13312.

Herdiana, H., Irnawati, I., Coutrier, F.N., Munthe, A., Mardiati, M., Yuniarti, T., Sariwati, E., Sumiwi, M.E., Noviyanti, R., Pronyk, P., Hawley, W.A., 2018. Two clusters of *Plasmodium knowlesi* cases in a malaria elimination area, Sabang Municipality, Aceh, Indonesia. Malar. J. 17, 186.

Hocking, S.E., Divis, P.C.S., Kadir, K.A., Singh, B., Conway, D.J., 2020. Population genomic structure and recent evolution of *Plasmodium knowlesi*, Peninsular Malaysia. Emerg. Infect. Dis. 26, 1749–1758.

Imwong, M., Madmanee, W., Suwannasin, K., Kunasol, C., Peto, T.J., Tripura, R., von Seidlein, L., Nguon, C., Davoeung, C., Day, N.P.J., Dondorp, A.M., White, N.J., 2019. Asymptomatic natural human infections with the simian malaria parasites *Plasmodium cynomolgi* and *Plasmodium knowlesi*. J. Infect. Dis. 219, 695–702.

Iwagami, M., Nakatsu, M., Khattignavong, P., Soundala, P., Lorphachan, L., Keomalaphet, S., Xangsayalath, P., Kawai, S., Hongvanthong, B., Brey, P.T., Kano, S., 2018. First case of human infection with *Plasmodium knowlesi* in Laos. PLoS Negl. Trop. Dis. 12, e0006244.

Jeslyn, W.P., Huat, T.C., Vernon, L., Irene, L.M., Sung, L.K., Jarrod, L.P., Singh, B., Ching, N.L., 2011. Molecular epidemiological investigation of *Plasmodium knowlesi* in humans and macaques in Singapore. Vector Borne Zoonotic Dis. 11, 131–135.

Jiang, N., Chang, Q., Sun, X., Lu, H., Yin, J., Zhang, Z., Wahlgren, M., Chen, Q., 2010. Co-infections with *Plasmodium knowlesi* and other malaria parasites, Myanmar. Emerg. Infect. Dis. 16, 1476–1478.

Jiram, A.I., Vythilingam, I., Noorazian, Y.M., Yusof, Y.M., Azahari, A.H., Fong, M.Y., 2012. Entomologic investigation of *Plasmodium knowlesi* vectors in Kuala Lipis, Pahang, Malaysia. Malar. J. 11, 213.

Jiram, A.I., Hisam, S., Reuben, H., Husin, S.Z., Roslan, A., Ismail, W.R.W., 2016. Submicroscopic evidence of the simian malaria parasite, *Plasmodium knowlesi*, in an Orang Asli community. Southeast Asian J. Trop. Med. Public Health 47, 591–599.

Jongwutiwes, S., Putaporntip, C., Iwasaki, T., Sata, T., Kanbara, H., 2004. Naturally acquired *Plasmodium knowlesi* malaria in human, Thailand. Emerg. Infect. Dis. 10, 2211–2213.

Jongwutiwes, S., Buppan, P., Kosuvin, R., Seethamchai, S., Pattanawong, U., Sirichaisinthop, J., Putaporntip, C., 2011. *Plasmodium knowlesi* malaria in humans and macaques, Thailand. Emerg. Infect. Dis. 17, 1799–1806.

Joveen-Neoh, W.F., Chong, K.L., Wong, C.M., Lau, T.Y., 2011. Incidence of malaria in the interior division of Sabah, Malaysian Borneo, based on nested PCR. J. Parasitol. Res. 2011, 104284.

Khim, N., Siv, S., Kim, S., Mueller, T., Fleischmann, E., Singh, B., Divis, P.C., Steenkeste, N., Duval, L., Bouchier, C., Duong, S., Ariey, F., Menard, D., 2011. *Plasmodium knowlesi* infection in humans, Cambodia, 2007-2010. Emerg. Infect. Dis. 17, 1900–1902.

Knowles, R., Das Gupta, B.M., 1932. A study of monkey malaria and its experimental transmission to man. Ind. Med. Gaz. 67, 301–320.

Kocken, C.H., Ozwara, H., Van Der Wel, A., Beetsma, A.L., Mwenda, J.M., Thomas, A.W., 2002. *Plasmodium knowlesi* provides a rapid in vitro and in vivo transfection system that enables double-crossover gene knockout studies. Infect. Immun. 70, 655–660.

Lapp, S.A., Geraldo, J.A., Chien, J.T., Ay, F., Pakala, S.B., Batugedara, G., Humphrey, J., Ma, H.C., De, B.J., Le Roch, K.G., Galinski, M.R., Kissinger, J.C., 2018. PacBio assembly of a *Plasmodium knowlesi* genome sequence with Hi-C correction and manual annotation of the Sicavar gene family. Parasitology 145, 71–84.

Lee, K.S., Cox-Singh, J., Singh, B., 2009. Morphological features and differential counts of *Plasmodium knowlesi* parasites in naturally acquired human infections. Malar. J. 8, 73.

Lee, K.S., Divis, P.C., Zakaria, S.K., Matusop, A., Julin, R.A., Conway, D.J., Cox-Singh, J., Singh, B., 2011. *Plasmodium knowlesi*: reservoir hosts and tracking the emergence in humans and macaques. PLoS Pathog. 7, e1002015.

Li, M.I., Mailepessov, D., Vythilingam, I., Lee, V., Lam, P., Ng, L.C., Tan, C.H., 2021. Prevalence of simian malaria parasites in macaques of Singapore. PLoS Negl. Trop. Dis. 15, e0009110.

Liedigk, R., Kolleck, J., Boker, K.O., Meijaard, E., Md-Zain, B.M., Abdul-Latiff, M.A., Ampeng, A., Lakim, M., Abdul-Patah, P., Tosi, A.J., Brameier, M., Zinner, D., Roos, C., 2015. Mitogenomic phylogeny of the common long-tailed macaque (*Macaca fascicularis fascicularis*). BMC Genomics 16, 222.

Lim, C., Hansen, E., Desimone, T.M., Moreno, Y., Junker, K., Bei, A., Brugnara, C., Buckee, C.O., Duraisingh, M.T., 2013. Expansion of host cellular niche can drive adaptation of a zoonotic malaria parasite to humans. Nat. Commun. 4, 1638.

Liu, Q., Zhu, S., Mizuno, S., Kimura, M., Liu, P., Isomura, S., Wang, X., Kawamoto, F., 1998. Sequence variation in the small-subunit rrna gene of *Plasmodium malariae* and prevalence of isolates with the variant sequence in Sichuan, China. J. Clin. Microbiol. 36, 3378–3381.

Lubis, I.N.D., Wijaya, H., Lubis, M., Lubis, C.P., Divis, P.C.S., Beshir, K.B., Sutherland, C.J., 2017. Contribution of *Plasmodium knowlesi* to multispecies human malaria infections in north Sumatera, Indonesia. J. Infect. Dis. 215, 1148–1155.

Luchavez, J., Espino, F., Curameng, P., Espina, R., Bell, D., Chiodini, P., Nolder, D., Sutherland, C., Lee, K.S., Singh, B., 2008. Human infections with *Plasmodium knowlesi*, the Philippines. Emerg. Infect. Dis. 14, 811–813.

Marchand, R.P., Culleton, R., Maeno, Y., Quang, N.T., Nakazawa, S., 2011. Co-infections of *Plasmodium knowlesi*, *P. falciparum*, and *P. vivax* among humans and *Anopheles dirus* mosquitoes, southern Vietnam. Emerg. Infect. Dis. 17, 1232–1239.

Mohring, F., Hart, M.N., Rawlinson, T.A., Henrici, R., Charleston, J.A., Diez Benavente, E., Patel, A., Hall, J., Almond, N., Campino, S., Clark, T.G., Sutherland, C.J., Baker, D.A., Draper, S.J., Moon, R.W., 2019. Rapid and iterative genome editing in the malaria parasite *Plasmodium knowlesi* provides new tools for *P. vivax* research. elife 8, e45829.

Molina-Cruz, A., Canepa, G.E., Alves, E.S.T.L., Williams, A.E., Nagyal, S., Yenkoidiok-Douti, L., Nagata, B.M., Calvo, E., Andersen, J., Boulanger, M.J., Barillas-Mury, C., 2020. *Plasmodium falciparum* evades immunity of anopheline mosquitoes by interacting with a PFS47 midgut receptor. Proc. Natl. Acad. Sci. U. S. A. 117, 2597–2605.

Moon, R.W., Hall, J., Rangkuti, F., Ho, Y.S., Almond, N., Mitchell, G.H., Pain, A., Holder, A.A., Blackman, M.J., 2013. Adaptation of the genetically tractable malaria pathogen *Plasmodium knowlesi* to continuous culture in human erythrocytes. Proc. Natl. Acad. Sci. U. S. A. 110, 531–536.

Moon, R.W., Sharaf, H., Hastings, C.H., Ho, Y.S., Nair, M.B., Rchiad, Z., Knuepfer, E., Ramaprasad, A., Mohring, F., Amir, A., Yusuf, N.A., Hall, J., Almond, N., Lau, Y.L., Pain, A., Blackman, M.J., Holder, A.A., 2016. Normocyte-binding protein required for human erythrocyte invasion by the zoonotic malaria parasite *Plasmodium knowlesi*. Proc. Natl. Acad. Sci. U. S. A. 113, 7231–7236.

Moyes, C.L., Shearer, F.M., Huang, Z., Wiebe, A., Gibson, H.S., Nijman, V., Mohd-Azlan, J., Brodie, J.F., Malaivijitnond, S., Linkie, M., Samejima, H., O'brien, T.G., Trainor, C.R., Hamada, Y., Giordano, A.J., Kinnaird, M.F., Elyazar, I.R., Sinka, M.E., Vythilingam, I., Bangs, M.J., Pigott, D.M., Weiss, D.J., Golding, N., Hay, S.I., 2016. Predicting the geographical distributions of the macaque hosts and mosquito vectors of *Plasmodium knowlesi* malaria in forested and non-forested areas. Parasit. Vectors 9, 242.

Naing, D.K.S., Anderios, F., Kin, Z., 2011. Geographic and ethnic distributions of *Plasmodium knowlesi* infection in Sabah, Malaysia. Int. J. Collab. Res. Intern. Med. Public Health 3, 9.

Nakazawa, S., Marchand, R.P., Quang, N.T., Culleton, R., Manh, N.D., Maeno, Y., 2009. *Anopheles dirus* co-infection with human and monkey malaria parasites in Vietnam. Int. J. Parasitol. 39, 1533–1537.

Ng, O.T., Ooi, E.E., Lee, C.C., Lee, P.J., Ng, L.C., Pei, S.W., Tu, T.M., Loh, J.P., Leo, Y.S., 2008. Naturally acquired human *Plasmodium knowlesi* infection, Singapore. Emerg. Infect. Dis. 14, 814–816.

Pain, A., Bohme, U., Berry, A.E., Mungall, K., Finn, R.D., Jackson, A.P., Mourier, T., Mistry, J., Pasini, E.M., Aslett, M.A., Balasubrammaniam, S., Borgwardt, K., Brooks, K., Carret, C., Carver, T.J., Cherevach, I., Chillingworth, T., Clark, T.G., Galinski, M.R., Hall, N., Harper, D., Harris, D., Hauser, H., Ivens, A., Janssen, C.S., Keane, T., Larke, N., Lapp, S., Marti, M., Moule, S., Meyer, I.M., Ormond, D., Peters, N., Sanders, M., Sanders, S., Sargeant, T.J., Simmonds, M., Smith, F., Squares, R., Thurston, S., Tivey, A.R., Walker, D., White, B., Zuiderwijk, E., Churcher, C., Quail, M.A., Cowman, A.F., Turner, C.M., Rajandream, M.A., Kocken, C.H., Thomas, A.W., Newbold, C.I., Barrell, B.G., Berriman, M., 2008. The genome of the simian and human malaria parasite *Plasmodium knowlesi*. Nature 455, 799–803.

Pinheiro, M.M., Ahmed, M.A., Millar, S.B., Sanderson, T., Otto, T.D., Lu, W.C., Krishna, S., Rayner, J.C., Cox-Singh, J., 2015. *Plasmodium knowlesi* genome sequences from clinical isolates reveal extensive genomic dimorphism. PLoS One 10, e0121303.

Pongvongsa, T., Culleton, R., Ha, H., Thanh, L., Phongmany, P., Marchand, R.P., Kawai, S., Moji, K., Nakazawa, S., Maeno, Y., 2018. Human infection with *Plasmodium knowlesi* on the Laos-Vietnam border. Trop. Med. Health 46, 33.

Putaporntip, C., Hongsrimuang, T., Seethamchai, S., Kobasa, T., Limkittikul, K., Cui, L., Jongwutiwes, S., 2009. Differential prevalence of *Plasmodium* infections and cryptic *Plasmodium knowlesi* malaria in humans in Thailand. J. Infect. Dis. 199, 1143–1150.

Putaporntip, C., Jongwutiwes, S., Thongaree, S., Seethamchai, S., Grynberg, P., Hughes, A.L., 2010. Ecology of malaria parasites infecting southeast Asian macaques: evidence from cytochrome b sequences. Mol. Ecol. 19, 3466–3476.

Putaporntip, C., Thongaree, S., Jongwutiwes, S., 2013. Differential sequence diversity at merozoite surface protein-1 locus of *Plasmodium knowlesi* from humans and macaques in Thailand. Infect. Genet. Evol. 18, 213–219.

Putaporntip, C., Kuamsab, N., Pattanawong, U., Yanmanee, S., Seethamchai, S., Jongwutiwes, S., 2021. *Plasmodium cynomolgi* co-infections among symptomatic malaria patients, Thailand. Emerg. Infect. Dis. 27, 590–593.

Siner, A., Liew, S.T., Kadir, K.A., Mohamad, D.S.A., Thomas, F.K., Zulkarnaen, M., Singh, B., 2017. Absence of *Plasmodium inui* and *Plasmodium cynomolgi*, but detection of *Plasmodium knowlesi* and *Plasmodium vivax* infections in asymptomatic humans in the Betong division of Sarawak, Malaysian Borneo. Malar. J. 16, 417.

Singh, B., Bobogare, A., Cox-Singh, J., Snounou, G., Abdullah, M.S., Rahman, H.A., 1999. A genus- and species-specific nested polymerase chain reaction malaria detection assay for epidemiological studies. Am. J. Trop. Med. Hyg. 60, 687–692.

Singh, B., Kim Sung, L., Matusop, A., Radhakrishnan, A., Shamsul, S.S., Cox-Singh, J., Thomas, A., Conway, D.J., 2004. A large focus of naturally acquired *Plasmodium knowlesi* infections in human beings. Lancet 363, 1017–1024.

Tan, C.H., Vythilingam, I., Matusop, A., Chan, S.T., Singh, B., 2008. Bionomics of *Anopheles latens* in Kapit, Sarawak, Malaysian Borneo in relation to the transmission of zoonotic simian malaria parasite *Plasmodium knowlesi*. Malar. J. 7, 52.

Tyagi, R.K., Das, M.K., Singh, S.S., Sharma, Y.D., 2013. Discordance in drug resistance-associated mutation patterns in marker genes of *Plasmodium falciparum* and *Plasmodium knowlesi* during coinfections. J. Antimicrob. Chemother. 68, 1081–1088.

UK Health Protection Agency, 2011. Imported Malaria Cases and Deaths, United Kingdom: 1992–2011. Health Protection Agency, London.

Ukegbu, C.V., Giorgalli, M., Tapanelli, S., Rona, L.D.P., Jaye, A., Wyer, C., Angrisano, F., Blagborough, A.M., Christophides, G.K., Vlachou, D., 2020. PIMMS43 is required for malaria parasite immune evasion and sporogonic development in the mosquito vector. Proc. Natl. Acad. Sci. U. S. A. 117, 7363–7373.

Van Den Eede, P., Van, H.N., Van Overmeir, C., Vythilingam, I., Duc, T.N., Hung Le, X., Manh, H.N., Anne, J., D'alessandro, U., Erhart, A., 2009. Human *Plasmodium knowlesi* infections in young children in Central Vietnam. Malar. J. 8, 249.

Vythilingam, I., Tan, C.H., Asmad, M., Chan, S.T., Lee, K.S., Singh, B., 2006. Natural transmission of *Plasmodium knowlesi* to humans by *Anopheles latens* in Sarawak, Malaysia. Trans. R. Soc. Trop. Med. Hyg. 100, 1087–1088.

Vythilingam, I., Noorazian, Y.M., Huat, T.C., Jiram, A.I., Yusri, Y.M., Azahari, A.H., Norparina, I., Noorrain, A., Lokmanhakim, S., 2008. *Plasmodium knowlesi* in humans, macaques and mosquitoes in peninsular Malaysia. Parasit. Vectors 1, 26.

Wong, M.L., Chua, T.H., Leong, C.S., Khaw, L.T., Fornace, K., Wan-Sulaiman, W.Y., William, T., Drakeley, C., Ferguson, H.M., Vythilingam, I., 2015. Seasonal and spatial dynamics of the primary vector of *Plasmodium knowlesi* within a major transmission focus in Sabah, Malaysia. PLOS Negl. Trop. Dis. 9, e0004135.

Yusof, R., Lau, Y.L., Mahmud, R., Fong, M.Y., Jelip, J., Ngian, H.U., Mustakim, S., Hussin, H.M., Marzuki, N., Mohd Ali, M., 2014. High proportion of knowlesi malaria in recent malaria cases in Malaysia. Malar. J. 13, 168.

Yusof, R., Ahmed, M.A., Jelip, J., Ngian, H.U., Mustakim, S., Hussin, H.M., Fong, M.Y., Mahmud, R., Sitam, F.A., Japning, J.R., Snounou, G., Escalante, A.A., Lau, Y.L., 2016. Phylogeographic evidence for 2 genetically distinct zoonotic *Plasmodium knowlesi* parasites, Malaysia. Emerg. Infect. Dis. 22, 1371–1380.

Zhang, X., Kadir, K.A., Quintanilla-Zarinan, L.F., Villano, J., Houghton, P., Du, H., Singh, B., Smith, D.G., 2016. Distribution and prevalence of malaria parasites among long-tailed macaques (*Macaca fascicularis*) in regional populations across Southeast Asia. Malar. J. 15, 450.

Zhu, H.M., Li, J., Zheng, H., 2006. Human natural infection of Plasmodium knowlesi. Zhongguo Ji Sheng Chong Xue Yu Ji Sheng Chong Bing Za Zhi 24, 70–71.

Ziegler, T., Abegg, C., Meijaard, E., Perwitasari-Farajallah, D., Walter, L., Hodges, J.K., Roos, C., 2007. Molecular phylogeny and evolutionary history of Southeast Asian macaques forming the *M. silenus* group. Mol. Phylogenet. Evol. 42, 807–816.

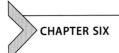

CHAPTER SIX

Epidemiology of the zoonotic malaria *Plasmodium knowlesi* in changing landscapes

Pablo Ruiz Cuenca[a,†], Stephanie Key[a,†], Amaziasizamoria Jumail[b], Henry Surendra[c,d], Heather M. Ferguson[e], Chris J. Drakeley[a], and Kimberly Fornace[a,e,*]

[a]Faculty of Infectious and Tropical Diseases, London School of Hygiene and Tropical Medicine, London, United Kingdom
[b]Danau Girang Field Centre, Kota Kinabalu, Malaysia
[c]Eijkman-Oxford Clinical Research Unit, Jakarta, Indonesia
[d]Centre for Tropical Medicine, Faculty of Medicine, Public Health and Nursing, Universitas Gadjah Mada, Yogyakarta, Indonesia
[e]Institute of Biodiversity, Animal Health and Comparative Medicine, University of Glasgow, Glasgow, Scotland, United Kingdom
[*]Corresponding author: e-mail address: Kimberly.Fornace@lshtm.ac.uk

Contents

1. Introduction	226
2. Ecological change and mechanisms of disease emergence and transmission	228
2.1 Biodiversity impacts on vector-borne and zoonotic diseases	228
2.2 Habitat fragmentation and zoonotic and vector-borne diseases	231
2.3 Physical changes to the environment and disease transmission	233
2.4 Socio-economic changes and development and disease risks	234
3. Distribution and burden of *Plasmodium knowlesi*	236
3.1 Spatial distribution of reported *P. knowlesi* incidence	237
3.2 Community-level spatial distribution of exposure and infection	239
3.3 Reporting bias and surveillance for *P. knowlesi*	240
3.4 Emergence of other zoonotic simian malarias in Southeast Asia	243
4. Landscape impacts on *P. knowlesi* disease dynamics	244
4.1 Environmental change in Southeast Asia	244
4.2 Impacts of environmental change on distribution of *P. knowlesi*	248
4.3 Human populations, movement and occupational risks	249
4.4 Simian host ecology and infection rates	251
4.5 Mosquito ecology, infection and bionomics	255
5. Transmission dynamics and potential for human to human transmission	257

[†] These authors contributed equally.

6. Designing surveillance and control measures for changing environments	259
6.1 Opportunities to improve surveillance for *P. knowlesi*	259
6.2 Management of wildlife populations	262
6.3 Land management strategies	265
7. Conclusions and future research priorities	266
References	267

Abstract

Within the past two decades, incidence of human cases of the zoonotic malaria *Plasmodium knowlesi* has increased markedly. *P. knowlesi* is now the most common cause of human malaria in Malaysia and threatens to undermine malaria control programmes across Southeast Asia. The emergence of zoonotic malaria corresponds to a period of rapid deforestation within this region. These environmental changes impact the distribution and behaviour of the simian hosts, mosquito vector species and human populations, creating new opportunities for *P. knowlesi* transmission. Here, we review how landscape changes can drive zoonotic disease emergence, examine the extent and causes of these changes across Southeast and identify how these mechanisms may be impacting *P. knowlesi* dynamics. We review the current spatial epidemiology of reported *P. knowlesi* infections in people and assess how these demographic and environmental changes may lead to changes in transmission patterns. Finally, we identify opportunities to improve *P. knowlesi* surveillance and develop targeted ecological interventions within these landscapes.

1. Introduction

The zoonotic malaria, *Plasmodium knowlesi*, is an emerging disease driven by changing patterns of land use. Carried by long- and pig-tailed macaques (*Macaca fascicularis* and *M. nemestrina*) and transmitted by the *Anopheles* Leucosphyrus Group of mosquitoes, the geographical range of *P. knowlesi* is limited by the distribution of the mosquito vectors and simian hosts (Moyes et al., 2014, 2016). *P. knowlesi* was first described in macaques in the 1930s with only one naturally acquired human infection reported in the twentieth century (Chin et al., 1965; Knowles and Das Gupta, 1932). However, in 2004, the use of molecular diagnostics identified a large number of human infections with *P. knowlesi* in Malaysian Borneo which were previously misdiagnosed by microscopy (Singh et al., 2004). Since detection of this cluster, reported incidence of *P. knowlesi* has increased markedly, with *P. knowlesi* now the most common cause of human malaria in Malaysia and identified across Southeast Asia (Singh et al., 2004; William et al., 2013, 2014). These rising numbers of human *P. knowlesi* cases correspond to a period of rapid and extensive environmental change within endemic areas. Land use changes, such as deforestation and agricultural expansion, may increase spatial overlap between people, macaques and mosquitoes and have been proposed as the main driver of this emergence (Lee et al., 2011; Moyes et al., 2016; Singh and Daneshvar, 2013).

These changing disease dynamics threaten to undermine regional malaria elimination efforts. The potential threat of simian malaria to malaria elimination has been recognised since the first Global Malaria Eradication campaign in the 1960s (Coatney, 1963). This is most pronounced in Malaysia where *P. knowlesi* emergence has reversed decades of progress in reducting malaria cases (Barber et al., 2017). The first malaria eradication programme in Malaysia began in 1961, with a focus on reducing transmission of non-zoonotic malaria species primarily through vector control. This led to a precipitous decline in transmission from the 1980s onwards, culminating in Malaysia moving to the elimination phase in 2011 (Chin et al., 2020). While Malaysia has not reported any indigenous cases of human malaria since 2017, thousands of human *P. knowlesi* cases are reported in Malaysia annually (Chin et al., 2020). The World Health Organization has recently recognised the regional importance of *P. knowlesi* to malaria elimination and instigated the formation of an Evidence Review Group to identify key knowledge gaps and possible interventions (World Health Organisation Regional Office for Western Pacific, 2017). Critical to these initiatives is understanding how deforestation and other ecological changes may alter future *P. knowlesi* transmission dynamics and human risks.

Anthropogenic environmental changes affect the distribution of people, animal reservoirs and disease vectors, impacting infectious disease risks (Gottdenker et al., 2014; Kilpatrick and Randolph, 2012). These have been linked to altered dynamics and geographical distribution of malaria and other zoonotic and vector-borne diseases globally (Guerra et al., 2006; Hahn et al., 2014; Yasuoka and Levins, 2007). Current levels of landscape change are unprecedented, with pathogen emergence from wildlife populations in altered ecosystems threatening global health. Understanding how ecological changes driven by human activity can modify the epidemiology of these diseases is vital to predicting future disease risks and designing effective public health measures. In addition to posing a major threat to malaria elimination, *P. knowlesi* exemplifies an emerging disease driven by environmental change. Here, we review how ecological changes impact disease emergence, describe spatial distribution of human *P. knowlesi* infections, define the extent of landscape change across Southeast Asia and examine mechanisms through which landscape impacts *P. knowlesi* risks. We additionally assess potential future changes in transmission pathways and opportunities to improve surveillance and control for this emerging zoonotic malaria species within these rapidly changing landscapes.

2. Ecological change and mechanisms of disease emergence and transmission

Deforestation has been identified as one of the key drivers of *P. knowlesi* emergence and likely to shape changing risks of *P. knowlesi* and other simian malarias. There is an increasing body of evidence documenting the complex relationship between land use and land cover changes and disease emergence; changes in human disease risk as a result of forest clearance is governed by a multitude of factors including physical changes to the environment, knock-on effects to ecological communities and by human behaviours and activity in areas where land use change occurs (Table 1). Within this section, we review the key mechanisms through which landscape change impacts disease transmission in relation to *P. knowlesi*.

2.1 Biodiversity impacts on vector-borne and zoonotic diseases

High biodiversity areas like tropical forests are often considered "hotspots" for emerging diseases due to the large pool of novel enzootic pathogens. However, the impacts of biodiversity on infectious disease are difficult to generalise, and have caused a great deal of debate. Attempts to establish a general unifying theory have been thwarted by contrasting evidence of both dilution and amplification effects being associated with high levels of biodiversity. There is evidence that in different circumstances high biodiversity can limit or increase the transmission of infectious diseases, whether emerging or established (Luis et al., 2018).

Spread of pathogens with density-dependent transmission may be amplified when species diversity is high if there is no compensatory reduction in abundance of a host species (Dobson, 2004). However, high host diversity in frequency-dependent and vector-mediated pathogens can in some circumstances buffer disease spread as infection rates within species populations remain relatively low (Dobson, 2004). Transmission of most vector-borne diseases is considered to be frequency-dependent as it is reliant on the actions of the vector (e.g. biting rate); high diversity is predicted to reduce disease risk in frequency dependent scenarios, due to differences in host competence between species (Ferrari et al., 2011).

Table 1 Examples of effects of land use change on infectious disease risk.

Environmental changes		References
Deforestation	Biodiversity loss caused by deforestation may be followed by colonization or domination by more efficient vectors and hosts of disease, e.g., malaria, hantavirus, Chagas disease.	Guerra et al. (2006), Roque et al. (2008), Durnez et al. (2013), Prist et al. (2017)
	Changes in vector habitat suitability are linked with forest disturbance, including for *Aedes*, *Culex*, and *Anopheles* mosquitoes.	Brant (2011), Loaiza et al. (2017)
	Changes in ecological structure and biodiversity can increase or decrease density and infection rates in hosts and vectors and availability of blood meals for vectors, influencing disease risks, e.g., malaria, trypanosomiasis, Lyme disease, hantaviruses.	Leonardo et al. (2005), Randolph and Dobson (2012), Mweempwa et al. (2015), Halsey and Miller (2020)
Agricultural expansion	Irrigation systems provide habitat for disease vectors and hosts including; anopheline & culicine mosquitoes incriminated in transmission of diseases such as malaria, Japanese encephalitis, and filiariasis, and intermediate snail hosts of schistosomiasis.	Madsen et al. (1987), Keiser et al. (2005a), Leonardo et al. (2005)
	Rubber plantations associated with vector-borne diseases (including malaria, chikungunya, dengue, JEV, filiariasis), with increased density of mosquitoes & their breeding sites.	Yasuoka and Levins (2007), Tangena et al. (2016), Jones et al. (2013), de Andrade et al. (2016)
	Introduction of livestock to forest fringe areas increases opportunity for pathogen spillover from wild to domestic animals and farm workers, e.g., transmission of rabies to cattle and humans by vampire bats in South America has been associated with proximity of large cattle herds to deforesting activities.	
Socio-demographic changes		
Population at risk	Influx of susceptible populations into endemic areas in response to increased economic opportunity can increase prevalence of diseases to which local people have gained some immunity, e.g., malaria, leishmaniasis, Oropouche fever.	Desjeux (2001), Barbieri et al. (2005), Sakkas et al. (2018), Pindolia et al. (2014)
	Economic opportunities increase numbers and movement of migrant worker populations: in the Amazon and Southeast Asia this has been linked to malaria; seasonal fluctuations of urban-rural migration for agriculture drive measles outbreaks in Niger; schistosomiasis prevalence and spread in Tanzania.	Bruun and Aagaard-Hansen (2008), Hansen et al. (2008), Ferrari et al. (2010), Sativipawee et al. (2012), Wai et al. (2014)

Continued

Table 1 Examples of effects of land use change on infectious disease risk.—cont'd

Environmental changes		References
	Occupational changes, such as forestry, farming, and extraction activities bringing people into habitats where they are more likely to interact with vectors of diseases such as malaria and Yellow Fever, and wildlife disease hosts like non-human primates and rodents.	Norris (2004), de Castro et al. (2006), Basurko et al. (2013), Gibb et al. (2017), Bloomfield et al. (2020)
Socioeconomic status	Increased income following agricultural development leading to decrease in disease risks and improved health outcomes, e.g., improved house structure mitigating malaria risk.	Tusting et al. (2017), Tusting et al. (2015), Tusting et al. (2013)
Wildlife reservoirs		
Origin of disease	60% Emerging infectious diseases thought to have zoonotic origin, with three quarters of these having wildlife origins. E.g., *P. falciparum* originated from non-human primates; bats have been implicated in emergence of multiple viruses affecting humans; HIV thought to have evolved from SIV infecting chimpanzees South Cameroon.	Liu et al. (2010), Sharp and Hahn (2011)
Spatial overlap with wildlife hosts	Increased contact between people and non-human primates hypothesised as main driver of human infections with: *P. knowlesi* and *P. cynomolgi* in Asia; *P. simium* and *P. brasilianum* in South America; thought to have a role in Ebola transmission in Africa. Habitat loss driving fruit bats to feed from cultivated orchards and increasing contact with livestock and/or humans implicated in emergence & outbreaks of Nipah and Hendra viruses.	Imai et al. (2014), Guimaraes et al. (2012), Brasil et al. (2017), Olivero et al. (2017), Looi and Chua (2007), Giles et al. (2018)
Maintenance of infections	Pathogens causing human disease can be maintained in wild animal populations, e.g., human malaria species circulating in great apes and gorillas in West and Central Africa; wild chimpanzees in the Cote d'Ivoire harbour human metapneumovirus (HMPV) and human respiratory syncytial virus (HRSV).	Kondgen et al. (2010), Sundararaman et al. (2013), Boundenga et al. (2015)

Shifts in community structures as a result of environmental change could be more important than natural biodiversity gradients. For example, inconsistencies in observation of a "dilution effect" may be attributed to these effects being more likely to be observed where biodiversity levels have fallen due to ecological disruption, including through land use and land cover change, than in areas where low biodiversity is a result of community assembly and ecological drift (Halliday et al., 2020). Biodiversity loss in degraded ecological communities tends to be non-random. The species that survive or are able to recolonise areas after events leading to biodiversity loss usually have fast life history strategies that prioritise reproduction, growth and dispersal rather than protection against disease, and often therefore have disproportionate roles in pathogen spread (Lacroix et al., 2014). For example, predicted biodiversity loss caused by sugarcane expansion and subsequent dominance of generalist rodents in Sao Paolo is expected to increase risk of Hantavirus pulmonary syndrome from 1.3% to 1.5% and place 20% more people at risk of contracting the disease (Prist et al., 2017).

The loss of the preferred host of a vector can change their feeding behaviours, including shifts towards human hosts. For example, in Kenya, experimental plots with large herbivores excluded were associated with elevated human biting rates of *Aedes mcintoshi,* a primary vector of Rift Valley Fever virus; however, when evaluated with a decline in abundance of the vector, overall vectorial capacity in exclusion zones was half of that in plots populated by large herbivores (Tchouassi et al., 2021). This illustrates the complex effects arising from changes to community structure are not uniform in their influence and should be evaluated in combination when evaluating overall changes to disease risk. Land use and land cover change can also facilitate the arrival and establishment of invasive species that may bring new disease risks. Not only do invasive species often cause a decline in species richness, but they can introduce novel pathogens or strains of a disease to immunologically-naive local populations (Crowl et al., 2008). Invasive species also provide the opportunity for pathogen host-switching, amplifying the transmission of disease and potentially increasing pathogen evolution speed, which is hypothesized to be greater where multiple transmission cycles exist and interact (Jacquot et al., 2016; Parrish et al., 2008; Wilcox and Ellis, 2006).

2.2 Habitat fragmentation and zoonotic and vector-borne diseases

Habitat fragmentation is often defined as the breaking up of an expansive landscape to form several, smaller patches of habitat separated by an unlike matrix (Wilcove et al., 1986). It can influence the spread of disease by altering the physical structure of a landscape, as well as the diversity, composition, and dynamics of its community (Collinge, 1996). Habitat fragmentation has been linked to increased infection rates in vectors and hosts, vector prevalence, and frequency of spillover events (Barros and Honorio, 2015; Rulli et al., 2017).

Habitat fragmentation alters conditions within the forest structure and increases the amount of "edge" habitat where the environment and micro-climate is different from intact forest, graduating from the patch's edge to its primary forest core (Laurance and Yensen, 1991). Edge effects change abiotic variables such as light, airflow, temperature, humidity, and soil moisture which are evident at different distances into forest interiors. For example, there is evidence of airflow differences reaching 240 m in, whereas it is difficult to detect changes in humidity, temperature and light far beyond 50 m (Chen et al., 1995, 1999). The differing degrees to which these factors reach into the forest and interact with each other makes it difficult to disentangle their effects, but there is still evidence that altered environmental conditions can influence factors related to the spread of zoonotic disease. These transitional zones between ecosystems are known as ecotones and when connecting wild spaces to manmade or settled environments are often areas of increased contact between pathogens, hosts and vectors.

Fragmentation creates smaller, isolated habitat patches with less "core" area in favour of "edge", increasing likelihood of interactions between animals and vectors living within the forest, and humans living on its outskirts (Wilkinson et al., 2018). Yellow fever virus is an example of a pathogen associated with forest ecotone environments. In non-urban areas the virus typically transmits enzootically between non-human primates and mosquitoes in a canopy-level sylvatic cycle deep in the forest (Valentine et al., 2019). However, human encroachment and settlement in forest fringes has created habitat that supports *Aedes* mosquitoes able to bridge the ecological gap between sylvatic and peri-urban transmission cycles (Couto-Lima et al., 2017).

In the Brazilian Amazon, Barros and Honorio (2015) found that larval "hotspots" for *A. darlingi* are associated with aquatic habitats at forest fringes, leading to high malarial rates in those living in proximity to forest fragment fringes. Those living within 400 m of a hotspot had a 2.6 times higher risk of malaria; these people were often recent settlers who resided in closest proximity to the forest fringe ecotone (Barros and Honorio, 2015).

Exacerbated disease risk in forest edge environments has been attributed to more frequent encroachment of forest by people living in these areas, but interactions and mixing between humans, hosts, vectors and pathogens in the ecotones themselves are also likely to be related to spillover risk (Despommier et al., 2006).

Fragmentation can have conflicting influences on vector-borne diseases. For example, the abundance of tsetse flies responsible for the spread of human and animal trypanosomiasis in Eastern Zambia are lowest in numbers in areas with the greatest amount of fragmentation (Ducheyne et al., 2009). Additionaly, in Malawi, tsetse flies are near-absent outside of protected areas where natural vegetation has not been cleared (Van den Bossche et al., 2000). However, this reduction in vector abundance does not necessarily translate into decreased risk of trypanosomiasis; tsetse flies in fragmented areas live longer and are more likely to be infected. A study on impact of habitat fragmentation on tsetse fly populations by Mweempwa et al. (2015) found that infection rates were highest in the most fragmented site (14.5%), followed by the least fragmented (7.6%), and lowest at an intermediate level of fragmentation (4.8%). Combined with the enhanced longevity of flies in the most fragmented areas, trypanosomiasis infection risk was not significantly different in the least and most fragmented sites, despite an eight-fold reduction in tsetse density between the two (Mweempwa et al., 2015). In European bank voles, carriage of Puumala hantavirus is higher in animals living in larger more connected environments than smaller areas isolated from other suitable habitat, implying fragmentation would reduce prevalence of the disease in this species (Guivier et al., 2011). The effect of environmental change on disease transmission is complex and dependent on the response of vector and host species; understanding the ecology of animals involved in the transmission cycle is vital in order to predict how altering a landscape will impact disease dynamics.

2.3 Physical changes to the environment and disease transmission

Altering landscapes can change the physical characteristics of an environment. This can include very localised changes in variables such as temperature, wind flow and the chemical composition of water, soil and air, or act on a greater scale: regional weather patterns can be affected in the long term by land cover conversion, especially in tropical areas (Feddema et al., 2005). Land use and land cover change can significantly influence surface fluxes of heat and water vapour, as well as result in greenhouse gas emissions and changes in carbon sink availability, and is an important climate forcing particularly in regional projection models (Quesada et al., 2017).

Logging can alter environmental conditions within a forest to different degrees depending on the intensity of the operation and the method used, and create novel habitats conducive to the spread of zoonotic diseases (Inada et al., 2017; Walsh et al., 1993). Removing trees reduces the number of leaves falling into ponds and streams, and without the tannins released during decomposition of the organic matter, acidity is decreased and turbidity increased, enhancing algal growth (Herrera-Silveira and Ramirez-Ramirez, 1996). Many mosquito larvae feed on algae; combined with greater sunlight and warmth from decreased canopy cover, these conditions create favourable breeding sites for mosquitoes (Kweka et al., 2016; Tuno et al., 2005).

The mosquito *Anopheles gambiae*, the primary vector of malaria in sub-Saharan Africa, is an example of a vector whose larval habitats are enhanced by deforestation. Decreased canopy cover is associated with increased abundance of *A. gambiae* larvae; artificial experiments by Afrane et al. revealed much higher larval survivorship in sunlit pools than in the shaded conditions associated with intact forest (Afrane et al., 2006). Similarly, Vittor et al. found that biting rates of *Anopheles darlingi,* an important vector for malaria in the Americas, were 278-times higher (after controlling for human population) in areas in the Amazon basin that have experienced over 80% deforestation than areas where deforestation was lower than 30% (Vittor et al., 2009).

Changes to the physical environment can also reduce disease risk. The black fly, *Simulium woodi*, is a vector for human onchocerciasis (river blindness). The Tanzanian population of black flies rapidly declined between 1963 and 1985, with the mean-biting catch falling by 87% in this time. Muro & Raybould, attributed this to a loss of suitable, cool, shaded breeding habitat due to deforestation. This period also saw a reduction in the percentage of mature *S. woodi* infected with the disease-causing agent, the nematode *Onchocerca volvulus,* from 17% to 3% (Muro and Raybould, 1990). While this decline plateaued, 25 years later populations had not recovered, suggesting deforestation in the area had a significant and long-term impact on vector numbers (Kalinga and Post, 2011).

2.4 Socio-economic changes and development and disease risks

Land use and land cover change, especially for extractive industries and conversion to agriculture, creates economic opportunity and can attract large numbers of migrant workers and settlers. When this economic migration introduces a novel population of immunologically naive humans to an area, increased levels of some diseases can be observed, especially in the early stages of settlement and forest clearance. Yellow fever outbreaks in the Angola and Democratic Republic of Congo have been associated with high population mobility combined with low vaccine coverage, for example (Kraemer et al., 2017). This dynamic has also been used to explain the meteoric rise in malaria cases associated with development in the Brazilian Amazon (dubbed "frontier malaria"), from around 8,000 cases per annum in 1970 to 615,000 in 2000 (Barbieri et al., 2005). Patterns of initial increased disease risk followed by reduction in infection have been explained by the different landscape patterns and human behaviour associated with early as compared to late stages of land cover change. Initial encroachment tends to involve small-scale agriculture and resource extraction, creating large amounts of forest-edge and increasing human exposure to pathogens, hosts and vectors, as more time is spent in forest and forest edge (MacDonald and Mordecai, 2019). As settlements become more established, they often grow in size and distance from forest habitat and develop stronger social institutions with better access to healthcare and disease prevention measures (de Castro et al., 2006). Additionally, forest edge habitat decreases as agricultural land is consolidated and intensification begins to take precedence over expansion, reducing deforestation rates (MacDonald and Mordecai, 2019).

Land use change is often accompanied by the building of infrastructure that can influence disease risks; this is particularly well documented for roads and for water management systems such as irrigation and dams. These can exacerbate fragmentation, create environmental conditions and novel habitats that may be suitable for vectors of disease, and facilitate the spread of people, animals and pathogens (Wilcox and Ellis, 2006; Wolfe et al., 2005). For example, trenches formed along roadsides can increase the amount of standing water and therefore breeding sites for mosquito vectors; the obstruction of natural water drainage is also associated with increased leptospirosis, as waterlogging forces rodents to leave their burrows and saturated agricultural fields become contaminated with urine, exposing farm workers to infection (Dubey et al., 2021). Logging roads designed to bring timber workers deeper into forest environments can increase likelihood of human contact with novel pathogens, and allow hunting activities to take place from any location along these rapidly expanding networks rather than within a radius of a settlement (Laurance et al., 2006); logging practices have been linked to elevated bushmeat demand, the hunting and consumption of which are associated with blood-borne and ingestion pathways of zoonotic spillover (Karesh and Noble, 2009; Poulsen et al., 2009). Roads also importantly facilitate increased movement of people, goods, livestock, and wildlife including invasive species and animals captured for the international wildlife trade, which can lead to establishment of diseases in new areas. Dengue is thought to have been transported to some areas through the international trade of used tyres harbouring infected *Aedes* species (Bennett et al., 2019). In Morocco, foci of anthroponotic cutaneous leishmaniasis are aligned geographically and temporally with the construction of road networks (Kahime et al., 2014). Areas of forest converted for agricultural use are often irrigated; the creation of novel freshwater habitats have been associated with increases in mosquito-borne and water-borne diseases. Risk of Japanese encephalitis virus (JEV), a mosquito-borne disease maintained zoonotically in wild birds, is elevated in irrigated areas (especially where pigs are kept as livestock and provide a domestic animal reservoir) (Pearce et al., 2018); this has been attributed to the proliferation of the primary vector *Culex tritaeniorhynchus* in habitat created by irrigation (Keiser et al., 2005b).

Different types of land cover change can be associated with different risks. For example: clear cutting of forest has a greater impact on biodiversity and the physical environmental conditions of a landscape, while individual exposure risk may be greater in selective logging due to more time spent in the forest environment (Wilcox and Ellis, 2006). Similarly, in rice-farming areas of the Philippines, *S. japonicum* is more prevalent in males of working age than other demographics (Tarafder et al., 2006). In South America and Southeast Asia, miners are at high risk from malaria, likely a combination of the high population mobility and minimal infrastructure of small-scale mining camps (Douine et al., 2020). Additionally, wildlife pathogens can infect livestock, and animal agriculture is associated with enhanced risk of zoonotic spillover and the potential for pathogen mixing and emergence (Jones et al., 2013). The effects of deforestation on disease emergence are not uniform, are highly dependent on how settlers and workers in frontier areas interact with and further alter their environments and are subject to change over time.

3. Distribution and burden of *Plasmodium knowlesi*

One of the critical limitations to understanding the role of these ecological changes on *P. knowlesi* transmission is data on the distribution of *P. knowlesi* infections in humans. While infection with *P. knowlesi* can cause severe and fatal disease in people, there are frequent asymptomatic infections and diagnostic limitations (Barber et al., 2013a; Daneshvar et al., 2009;

Grigg et al., 2016; Rajahram et al., 2012; William et al., 2011). Designing effective control programmes requires detailed information on the spatial epidemiology of *P. knowlesi* as well as an understanding of how environmental changes are likely to impact this distribution. Within this section, we review the spatial distribution of clinical and community-based *P. knowlesi* infections and associated reporting biases and describe reports of other simian malaria species.

3.1 Spatial distribution of reported *P. knowlesi* incidence

Molecular studies indicate *P. knowlesi* is not a newly emergent malaria species and likely pre-dates human settlement in Southeast Asia (Lee et al., 2011). *P. knowlesi* was first described in macaques in the 1930s and the first naturally acquired human case was reported in 1965 in peninsular Malaysia (Chin et al., 1965; Knowles and Das Gupta, 1932). Subsequent epidemiological investigations of people residing within the area where this individual was infected did not identify any additional human *P. knowlesi* cases, although *P. knowlesi* was detected in two out of the four long-tailed macaques screened (Warren et al., 1970). No further natural infections were reported until 2004, when the application of molecular diagnostic tools identified a large focus of *P. knowlesi* infections in the Kapit division of Sarawak in Malaysian Borneo (Singh et al., 2004). Retrospective studies have since detected *P. knowlesi* infections from archival blood films collected in the mid-1990s in Malaysia and Thailand, suggesting that previous human infections were misdiagnosed as other species by microscopy (Jongwutiwes et al., 2011; Lee et al., 2009a).

Since 2004, human *P. knowlesi* infections have been reported from a number of Southeast Asian countries (Moyes et al., 2014; Shearer et al., 2016). While sporadic cases have been reported from countries including the Philippines, Thailand, Vietnam, Cambodia, Laos, Myanmar, Singapore, Brunei, India, Indonesia and China, *P. knowlesi* is now the most common cause of human malaria in Malaysia (Barber et al., 2012; Cox-Singh et al., 2008; Figtree et al., 2010; Iwagami et al., 2018; Jiang et al., 2010; Jongwutiwes et al., 2004; Khim et al., 2011; Lee et al., 2009c; Luchavez et al., 2008; Ninan et al., 2012; Putaporntip et al., 2009; Sermwittayawong et al., 2012; Tyagi et al., 2013; Van den Eede et al., 2009; William et al., 2013, 2014; Zhou et al., 2014) (Fig. 1). In the Malaysian state of Sabah, despite an overall decrease in malaria notifications following successful malaria control measures, the percentage of suspected *P. knowlesi* notifications increased from 2% (59/2741) of all malaria notifications in 2004 to 62% (996/1606) of reported malaria cases in 2013 (William et al., 2013, 2014). Similar trends have

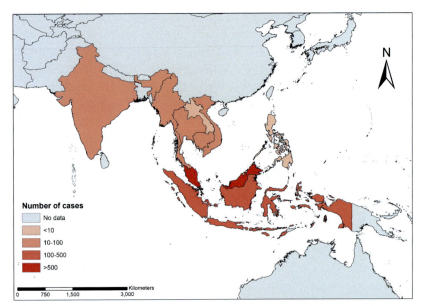

Fig. 1 Reports of PCR confirmed *P. knowlesi* infections in people by country from 1996 to 2021 by published literature (Ruiz Cuenca et al., 2021).

been reported in the neighbouring state of Sarawak, where suspected *P. knowlesi* accounted for the majority of reported malaria cases over the previous decade (Singh and Daneshvar, 2010). While Malaysia has not reported any indigenous malaria cases since 2018 and is currently under review for malaria elimination, increasing numbers of *P. knowlesi* cases continue to be reported, including over 4100 confirmed human infections with *P. knowlesi* in 2018 (Chin et al., 2020).

However, the true burden of *P. knowlesi* remains poorly understood due to frequent misidentification as other human malaria species by microscopy and the limited availability of *P. knowlesi*- specific molecular diagnostic capabilities. *P. knowlesi* appears microscopically similar to the human malaria species *P. malariae* but also can be misdiagnosed as *P. falciparum* and *P. vivax* (Barber et al., 2013c; Lee et al., 2009b; Singh and Daneshvar, 2013). Rapid diagnostic tests (RDTs) developed for other malaria species are also insufficiently sensitive to detect *P. knowlesi* and can lead to misdiagnosis as other species (Barber et al., 2013b; Foster et al., 2014; Grigg et al., 2014). While it is difficult to determine whether there is a genuine increase in human cases rather than improved detection, evidence of a significant increase in numbers and proportions of *P. knowlesi* malaria suggests transmission of *P. knowlesi* is rising in areas of Malaysia (Joveen-Neoh et al., 2011; William et al., 2013, 2014; Yusof et al., 2014).

3.2 Community-level spatial distribution of exposure and infection

Despite increasing amounts of data available for symptomatic *P. knowlesi* cases presenting at hospital facilities, there remain substantial knowledge gaps on patterns of infection and exposure in the community. The development and implementation of molecular diagnostic tools such as PCR has greatly contributed to the increasing detection of human *P. knowlesi* infection throughout Southeast Asia (Anstey and Grigg, 2019). Previous studies in Malaysia suggested that *P. knowlesi* infections were likely to be misdiagnosed as *P. malariae* by routine microscopy reading due to their similar morphological features (Kantele and Jokiranta, 2011; Lee et al., 2009b; Singh et al., 2004). In Indonesia, *P. knowlesi* has been universally misdiagnosed by microscopy, with no notifications of *P. knowlesi* made using standard national malaria reporting systems. However, a study in Indonesia identified an asymptomatic *P. knowlesi* case through a reactive case detection programme and *P. knowlesi* has been reported from specific research studies, confirming the presence of *P. knowlesi* in Indonesia (Herdiana et al., 2016).

The burden of *P. knowlesi* cannot be revealed in the absence of sensitive and specific diagnostic tools such as PCR. Molecular detection methods will also be vital to accurately demonstrate elimination of human–only malaria species in countries approaching this goal, given current malaria rapid diagnostic tests also lack specificity to differentiate *P. knowlesi* (Grigg et al., 2014; Singh and Daneshvar, 2013). In addition, understanding the true prevalence of zoonotic *Plasmodium* species requires sensitive detection of submicroscopic and/or asymptomatic infections, now increasingly reported to be present from molecular surveys conducted in Malaysia (Fornace et al., 2016b; Siner et al., 2017), Indonesia (Lubis et al., 2017), Cambodia (Imwong et al., 2019) and Myanmar (Ghinai et al., 2017). Population-based cross-sectional surveys are required to understand the prevalence of these infections in different settings and understand spatial patterns of disease infection.

The distribution of community-level exposure can also be assessed by prevalence of antibodies to species-specific malaria antibodies, reflecting previous exposure to malaria (Bousema et al., 2010; Corran et al., 2007; Wilson et al., 2007). Age-specific prevalence of these antibodies can be used to calculate seroconversion rates and evaluate changes in transmission over time; this measure has been shown to be closely correlated with other indicators of malaria transmission intensity such as parasite prevalence or entomological inoculation rates (Drakeley et al., 2005). Serological indices of exposure also have increased utility in low transmission settings where the probability of detecting infections is very low (Bousema et al., 2010; Cook et al., 2010).

While numerous antigens have been described for *P. falciparum* and *P. vivax*, species-specific antigens for *P. knowlesi* have only relatively recently been developed (Herman et al., 2018). This *P. knowlesi*-specific panel of novel recombinant antigens has allowed surveillance of selected endemic communities and has demonstrated that exposure to *P. knowlesi* is more widespread in women and children as well as male agricultural workers in Malaysia than previously thought and has also allowed evaluation of differences in spatial patterns of zoonotic versus non-zoonotic malaria (Fornace et al., 2018a, 2019b). Integrating both serological and molecular diagnostic tools is the most promising approach to characterise community-level *P. knowlesi* risks and to identify how environmental changes are shaping these risks.

3.3 Reporting bias and surveillance for *P. knowlesi*

Since the identification of a large number of *P. knowlesi* cases in Sarawak, Malaysia in 2004, research and surveillance efforts for *P. knowlesi* have been concentrated in Malaysia. Of 26 research projects on *P. knowlesi* identified between 2004 and 2021, 14 projects focused on Malaysia and another 10 projects focused solely on laboratory studies conducted in the United States, United Kingdom or Australia (MESA Track, 2021). This is broadly reflected in the published literature as well, with the number and amount of research publications addressing *P. knowlesi* dramatically increasing after 2004 (Fig. 2). Similarly, the identification of human

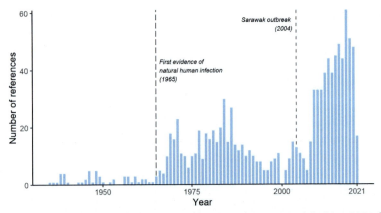

Fig. 2 Number of peer-reviewed papers on *P. knowlesi* retrieved in May 2021 from MEDLINE by year. Vertical dotted lines represent 2 key points in time, the first report of natural human infection with *P. knowlesi* and the identification of a *P. knowlesi* outbreak in Sarawak, Malaysian Borneo (Ruiz Cuenca et al., 2021).

infections with *P. knowlesi* has been predominantly concentrated within Malaysia despite identification of cases across Southeast Asia. This is a product of both the increased focus of research studies within Malaysia as well as changes to policies for malaria diagnosis and surveillance within Malaysia, particularly around the use of molecular methods (Table 2).

Diagnostic limitations are one of the key barriers to understanding the burden of *P. knowlesi* across Southeast Asia. WHO recommends countries confirm *P. knowlesi* infections by PCR and standardize case definition and investigation procedures but this is not routinely applied across all settings (World Health Organisation Regional Office for Western Pacific, 2017). Malaria has been a notifiable disease in Malaysia since 1988 and updated to include *P. knowlesi* specifically in 2010. (Fig. 3) As of 2017, malaria was routinely diagnosed in Malaysia by microscopy. Cases diagnosed as *P. falciparum*, *P. vivax* and *P. ovale* were quality controlled with all cases diagnosed as *P. malariae* or *P. knowlesi* confirmed by PCR. Within Sabah, Malaysia, a *P. knowlesi* foci, all human malaria cases were screened with molecular

Table 2 Number of studies reporting cases of human *P. knowlesi* infections by country and period within published scientific literature (Ruiz Cuenca et al., 2021). Numbers in brackets represent total number of cases. These totals excludes routinely collected malaria surveillance data.

	<2000	2000–2004	2005–2009	2010–2014	2015–2020
Brunei	0	0	0	0	1 (73)
Cambodia	0	0	3 (4)	2 (2)	1 (6)
India	0	0	0	0	9 (19)
Indonesia	0	0	2 (2)	13 (414)	0
Laos	0	0	0	0	1 (1)
Malaysia	1 (1)	4 (120)	63 (1167)	42 (1699)	26 (1401)
Myanmar	0	0	4 (32)	2 (17)	1 (1)
Philippines	0	0	2 (4)	0	2 (2)
Singapore	0	0	3 (5)	0	0
Thailand	1 (1)	1 (1)	5 (13)	3 (3)	20 (34)
Vietnam	0	2 (5)	3 (32)	0	0
South-East Asia[a]	0	0	1 (1)	1 (1)	1 (1)

[a]Studies identifying human cases but unable to specify which country infection took place in.

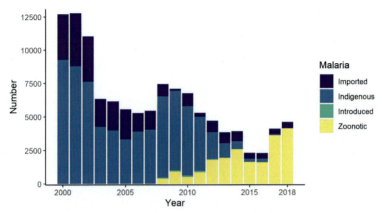

Fig. 3 Routinely collected malaria surveillance data of clinical malaria cases detected at health facilities from Malaysia (Chin et al., 2020b).

methods (World Health Organisation Regional Office for Western Pacific, 2017). With a move towards malaria elimination and the substantial decrease in non-zoonotic species, increased effort has been focused on diagnosing *P. knowlesi* in Malaysia (Chin et al., 2020).

Despite increasing data on *P. knowlesi* from Malaysia, there are notably fewer *P. knowlesi* reports from neighbouring Indonesia. All species of *Plasmodium* have been reported in Indonesia, with increasing number of human cases of *P. knowlesi* malaria being reported by several studies in the province of South Kalimantan (Sulistyaningsih et al., 2010), Central Kalimantan (Setiadi et al., 2016), North Sumatera (Lubis et al., 2017), and in Aceh (Herdiana et al., 2016, 2018). The limited evidence of *P. knowlesi* infection in Indonesia was partly due to limited diagnosis capacity of the existing malaria surveillance and control programme (Coutrier et al., 2018; Sulistyaningsih et al., 2010). Although most of the current evidence of *P. knowlesi* infections in Indonesia came from studies in the island of Kalimantan and Sumatera, a geospatial modelling study has also estimated several other areas in Java and Sulawesi islands as areas with moderate to high risk of *P. knowlesi* malaria (Shearer et al., 2016). These areas were identified as priority areas for surveillance based on regions with sparse data and high estimated risk. As evidence of *P. knowlesi* risk becomes more prominent, the Indonesian national malaria control programme has developed a molecular surveillance approaches for *P. knowlesi* malaria that will be piloted in several areas in Kalimantan, Sumatera, and in Java island [personal communication with a member of national malaria committee]. Whilst there are ongoing cross-sectional surveys to assess molecular and seroprevalence of *P. knowlesi* in Kalimantan and North Sumatera, there is a need to expand these activities to other areas such as in Java and Sulawesi island, where knowlesi tranmission may be likely.

To date, reports of naturally acquired *P. knowlesi* are limited to Asia. Isolated cases of human *P. knowlesi* infections have been reported in Europe, North America, Japan, Australia and New Zealand but all reported individuals had histories of travel to Southeast Asia (Orth et al., 2013; Berry et al., 2011; Bronner et al., 2009; Cordina et al., 2014; De Canale et al., 2017; Hoosen and Shaw, 2011; Kantele et al., 2008; Mackroth et al., 2016; Nowak et al., 2019; Ozbilgin et al., 2016; Roe et al., 2020; Seilmaier et al., 2014; Ta et al., 2010; Takaya et al., 2018; Tanizaki et al., 2013). There have been no published *P. knowlesi* reports in travellers or other individuals in Africa or South America, potentially due to diagnosis as other malaria species in endemic regions. Although other simian malarias are reported in these regions, *P. knowlesi* distribution currently only extends to Southeast Asia and India. Within these regions, substantial spatial heterogeneities in reported disease burden remain, raising key questions about the mechanisms underlying these differences in *P. knowlesi* transmission.

3.4 Emergence of other zoonotic simian malarias in Southeast Asia

Although *P. knowlesi* is the most widely reported zoonotic malaria species globally, other simian malaria species can cause human infections. *P. cynomolgi*, a simian malaria parasite widely distributed in macaques in Southeast Asia, was first shown to be transmissible to people accidentally in laboratory studies conducted in the United States in 1960 (Eyles et al., 1960). Subsequent studies in experimentally infected human volunteers with *P. cynomolgi* demonstrated potential for non-zoonotic transmission through mosquito vectors (Contacos et al., 1962; Schmidt et al., 1961). Further studies also demonstrated the potential for human infection with the simian malaria *P. inui* in laboratory settings (Coatney et al., 1966). Recently, natural asymptomatic *P. inui* infections have been identified in people in Malaysia, although the extent and the public health importance of these infections remains unknown (Liew et al., 2021).

Despite this early experimental evidence of zoonotic potential, the first naturally acquired human infection with *P. cynomolgi* was only identified in 2011. An adult residing in a malaria-free area of peninsular Malaysia reported to a clinic with symptomatic malaria molecularly identified as *P. cynomolgi*

(Ta et al., 2014). Subsequently, asymptomatic infections with *P. cynomolgi* have been identified in Malaysian Borneo and Cambodia (Grignard et al., 2019; Imwong et al., 2019). A retrospective review of blood samples from symptomatic malaria patients in Sarawak, Malaysia additionally identified 6 *P. cynomolgi/ P. knowlesi* co-infections (Raja et al., 2020). These isolated studies and the high prevalence of *P. cynomolgi* detected in both macaques and mosquito vectors suggest transmission of *P. cynomolgi* to people is almost certainly occurring more frequently than detected. There remains little evidence that *P. cynomolgi* currently causes significant public health impacts; however, monitoring transmission of other simian malarias is a priority for malaria surveillance in this region.

4. Landscape impacts on *P. knowlesi* disease dynamics

Land use changes, and associated ecological and social changes, have been proposed as the main drivers of the apparent emergence of human *P. knowlesi* and may impact risks of other simian malaria species (Cox-Singh and Singh, 2008; Lee et al., 2011). While many of the mechanisms through which land use change influences *P. knowlesi* transmission are less well characterised than for other diseases, deforestation and other landscape changes are known to impact the distribution, behaviour and susceptibility of human, macaque and mosquito populations. Southeast Asia is one of the most rapidly changing environments on the planet and has been identified as a global hotspot of disease emergence (Allen et al., 2017). Within this section, we review the drivers and extent of environmental change in Southeast Asia, identifying links between landscape change and *P. knowlesi* risks and describe evidence of how landscape change impacts human populations, wildlife reservoirs and vector dynamics.

4.1 Environmental change in Southeast Asia

Southeast Asia contains around 15% of the world's tropical forest, encompassing a range of important and diverse habitats, including montane and lowland rainforests, dry deciduous forests, swamp forests and mangroves (Stibig et al., 2014). At least 4 of the globe's 25 most important biodiversity hotspots can be found in the region, home to endemic species found nowhere else (Sodhi et al., 2010). Tropical forests are also important carbon sinks, mitigating greenhouse gas emissions and providing a crucial buffer against climate change (De Deyn et al., 2008).

However, this region has experienced one of the highest rates of deforestation globally, losing an average of 1.6 million hectares of forest per year between 1990 and 2010 (Fig. 4) (Stibig et al., 2014). Between 1990 and 2020, the region's forest cover declined by 376,000 km^2, with rates differing between constituent countries (FAO, 2020) (Table 3). A substantial proportion of deforestation has occurred within protected conservation areas and led to predictions that up to 85% of the region's biodiversity could be lost by 2100 (Sodhi et al., 2010). Commodity-driven deforestation is the cause of over 75% of forest loss in Southeast Asia since 2000, with smaller losses attributable to smallholder shifting agricultural practices and forestry (Curtis et al., 2018). These forest losses are a major source of anthropogenic carbon emissions and are the focus of on-going national and international climate change initiatives (Estoque et al., 2019).

Within Southeast Asia, there are substantial heterogeneities in land use change, drivers and policy responses. Malaysia and Indonesia have been named as global hotspots of forest loss and degradation due the rapid conversion of land for industrial oil palm plantations and other agricultural activities (Bryan et al., 2013; Danylo et al., 2021; Gaveau et al., 2016).

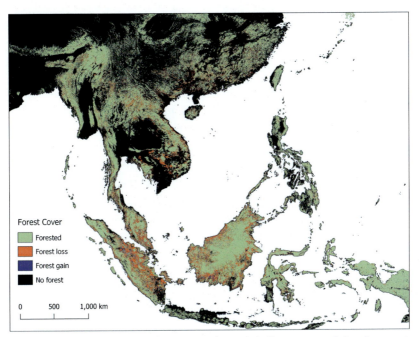

Fig. 4 Forest loss from 2000 to 2019 in Southeast Asia (forest cover defined as greater than 50% canopy cover, obtained from (Hansen et al., 2013)).

Table 3 Change in forest area in Southeast Asian countries between 1990 and 2020 (FAO, 2020). While most underwent net forest loss in this time period, some countries which saw significant deforestation prior to this time period have entered a reforestation phase; concentrated efforts towards restoring historical levels of forest cover in Vietnam have been implemented since the 1990s, for example (McElwee, 2009).

Country	Forest area (1000 ha)			
	1990	2020	Change	Cover change (%)
Myanmar	39,218.48	28,543.89	−10,674.59	−27.22
Cambodia	11,004.79	8068.37	−2936.42	−26.68
Indonesia	118,545.00	92,133.20	−26,411.80	−22.28
Brunei	413.00	380.00	−33.00	−7.99
the Philippines	7,778.81	7188.59	−590.22	−7.59
Malaysia	20,618.50	19,114.04	−1504.46	−7.30
Laos	17,843.00	16,595.50	−1247.50	−6.99
Timor-Leste	963.10	921.10	−42.00	−4.36
Thailand	19,361.00	19,873.00	512.00	2.64
Singapore	14.83	15.57	0.74	4.99
Vietnam	9375.96	14,643.09	5267.13	56.18

While both industrial and smallholder agricultural practices contribute to deforestation, industrial plantations have been associated with over three times the amount of forest conversion and are a main driver of loss in old growth forests (Gaveau et al., 2021). Increases in land used for industrial oil palm plantations are driven by global increases in crude palm oil prices, primarily due to the expanding markets for biofuels (Li et al., 2020). In 2011, Indonesia enacted a moratorium prohibiting conversion of primary forests and peat lands to tree plantations as part of a strategy to reduce emissions from deforestation (Busch et al., 2015). Malaysia has introduced similar restrictions on forest conversion and corporate commitments to reduce deforestation and promote sustainable palm oil development now cover the majority of industrial production in Malaysia and Indonesia (Weisse and Goldman, 2021). Although spikes in deforestation occurred in 2015 following widespread droughts and fires, rates of primary forest loss have consistently decreased in Malaysia and Indonesia from 2017—2020 following these policy changes (Weisse and Goldman, 2021).

In mainland Southeast Asia, commodity production has also driven forest loss. Between 1998 and 2018, over 50% of lowland forest cover was lost in Vietnam, Thailand, Cambodia, Laos, Peninsular Malaysia and Myanmar. This included a 50% loss of lowland forests within protected areas (Namkhan et al., 2021). Notably, Cambodia has lost over 1.1 million hectares of primary forest and over 24% of the country's tree cover since 2002 (Hansen et al., 2013). In contrast to Malaysia and Indonesia, expansion of rubber plantations is the primary driver of Cambodian forest conversion, with forest loss highly correlated with global rubber prices (Grogan et al., 2019). Within the Greater Mekong basin, small-scale shifting agriculture and local timber use have transformed areas into a patchwork of fragmented forests and cropland (Curtis et al., 2018; Namkhan et al., 2021). Swidden farming practices, in which land is cultivated for a short fertile period and then abandoned, are also an important driver of deforestation, especially in Northern Vietnam (Weisse and Goldman, 2021). Deliberate slash-and-burn agriculture and the draining of peat-swamps for farming are also associated with drought and wildfires that exacerbate direct deforestation effects (Page and Hooijer, 2016; Sloan et al., 2017). The majority (90%) of lowland forests within mainland Southeast Asia have been identified as severely threatened and vulnerable to deforestation (Namkhan et al., 2021). Further increases in deforestation and losses of biodiversity are predicted within this area following extensive infrastructure development for the Belt and Road Initiative (Ng et al., 2020).

Logging is also a lucrative industry in Southeast Asia and accounts for 19% of forest loss; its dipterocarp forests are one of the globe's most important sources of tropical hardwood (Kettle, 2009). Clear cutting operations fell all trees in an area, thereby completely deforesting it. Selective and reduced-impact logging extract only high-value trees, leaving most of the forest intact, and may involve additional measures to minimise forest degradation. For example, pre-harvest assessments and identification of crop trees ahead of time allow for carefully planned road and skid trail construction so as to minimise the number and destructive effects of these routes, while lianas and vines connecting tree crowns of non-target trees to crop trees and directional felling prevent non-target trees being pulled down or weakened (Putz et al., 2008). While licensed selective timber extraction is less ecologically disruptive, Southeast Asia (especially Indonesia) sees high rates of illegal logging usually employing more destructive measures (Weisse and Goldman, 2021).

These changes in forest cover have occurred in parallel to wider population and climatic changes. An overall increase in temperature as well as increases in temperature extremes have been observed across Southeast Asia over the past century. These have been accompanied with increased variability of precipitation and resulting challenges in water scarcity and food insecurity (Hijioka et al., 2014). These changes are likely to interact with wider landscape and demographic changes to pose substantial challenges to sustainable development and public health. Consistent with global trends, populations in Southeast Asia have becoming increasingly urbanised. Across Southeast Asia, the proportion of populations living in urban areas increased from 15.6% in 1950 to over 50% in 2020, with 66% of the population projected to live in cities by 2050 (United Nations Department of Economic and Social Affairs Population Division, 2018). Despite rapidly growing urban centres, increasing urbanization has mainly corresponded to increased population density and less than 1% of deforestation is due to urban expansion (Curtis et al., 2018).

4.2 Impacts of environmental change on distribution of *P. knowlesi*

Since the first identification of a large number of human *P. knowlesi* cases in forest and plantation workers, the recent increases in *P. knowlesi* incidence have widely been attributed to deforestation and land use change. Mathematical models of simulated data were first used quantitatively to examine the role of land use change in *P. knowlesi* transmission. Imai et al. used multi-host transmission models to assess the role of mixing between human and macaque populations in different ecological settings and demonstrate how deforestation may drive transmission by bringing these populations in closer proximity (Imai et al., 2014). Using empirical data, statistical associations between deforestation and human *P. knowlesi* incidence were first confirmed in Northern Sabah, Malaysia. Analysing hospital-based reports adjusted for diagnostic uncertainty and remotely sensed data on land cover, village-level *P. knowlesi* incidence was positively associated with both forest cover and historical forest loss (Fornace et al., 2016a). Subsequent studies in the same region identified strong associations between forest cover, fragmentation and deforestation with household level *P. knowlesi* risks. These factors were most predictive at different spatial scales, highlighting the complex role of land cover in transmission of multi-host vector-borne diseases (Brock et al., 2019).

At regional levels, spatial modelling studies identified similar associations between different forest types, deforestation and *P. knowlesi* presence across Southeast Asia (Shearer et al., 2016). These patterns were consistent with the distribution of the main *P. knowlesi* reservoirs and vectors across Southeast Asia (Moyes et al., 2016). Further mapping studies have demonstrated human infection risks are associated with specific agricultural practices in addition to deforestation. A cross-sectional survey across four districts in Northern Sabah, Malaysia identified positive associations between recent exposure to *P. knowlesi* (as measured by serology) and proportions and configuration of irrigated farming, pulpwood and oil palm plantations. This study additionally showed protective effects of intact, old-growth forests (Fornace et al., 2019b). A study examining reported incidence of symptomatic *P. knowlesi* cases in this region similarly identified associations between oil palm plantations and forest fragments (Sato et al., 2019). Although not specifically assessing the role of land cover, another study found significant spatial and temporal heterogeneity in reported cases in Peninsular Malaysia (Phang et al., 2020). Elsewhere in Southeast Asia, *P. knowlesi* infections have been detected during malaria surveys but at a frequency insufficient for analysis of environmental risk factors (e.g. (Shimizu et al., 2020)).

4.3 Human populations, movement and occupational risks

Landscape changes bring humans into closer contact with disease reservoirs and vectors as new areas are settled and agricultural and forest activities are undertaken. Individual human movement patterns influence the exposure to disease vectors and wildlife reservoirs within different environments (Hausermann et al., 2012; Stoddard et al., 2009). These movements occur on different spatial and temporal scales, from long term migrations to daily movements in areas surrounding households (Pindolia et al., 2012, 2014). Regional migration can lead to immunologically naïve individuals moving to areas of disease transmission or introduce infected individuals to areas previously free from disease (Wesolowski et al., 2012). On a local scale, deforestation has been associated with higher levels of human activities in forest areas and increased exposure to anopheline malaria vectors (Barbieri et al., 2005; de Castro et al., 2006). Other forest-related occupational activities, such as logging, rubber tapping and mining, have also been linked to higher malaria risks (Basurko et al., 2013; Hahn et al., 2014; Satitvipawee et al., 2012; Wai et al., 2014).

In Kapit, Sarawak, the majority (83%; 93/107) of molecularly confirmed *P. knowlesi* patients reported some type of forest exposure (Daneshvar et al., 2009). Similarly, a study of patients from a referral hospital in Sabah found that most *P. knowlesi* cases (92%, 119/130) had spent time in a forest or plantation the previous month (Barber et al., 2013a). However, reports from a district hospital in the largely deforested area of Kudat in Northwest Sabah describe a wide age distribution of *P. knowlesi* cases (0.7–89 years) and lack of association with forest activities (Barber et al., 2012). A subsequent case control study conducted within Kudat and Kota Marudu districts found a similarly wide age distribution (3–85 years), with 9% of cases occurring in children under the age of 15 (Grigg et al., 2017). This study also identified plantation work, forest activities and sleeping outside overnight as associated with increased *P. knowlesi* risk, however, a minority of cases, including children, had no reported farm or forest activities, suggesting the possibility of peri-domestic transmission. The protective effects of indoor residual spraying (IRS) and associations between risk and vegetation surrounding the household provide additional evidence for transmission around the household. Community-based studies similarly found high proportions of women and children with evidence of asymptomatic infections and exposure to *P. knowlesi* and raises questions on the role and importance of peri-domestic transmission (Fornace et al., 2018a, 2019b).

The increasing availability of technology offers new opportunities to characterise human movement patterns and behaviours. While mobile phone records can be used to track long-range human migration and movement patterns, GPS trackers and other devices allow fine-scale examination of how people use landscapes (Pindolia et al., 2012). A large-scale GPS tracking study in Northern Sabah, Malaysia identified substantial heterogeneities in routine individual space use patterns not strongly correlated with demographic characteristics or reported occupational activities. By integrating movement data with spatiotemporal models of mosquito biting and infection rates, this study demonstrated over 90% of infectious bites with *P. knowlesi* were likely to occur in areas close to households at forest edges despite higher biting rates in interior forested areas (Fornace et al., 2019a). Along the Thai-Myanmar border, entomological and human movement data were similarly integrated to identify likely areas of exposure, using repeated transect walks to estimate human population density. Results demonstrated the importance of farm huts and temporary dwellings in malaria transmission, notably identifying behaviour changes, including the reduced use of insecticide treate- bed nets, within these forested areas

(Edwards et al., 2019). An anthropological study in Cambodia also identified high variability in human behaviour and use of vector control methods within these different environments (Gryseels et al., 2015).

These behavioural patterns are likely also to impact access to healthcare and corresponding immunity and susceptibility to infections. In addition to changing the physical environment, deforestation and other land use changes transform socio-economic and demographic practices (Fornace et al., 2021). Frontier communities involved in forestry or plantation activities often have reduced access to health systems; these dynamics may change over time as communities become more established and implement public health measures in response to outbreaks (Baeza et al., 2017). Individuals living within endemic areas are additionally more likely to acquire clinical immunity to malaria over time. In a frontier settlement in the Amazon, malaria risks were strongly associated with land clearing and agricultural activities; however, risks of clinical malaria sharply decreased after continued residence in this area (da Silva-Nunes et al., 2008). These infections are also much less likely to be detected by passive surveillance systems. In the Philippines, residence near intact forests was associated with decreased detection at health clinics, increased malaria infection risks detected by molecular methods and decreased risks of clinical malaria (Fornace et al., 2020). While the role of immunity to *P. knowlesi* through previous exposure or exposure to other malaria species is largely unknown, landscape change is likely to alter the susceptibility of human populations to *P. knowlesi* infections through both biological and social mechanisms.

4.4 Simian host ecology and infection rates

Changing habitats are likely to have similar effects on the distribution and density of the simian hosts (Table 4). The main natural hosts of *P. knowlesi* are long-tailed macaques (*Macaca fascicularis*) and pig-tailed macaques (*Macaca nemestrina*) (Coatney et al., 1971). A report in peninsular Malaysia identified a banded leaf monkey (*Presbytis melalophos*) infected by *P. knowlesi* (Eyles et al., 1962) and a study in Thailand reported an infection of the parasite in dusky leaf monkey (*Semnopithecus obscurus*) (Putaporntip et al., 2010). A recent study by Fungfuang et al. (2020), first documented natural infections of stump-tailed macaques (*Macaca arctoides*) with *P. knowlesi* (Fungfuang et al., 2020). Other primate species identified as susceptible to *P. knowlesi* infection in laboratory studies include *Callithrix jacchus, Cebus* spp., *Cercocebus fuliginosus, Cercophitecus cephus, Cynochepalus papio, Hoolock*

Table 4 Hosts with confirmed evidence of *P. knowlesi* infections, separated into confirmed hosts, possible hosts (single case reports of infections in wild) and laboratory infections.

Confirmed hosts			Possible hosts			Experimental infections		
Long-tailed macaque	*Macaca fascicularis*	Coatney et al. (1971)	Stump-tailed macaque	*Macaca arctoides*	Fungfuang et al. (2020)	Common marmoset	*Callithrix jacchus*	Coatney et al. (1971)
Pig-tailed macaque	*Macaca nemestrina*	Coatney et al. (1971)	Banded leaf monkey	*Presbytis melalophos*	Eyles et al. (1962)	White-eyelid mangabey	*Cercocebus fuliginosus*	Coatney et al. (1971)
			Dusky leaf monkey	*Semnopithecus obscurus*	Putaporntip et al. (2010)	Moustached guenon	*Cercophitecus cephus*	Coatney et al. (1971)
						Yellow baboon	*Cynocephalus papio*	Coatney et al. (1971)
						Western hoolock gibbon	*Hoolock hoolock*	Coatney et al. (1971)
						Bonnet macaque	*Macaca radiata*	Coatney et al. (1971)
						Assam macaque	*Macaca assamensis*	Dutta et al. (1978)
						Dog face baboon	*Papio doguera*	Coatney et al. (1971)
						Baboon	*Papio jubilaeus*	Coatney et al. (1971)
						Guinea baboon	*Papio papio*	Coatney et al. (1971)
						Silvered leaf-monkey	*Presbytis cristatus*	Coatney et al. (1971)
						Common squirrel monkey	*Saimiri sciureus*	Coatney et al. (1971)
						Gray langur	*Semnopithecus entellus*	Coatney et al. (1971)

hoolock, Macaca radiata, Macaca arctoides, Papio doguera, Papio jubilaeus, Papio papio, Presbytis cristatus, Saimiri sciureus and *Semnopithecus entellus* (Coatney et al., 1971). Of these potential reservoirs, macaques are ecologically diverse and are the most widely distributed genus of nonhuman primates. Some macaques are prone to various infectious agents including viruses and parasites, and therefore could be the causes of emerging or re-emerging zoonotic diseases in humans (Wolfe et al., 1998). In particular, long-tailed macaques have substantial interfaces with humans, primarily with local populations but also with tourists visiting macaque habitats. This interface can lead to mutual disease transmission.

Previous studies have indicated a relatively high proportion of macaques are infected with *P. knowlesi* and genetic studies of human infections have identified two distinct parasite populations associated with long-tailed and pig-tailed macaque reservoir species (Divis et al., 2015; Lee et al., 2011). While the possibility of human to human transmission of *P. knowlesi* has been demonstrated experimentally, the high parasite diversity found within macaques suggests transmission remains primarily zoonotic (Assefa et al., 2015; Chin et al., 1968; Divis et al., 2015). Little data exist about the prevalence or infectiousness in macaque hosts. Identification of infections in macaques is limited by the same diagnostic challenges as in human samples, further complicated by the difficulty of obtaining macaque blood samples or isolating *Plasmodium* from faecal samples (Siregar et al., 2015; Stark and Salgado-Lynn, 2014). Collecting additional data on macaque populations is challenged by both logistical difficulties in catching, sampling and detecting macaques as well as strict ethical guidelines on the sampling of non-human primates, both from local and international guidelines (e.g. CITES, the Convention on International Trade in Endangered Species of Wild Fauna and Flora). Although little is known about the pathology of *P. knowlesi* infections in macaques, the identification of large proportions of macaque populations as infected suggests that infections are likely to be long term (Lee et al., 2011). Available evidence suggests most monkey species are asymptomatic when infected with *P. knowlesi* and have low parasitaemia levels, with the notable exception of rhesus macaques (*M. mulatta*) in which *P. knowlesi* infections are typically fatal (Baird, 2009; Vadivelan and Dutta, 2014).

Substantial gaps remain in the understanding of infection dynamics within wild primates and how these are likely to respond to habitat changes. *P. knowlesi* transmission and prevalence can be affected by ecosystem changes by changing the ecology (abundance and behaviour) of reservoir hosts or by compromising immune function through stress (Keesing et al., 2010). These changes are likely to lead to geographical differences in the prevalence of malaria parasites in macaque species. Within the major *P. knowlesi* transmission focus of Sabah, Malaysia, human cases of *P. knowlesi* are mainly reported from the interior mountainous and more densely forested districts that lie along the Crocker range, which stretches along the southwest-northeast axis of Sabah from Tenom to Ranau. On the contrary, incidence in the more cultivated low-lying districts along the West and East coast has remained relatively low (William et al., 2014). The spatial distribution of *P. knowlesi* cases across Sabah is consistent with forest or forest-edge exposure being a likely risk factor for human infection and spillover occurring in forest edges or farms where both humans and macaques are present (Cox-Singh and Singh, 2008; Imai et al., 2014). Studies of pig-tailed and long-tailed macaques within similar environments in Sarawak, Borneo identified a high proportion were infected with *Plasmodium species*, including 78% with *P. knowlesi* (Lee et al., 2011). In Thailand, a study demonstrated that malaria was prevalent in macaques living in mangrove forests, but no malaria infections were found in macaques living in urban areas (Seethamchai et al., 2008). Similarly, studies by Vythilingam et al. (2008) and Gamalo et al. (2019) also found no parasites in long-tailed macaques living in urban areas, however, monkeys caught in forested areas were infected with simian malaria parasites (Gamalo et al., 2019; Vythilingam et al., 2008).

These patterns of macaque infection and distribution may be changing due to increasing human encroachment into forests, high rates of construction and development, and the presence of secondary rainforests in the locality of urban and suburban residences which offer suitable habitats for monkeys that can harbour various species of simian malaria parasites (Braima et al., 2013). Deforestation converts primary forest to anthropogenic land uses and also fragments forest into smaller patches creating boundaries between small, disconnected islands of forest (Cushman et al., 2017; Taubert et al., 2018). Wildlife populations and individual primate species respond differently to the physical and biotic changes that arise as a result of disturbance of forest edge margins (Laurance et al., 2018). This habitat disturbance can influence primate disease transmission by altering ranging patterns, increasing density or crowding within forest patches or weakening immunity through exposure to other pathogens e.g. (Gillespie and Chapman, 2006; Kowalewski et al., 2011; Mbora et al., 2009; Nunn et al., 2003, 2014; Young et al., 2013). Macaques are also frequently found in close contact to human settlements and in highly disturbed environments, where loss of natural habitat may lead to increased dependence on anthropogenic food sources and closer contact with people (Fooden, 1995; Moyes et al., 2016; Young et al., 2013). Deforestation may cause macaques to use the remaining forest patches, spend more time on the ground and change their ranging behaviour and micro-habitat use (Chapman et al., 2005, 2006; Riley, 2008; Singh et al., 2001). Macaques may also go out to human settlements to raid crops or forage around houses, bringing them in contact with humans (Hambali et al., 2012).

Within Sabah, Malaysia, a case study report of a GPS-collared macaque troop suggests that macaque ranging behaviour is disturbed by deforestation events, with macaques moving in close proximity to houses where symptomatic human *P. knowlesi* cases were detected (Stark et al., 2019). Within this same geographic area, phylogenetic analysis provided further evidence of common *P. knowlesi* isolates between macaques, human cases and *An. balabacensis* mosquitoes in this region (Chua et al., 2017). A study by Brock et al. (2019) demonstrated that landscape fragmentation caused by deforestation influences *P. knowlesi* spillover into humans regionally, with the most predictive spatial scale of fragmentation influence on *P. knowlesi* transmission within 4 and 5 km of households. As macaques move distances up to 5 km in response to fragmentation, therefore, they may respond to deforestation on this emergent scale (Stark et al., 2019).

The transmission dynamics of *P. knowlesi* are almost certainly altered due to deforestation and changes in macaque populations and behaviour (Cox-Singh and Singh, 2008). Although Southeast Asian macaques harbour many parasites species, little is known about their distribution and epidemiology (Amir et al., 2020). It is critical to gather more information on the distribution and abundance of macaques as well as vectors of the parasite and assess how these may be influenced by rapidly changing landscapes over time. This information is essential to inform models of *P. knowlesi* transmission to target transmission hotspots and identify strategies for prevention and treatment.

4.5 Mosquito ecology, infection and bionomics

Physical changes in the environment, such as changes in vegetation, micro-climate and soil, can affect the species composition and abundance of vector populations (Yasuoka and Levins, 2007). For example, deforestation has been shown to create environmental conditions favourable for larval breeding sites of malaria vectors (Vittor et al., 2009). Within Southeast Asia, agriculture such as rubber plantations and rice paddies have been associated with increased anopheline densities as well as increases in malaria incidence (Yasuoka and Levins, 2007). In some cases, deforestation has been reported to cause initial depletion of forest dwelling vectors followed by colonisation of the area by more efficient vector species and overall increases in malaria transmission (Durnez et al., 2013; Guerra et al., 2006). Deforestation may also alter the importance of sylvatic and peri-domestic transmission cycles, as seen in yellow fever dynamics (Valentine et al., 2019).

Entomological dynamics of *P. knowlesi* are undoubtedly complex, with numerous vectors implicated in sylvatic and zoonotic transmission. The main *P. knowlesi* vectors are members of the *Anopheles* Leucosphyrus group of mosquitoes; *P. knowlesi* sporozoites and ooycsts have been identified in *An. latens*, *An. cracens, An. balabacensis, An. dirus* and *An. introlatus* (Chinh et al., 2019; Sallum et al., 2005; Vythilingam et al., 2006; Wong et al., 2015a). The geographical distribution of the Leucosphyrus group of mosquitoes extends across Southeast Asia, with these species commonly reported to be associated with forest environments (Moyes et al., 2016). Molecular evidence additionally identified *P. knowlesi* within members of the Barbirostris and Umbrosus groups and the Sundaicus complex; although the presence of oocysts and sporozoites has not been confirmed within these groups. Further studies are needed to determine the role of mosquitoes outside the Leucosphyrus group in *P. knowlesi* transmission.

Previous studies on the main vectors of *P. knowlesi*, the primarily exophagic *Anopheles leucosphyrus* group of mosquitoes, found relatively high biting rates in both farm and forest edge areas (Tan et al., 2008; Vythilingam et al., 2008). Entomological studies in Kapit, Sarawak have incriminated *An. latens* as the main vector of *P. knowlesi* in this area and observed this species is both attracted to macaques in the canopy and humans on the ground (Tan et al., 2008; Vythilingam et al., 2006). Studies within Sabah have implicated *An. balabacensis* as the primary vector of *P. knowlesi* in Northwest Sabah; this species was also historically the main vector of human malaria species within the region and has been experimentally shown to be able to transmit *P. knowlesi* (Collins et al., 1967; Hii, 1985; Wong et al., 2015b). Notably, the peak biting times of *An. balabacensis* and other mosquitoes from the Leucosphyrus group are in the early evening (6–10 pm) when people are unlikely to be using bed nets (De Ang et al., 2021; Wong et al., 2015a). Other possible vectors have been reported biting during the day time (7–11 am) which poses substantial challenges for vector control and prevention (De Ang et al., 2021).

Deforestation is likely to be impacting the distribution of *P. knowlesi* vectors. A study of mosquito ecology across a forest disturbance gradient in Sabah found abundance of *An. balabacensis* was higher in previously logged forests compared with primary forests. This vector was present at both ground and canopy levels, suggesting the potential for this mosquito to transmit *P. knowlesi* between canopy-dwelling primates and people at ground level (Brant et al., 2016). Additional investigations of anopheline mosquito densities within villages reporting *knowlesi* cases found higher densities of *An. balabacensis* in environments around cases households and identified vectors infected with simian malarias in peridomestic settings (Manin et al., 2016). Other studies have found higher *An. balabacensis* biting rates at both forest edges and farm or plantation areas (Brown et al., 2020; Hawkes et al., 2019). Despite this association with forest edges, the role of fragmentation in *P. knowlesi* vector ecology remains largely unknown; while fragmentation was not associated with increased *An. balabacensis* biting rates, fragmentation was associated with changes in vector composition and increases in density of secondary vectors in Sabah (Hawkes et al., 2019). *An. balabacensis* have reported breeding in shallow, muddy pools in farms and at forest edges, raising the question of whether fragmentation may be creating new breeding sites (Rohani et al., 2019). Key questions remain on how landscape changes will impact adult vector distributions, larval ecology and biting preferences. However, together, these data indicate that changing land use patterns are affecting the distribution and behaviour of mosquito vectors and that conversion of previously intact forests to agricultural land may increase the abundance of these vectors.

5. Transmission dynamics and potential for human to human transmission

While data anecdotally support the theory that transmission remains primarily zoonotic and driven by increased spatial overlap between people, macaques and mosquitoes in response to land use change, the possibility of human to human transmission cannot be ruled out. Zoonotic diseases have a number of barriers to overcome before they can cause human infections. Factors contributing to these include ecological drivers, pathogen characteristics and human factors. *P. knowlesi* has already overcome a significant number of these, causing multiple large-scale outbreaks in Malaysia.

For non-zoonotic transmission to occur, and indeed drive the increase in human cases, a number of conditions need to be met. Firstly, human-host interactions have to be close enough to cause the initial spillover event into human populations. Once this has occurred, infection has to take hold of a human host, invading red blood cells and replicating enough to produce a significant infectious dose for a mosquito to consume. Inside the mosquito, parasites have to complete their life-cycle for the next mosquito bite to become infectious to humans. Humans have to live in enough proximity to each other and within the mosquito range for the next mosquito bite to become infectious to humans.

Ecological and epidemiological studies have shown that macaque and human populations live in enough close proximity with enough strength of interactions for repeated spillover events to take place. Indeed, sighting macaques in peri-domestic environments has been identified as a risk factor for *P. knowlesi* (Moyes et al., 2016; Shearer et al., 2016). Experimental studies have shown that *P. knowlesi* can be transmitted from infected individuals to other people via suitable mosquito vectors, such as *An. balabacensis* (Chin et al., 1968). Parasite invasion of human red blood cells has been seen in laboratory experiments, with multiple proteins involved in different pathways (Moon et al., 2016; Tyagi et al., 2015). It has also been shown that *P. knowlesi* parasites can be maintained in laboratory settings using exclusively human blood, proving parasites are able to produce multiple generations without the need to infect macaques (Moon et al., 2013). Although experimental, this shows that there is biological plausibility for sustained human transmission to take place. Mathematical modelling studies have also identified specific scenarios under which this could be occurring (Brock et al., 2016; Imai et al., 2014). Although they concluded that sustained non-zoonotic transmission is unlikely to be occurring, conditions can be met for this to take place. Furthermore, there is evidence that this could have already occurred. Epidemiological studies have identified spatio-temporal clusters which are suggestive of sustained human to human transmission (Herdiana et al., 2018).

To better understand transmission, further research is needed to characterise fine-scale habitat preferences and densities of vectors and primate hosts. Currently available data are either too geographically limited to allow for extrapolation to other areas (e.g. (Stark et al., 2019, Wong et al., 2015a)) or too broadly aggregated at larger spatial scales to examine effects of changing movement patterns or habitat selection in response to land use change (Moyes et al., 2016). More detailed data on the densities of these populations would additionally allow exploration of vector biting preferences based on host availability in different environments. Incorporating detailed spatial data on host, vector and human populations would enable further insights into the mechanistic links between *P. knowlesi* incidence and land use change as well as quantification of the contribution of different populations to transmission and design of targeted control strategies.

6. Designing surveillance and control measures for changing environments

Despite increasing research on the role of landscape in *P. knowlesi* transmission, substantial knowledge gaps remain on *P. knowlesi* distribution regionally and how longer-term environmental changes are likely to shape human risks. One of the key barriers is lack of detailed information about spatial distributions of infections in the community due to detection bias from passive surveillance systems and diagnostic methods. Improving collection of spatial data on human infections enables detailed planning of control measures and can be integrated with environmental data to characterise these changing transmission patterns. Additionally, understanding the role of landscape in *P. knowlesi* transmission enables design of ecological interventions. As opposed to parasite-specific control strategies that focus on particular vector species or pathogens, wildlife and land management may provide a more general and sustainable strategy for controlling zoonotic malarias of current and future public health significance. Ecological interventions aim to prevent disease spillover by reducing pathogen flow between wildlife and human populations; this can include managing wildlife population sizes or pathogen prevalence, reducing contact between people, vectors and wildlife or targeted interventions to mitigate impacts of spillover (Sokolow et al., 2019). Within this section, we review potential surveillance and ecological control measures theoretically applicable to *P. knowlesi*.

6.1 Opportunities to improve surveillance for *P. knowlesi*

Heterogeneity of disease transmission occurs when a small proportion of the population is disproportionately affected and experiences the majority of the disease due to environmental, social or biological factors (Hay et al., 2013; Woolhouse et al., 1997). Capturing this heterogeneity is particularly critical for emerging diseases such as *P. knowlesi*, where the disease burdens are constantly shifting due to environmental change. To better target interventions, it is increasingly important to identify and target hotspots of transmission and understand the factors that may contribute to disease occurrence in these locations (Bannister-Tyrrell et al., 2017; Clements et al., 2013). However, assessment of transmission heterogeneity has been focused on national level estimates, mainly due to the availability of data. Previous studies reported that the detection of local level clusters of infection has an important role for improving understanding of the micro-epidemiological patterns of disease transmission, and to ensure that control strategies are tailored to the specific epidemiological characteristics in an area as much as is feasible (Bousema et al., 2012).

Adding data collection methods that enable surveillance to remotely capture spatial patterns of transmission at the micro epidemiological level are essential for strategic and operational planning of *P. knowlesi* surveillance and control programmes. Generally, the spatial analysis of disease transmission is based on address information automatically generated by geocoding software packages that can produce accurate spatial coordinate data for a large proportion of individuals (Carvalho and Nascimento, 2012; Dearwent et al., 2001). In circumstances where formal address data are unavailable, catchment areas of, for example, community pharmacies or general practitioners have been used for describing spatial patterns in disease occurrence (Florentinus et al., 2006; Han et al., 2013; Lash et al., 2012; Sturrock et al., 2013). However, this approach is likely to have less utility for resource-poor settings where formal address systems are commonly unavailable and where health-facility catchment areas are relatively large and poorly defined (Noor et al., 2009; Oduro et al., 2011; Stresman et al., 2014). An alternative geolocation method utilising mobile technology-based participatory mapping approaches utilising high-resolution offline maps has been validated to effectively improve spatial data collection for malaria surveillance activities in Asia (Indonesia and the Philippines) (Fornace et al., 2018b). A similar approach has also been used to assess human mobility traceability in rural offline populations with contrasting malaria dynamics in the Peruvian Amazon (Carrasco-Escobar et al., 2019). This approach is also being used in ongoing studies aimed at determining the spatial epidemiology of *P. knowlesi* in North Sumatera and South Kalimantan, Indonesia.

In addition to improving the collection of spatial data, one of the critical barriers to determining the spatial distribution of *P. knowlesi* is capturing infections occurring in communities which may not be reported to health centres. Malaria surveillance has traditionally focused on passive case detection of symptomatic cases at health facilities (Barclay et al., 2012; Cotter et al., 2013). However, information generated by passive case detection may not necessarily reflect the true burden of disease in areas where *P. knowlesi* cases are rare, frequently misdiagnosed and disproportionately affect high-risk populations who may not utilise public health facilities (Cotter et al., 2013). In addition, studies suggest that passive surveillance will miss a large proportion of asymptomatic and sub-microscopic *P. knowlesi* infections present in the community (Fornace et al., 2016b; Imwong et al., 2019).

Many countries conduct countrywide community-based surveys such as malaria indicator surveys (MaIS) to supplement the health facility-based reporting on malaria burden. The MaIS are useful to obtain information on the current malaria burden across the country. However, due to logistical difficulties, the MaIS are typically conducted sporadically and become less efficient for assessing malaria burden when transmission levels are low as they require large numbers of samples to achieve sufficient statistical power (Rabinovich et al., 2017; Stresman et al., 2012).

Alternatively, convenience sampling strategies such as health facility-based surveys recruiting all attendees instead of just suspected malaria cases (e.g. (Oduro et al., 2011, Reyes et al., 2021, Surendra et al., 2020)) and school-based surveys (e.g. (Druetz et al., 2020, Stevenson et al., 2013)) could provide more robust and reliable data compared to routine passive case detection, and are more operationally feasible than the large community-based strategies such as MaIS. For example, a study across different malaria transmission settings in the Philippines illustrated the utility of health facility–based surveys to augment surveillance data to increase the probability of detecting *P. knowlesi, P. falciparum, P. vivax,* and *P. malariae* infections in the wider community (Reyes et al., 2021). The use of the convenience sampling of health facility attendees markedly increased detection probabilities and spatial coverage of surveillance, particularly in rural populations living in forested areas (Fornace et al., 2020). In addition, health facility-based surveys conducted in Indonesia were able to capture heterogeneity of *P. falciparum* and *P. vivax* malaria transmission and identify areas still receptive to malaria in an elimination setting (52). However, the bias of such convenience sampling strategies for *P. knowlesi* malaria surveillance is not well characterized and requires further study.

Improving spatial data on the distribution of *P. knowlesi* additionally offers opportunities to examine how landscape changes impact *P. knowlesi* distribution, ideally leading to the design of early warning systems or targeted surveillance. Earth Observation data, typically collected by satellite or aerial methods, enables integration of data on landscape factors with spatial data on the distribution of *P. knowlesi* cases (Fornace et al., 2021). The quantity, types of data and spatial and temporal resolutions of free and commercially available Earth Observation data are rapidly expanding (Wimberly et al., 2021). Analysis-ready products, such as near real-time deforestation alerts, make these datasets increasingly accessible to health programmes (Hansen et al., 2016). Malaysia is now exploring the use of land cover data through incorporation of metrics of recent deforestation and recent construction activities into malaria foci investigations, in line with recent guidelines developed by the World Health Organization for defining malaria receptivity (Fornace et al., 2021; World Health Organisation, 2019). Increased data on relationships between land cover and *P. knowlesi* risks and developing sources of Earth Observation data offer new opportunities to develop environmentally targeted surveillance and control approaches for *P. knowlesi*.

6.2 Management of wildlife populations

In contrast to other human malaria species, there are fewer established control measures to reduce transmission of *P. knowlesi* following identification of high-risk areas. While vector control measures may limit human exposure to infectious bites, the zoonotic nature of *P. knowlesi* offers an opportunity to control transmission through management of macaque reservoir populations. In theory, this could include a variety of approaches ranging from population reduction, habitat segregation or even chemoprophylaxis directed at the macaque reservoir. To our knowledge, none of these approaches have been incorporated into *P. knowlesi* control strategies so far. Managing wildlife populations may offer opportunities to mitigate disruptions from environmental change on disease transmission by reducing the abundance or *P. knowlesi* prevalence in reservoirs. However, these interventions may have complex impacts on ecology, requiring further consideration and planning.

It has been speculated that reducing macaque population density via culling could be an effective means of reducing *P. knowlesi* spillover to humans, although ethical concerns and the unfeasible logistics prevent this strategy being adopted (Chin et al., 2020). Ethics and logistic feasibility are sound arguments against macaque culling, but even in their absence the scientific case for such an approach is unclear. The expected impact of a culling programme would depend on the strength of the relationship between the macaque population size and human infection risk. This has not been empirically estimated, but has been inferred through modification of standard, single-host models of malaria transmission incorporating human and macaque host population data (Yakob et al., 2010, 2018). Here, transmission is predicted to be positively associated with the ratio of vector to macaque population density, with the expectation of macaque density-dependent transmission (Yakob et al., 2010, 2018). However, other than the necessary requirement that macaques be locally available for transmission to occur, the contribution of macaque density to transmission is relatively small in comparison to the much larger effects of vector survival, feeding rates on macaques and humans respectively, and the parasite's extrinsic incubation period. Furthermore, as the effect of macaque density depends on corresponding vector density, there would be great uncertainty as to what level of macaque population reduction was required to prevent spillover in different ecological settings and seasons. Certainly, macaque culling in the absence of sustained vector control, including throughout the diverse forest and agricultural habitats where they occur, may be unlikely to have much impact.

In addition to these theoretical considerations, lessons can be learned from other zoonotic disease systems where wildlife culling has been employed for disease control. Worryingly, these provide several examples where culling either had no impact or increased transmission by changing aspects of the demographics and dispersal on the wildlife host population (Choisy and Rohani, 2006). Arguably the most poignant example is the controversial programme of badger culling implemented to reduce the transmission of bovine tuberculosis to livestock in the UK. Here, culling was not only found to be ineffective, but associated with increased infection risk in some settings because the repeated removal of badgers triggered inward migration of infected individuals from neighbouring areas (Bielby et al., 2014; Donnelly and Woodroffe, 2015). Similarly, the long-tailed and pig-tailed macaque reservoirs hosts of *P. knowlesi* are territorial, with habitat where individuals or troops have been removed likely to be recolonized (Fooden, 1995). Another zoonotic disease where culling has been extensively used as a control strategy is rabies. Rabies can be transmitted to humans by a variety of wildlife (e.g. foxes, bats) and domestic animals (dogs). Culling is often carried out in response to public concern when human cases occur, but review of evidence from large-scale culling programmes in Denmark, Indonesia and Korea found no impact on rabies incidence despite large reductions in dog population size. This was attributed to transmission being frequency rather than density-dependent, and/or that the degree of dog population reduction required to see any impact on human cases being beyond the feasibility of control programmes. Similarly, several countries in Latin America have carried out culling programmes for decades to control vampire-transmitted rabies. Despite these intensive efforts, transmission of bat rabies to livestock has persisted (Streicker et al., 2012). Again, this failure may be attributed to the unfeasibly high degree of wildlife population reduction required to see an impact on occasional spillover to livestock or human hosts. On the basis of theoretical and practical considerations, we argue that macaque culling is unlikely to be an effective strategy for *P. knowlesi* control.

Alternatively, the use of oral baits to distribute vaccines or drug treatments has been investigated and applied in a wide variety of wildlife populations (Abbott et al., 2012; Cross et al., 2007). Such programmes have been highly effective when used to control racoon-transmitted rabies in North America, and eliminate fox rabies in several European countries (Maki et al., 2017). Similar approaches have also been considered for control of Lyme disease in wildlife hosts (Bhattacharya et al., 2011). Three key criteria have been defined for development of effective oral vaccines for wildlife: an efficacious immunogen, an appropriate delivery vehicle, and a species-specific bait (Cross et al., 2007). As reviewed earlier, at present there are no vaccine candidates for *P. knowlesi* that could be adapted for use in wildlife programmes at present. However, oral baits could be considered for distribution of chemoprophylaxis to macaques in areas of high *P. knowlesi* human incidence should appropriate formulations and delivery systems be available.

The control of zoonoses through distribution of chemoprophylaxis to wildlife is likely to be more demanding than vaccines due to the likely higher frequency of distribution required to sustain infection reduction in reservoir populations. However, such an approach is not without precedence. A notable example is the tapeworm *Echinococcus multilocularis* which infects foxes (Comte et al., 2013). Humans can be exposed to this helminth through its presence in fox droppings, with infection leading to potentially fatal alveolar echinococcus (AE). Following the successful eradication of rabies from European fox populations, there has been a large rise in urban fox populations and an associated rise in human AE cases in several countries. There is no effective vaccine against *E. multilocularis*, however, the parasite is susceptible to the anti-helminthic drug praziquantel (Comte et al., 2013). Large-scale programmes have been implemented in several European countries and Japan where anti-helminthics have been disseminated to foxes in areas of high human exposure. A recent systematic review and meta-analysis of results of these programmes indicates they are generally successful in reducing environmental contamination with *E. multilocularis* and thus human exposure, although may not be sufficient for complete eradication (Umhang et al., 2019). In these programmes, the treatment frequency of oral baits ranged from monthly to every six months. Given the focalized nature of *P. knowlesi* incidence in humans, this frequency of application could be feasible within hotspots of human cases. Such programmes could exploit the presumable lack of drug resistance in malaria parasites that primarily infect wildlife, by using cheap and readily available antimalarials like chloroquine for which other human malaria parasites have become resistant.

6.3 Land management strategies

Despite the clear relevance of deforestation and conversion of land for agriculture to *P. knowlesi* spillover, the specific nature of these impacts are complex due to the involvement of interlinked social, environmental and economic drivers of risk (Fornace et al., 2020.). Instead of a straightforward relationship between deforestation and human disease incidence,recent work suggests that risk is determined by a more complex range of factors related to land use, symmetry and fragmentation that act at different scales. Effective environmental management of *P. knowlesi* will require consideration of the combined impacts of these diverse land use factors arising at different scales, and how they could be exploited to develop strategies for minimizing risk of human infection risk. This will require thorough understanding of transmission ecology, and how landscapes can be manipulated to reduce overlap between humans and the macaque reservoir. This could involve for example, better planning of deforestation and agricultural activities to build in larger continuous blocks of protected forest areas that could retain macaque populations, and/or the creation of buffer zones and habitat corridors that minimize contact between macaques, human settlements and agricultural workers. Such habitat management strategies have not been incorporated into *P. knowlesi* control, but may be the only way to achieve targets for malaria elimination.

Land management strategies and environmental modification have a long history of successfully reducing risks of non-zoonotic malaria species (Fornace et al., 2021). Famously, this includes an extensive long-term land management policy in Italy after the first World War which led to draining of marsh areas and agricultural development aimed at reduction of vector breeding habitats (Gachelin and Opinel, 2011). A systematic review of environmental management for malaria control found these interventions were highly effective in reducing malaria morbidity and mortality (Keiser et al., 2005c). Increasingly, global policy initiatives have focused on identifying co-benefits between health and climate interventions, integrating health into wider climate change mitigation policies (Workman et al., 2018). Climate mitigation strategies may already be having beneficial impacts in reducing *P. knowlesi* transmission, although it remains to be seen whether the recent changes in forest conservation policies in Malaysia and Indonesia aimed at reducing emissions will also lead to reductions in *P. knowlesi* burden (Weisse and Goldman, 2021). The recent COVID-19 pandemic has also led to renewed focus on landscape-based interventions to reduce pathogen spillover from wildlife; these interventions are essential for ensuring both human and ecosystem health (Reaser et al., 2021). While it remains unknown exactly how land management policies can reduce *P. knowlesi* risks, this is a priority for future research.

7. Conclusions and future research priorities

P. knowlesi exemplifies an emerging zoonotic disease driven by deforestation and other landscape changes. While substantial knowledge gaps exist on the true burden and distribution of *P. knowlesi*, increasing evidence illustrates how landscape impacts human, simian and mosquito populations and resulting *P. knowlesi* transmission between these populations. The identification of human *P. knowlesi* cases across Southeast Asia, particularly in areas where other human malaria species have been eliminated, highlights the urgent need to develop targeted control strategies for *P. knowlesi*. It is clear that for control of zoonotic malaria, much more innovative and intersectoral approaches are urgently needed to tackle the current public health problem of *P. knowlesi* now and emergence of other wildlife-dependent vector-borne diseases in the future.

Human exposure to zoonotic malaria is driven by a complex range of environmental, social and economic factors, acting across scales from individual, household, community up to landscape (Fornace et al., 2021). Correspondingly, effective control will require implementation of strategies acting at different scales; ranging from provision of personal protection measures to high risk groups, vector control and targeted chemoprophylaxis of macaques in high transmission foci, and land use management. Here, malaria control programmes can learn much from the experiences of other zoonotic disease control approaches that have successfully applied such comprehensive One Health approaches. Close intersectoral collaboration between public health, wildlife biologists, ecologists, social scientists, land use planners, communities and government policy makers will be crucial for successful development and implementation of such approaches. Additionally, this must be underpinned by more effective surveillance systems with capacity to incorporate data on environmental factors and land use

(Fornace et al., 2020). Such cross-disciplinary surveillance and control approaches will require substantial capacity strengthening and training to establish core research units and expertise within control programmes. Investments in this type of capacity strengthening will reap great benefits by enhancing the response not only to simian malaria, but the wider range of forest and agricultural-associated zoonoses and vector-borne diseases that have the potential to emerge as a consequence of increasing rates of land use change and deforestation in endemic countries (Plowright et al., 2021).

References

Abbott, R.C., Osorio, J.E., Bunck, C.M., Rocke, T.E., 2012. Sylvatic plague vaccine: a new tool for conservation of threatened and endangered species? Ecohealth 9, 243–250.

Afrane, Y.A., Zhou, G., Lawson, B.W., Githeko, A.K., Yan, G., 2006. Effects of microclimatic changes caused by deforestation on the survivorship and reproductive fitness of Anopheles gambiae in western Kenya highlands. Am. J. Trop. Med. Hyg. 74, 772–778.

Allen, T., Murray, K.A., Zambrana-Torrelio, C., Morse, S.S., Rondinini, C., Di Marco, M., Breit, N., Olival, K.J., Daszak, P., 2017. Global hotspots and correlates of emerging zoonotic diseases. Nat. Commun. 8, 1124.

Amir, A., Shahari, S., Liew, J.W.K., De Silva, J.R., Khan, M.B., Lai, M.Y., Snounou, G., Abdullah, M.L., Gani, M., Rovie-Ryan, J.J., Lau, Y.L., 2020. Natural Plasmodium infection in wild macaques of three states in peninsular Malaysia. Acta Trop. 211, 105596.

Anstey, N.M., Grigg, M.J., 2019. Zoonotic malaria: the better you look, the more you find. J Infect Dis 219, 679–681.

Assefa, S., Lim, C., Preston, M.D., Duffy, C.W., Nair, M.B., Adroub, S.A., Kadir, K.A., Goldberg, J.M., Neafsey, D.E., Divis, P., Clark, T.G., Duraisingh, M.T., Conway, D.J., Pain, A., Singh, B., 2015. Population genomic structure and adaptation in the zoonotic malaria parasite Plasmodium knowlesi. Proc. Natl. Acad. Sci. U. S. A. 112, 13027–13032.

Baeza, A., Santos-Vega, M., Dobson, A.P., Pascual, M., 2017. The rise and fall of malaria under land-use change in frontier regions. Nat. Ecol. Evol. 1, 108.

Baird, J.K., 2009. Malaria zoonoses. Travel Med. Infect. Dis. 7, 269–277.

Bannister-Tyrrell, M., Verdonck, K., Hausmann-Muela, S., Gryseels, C., Muela Ribera, J., Peeters Grietens, K., 2017. Defining micro-epidemiology for malaria elimination: systematic review and meta-analysis. Malar. J. 16, 164.

Barber, B.E., William, T., Dhararaj, P., Anderios, F., Grigg, M.J., Yeo, T.W., Anstey, N.M., 2012. Epidemiology of Plasmodium knowlesi malaria in north-east Sabah, Malaysia: family clusters and wide age distribution. Malar. J. 11, 401.

Barber, B.E., William, T., Grigg, M.J., Menon, J., Auburn, S., Marfurt, J., Anstey, N.M., Yeo, T.W., 2013a. A prospective comparative study of knowlesi, falciparum, and vivax malaria in Sabah, Malaysia: high proportion with severe disease from Plasmodium knowlesi and Plasmodium vivax but no mortality with early referral and artesunate therapy. Clin. Infect. Dis. 56, 383–397.

Barber, B.E., William, T., Grigg, M.J., Piera, K., Yeo, T.W., Anstey, N.M., 2013b. Evaluation of the sensitivity of a pLDH-based and an aldolase-based rapid diagnostic test for diagnosis of uncomplicated and severe malaria caused by PCR-confirmed Plasmodium knowlesi, Plasmodium falciparum, and Plasmodium vivax. J. Clin. Microbiol. 51, 1118–1123.

Barber, B.E., William, T., Grigg, M.J., Yeo, T.W., Anstey, N.M., 2013c. Limitations of microscopy to differentiate Plasmodium species in a region co-endemic for Plasmodium falciparum, Plasmodium vivax and Plasmodium knowlesi. Malar. J. 12, 8.

Barber, B.E., Rajahram, G.S., Grigg, M.J., William, T., Anstey, N.M., 2017. World Malaria Report: time to acknowledge Plasmodium knowlesi malaria. Malar. J. 16, 135.

Barbieri, A.F., Sawyer, I.O., Soares-Filho, B.S., 2005. Population and land use effects on malaria prevalence in the southern brazilian amazon. Hum. Ecol. 33, 847–874.

Barclay, V.C., Smith, R.A., Findeis, J.L., 2012. Surveillance considerations for malaria elimination. Malar. J. 11, 304.

Barros, F.S., Honorio, N.A., 2015. Deforestation and malaria on the amazon frontier: larval clustering of anopheles darlingi (Diptera: Culicidae) determines focal distribution of malaria. Am. J. Trop. Med. Hyg. 93, 939–953.

Basurko, C., Demattei, C., Han-Sze, R., Grenier, C., Joubert, M., Nacher, M., Carme, B., 2013. Deforestation, agriculture and farm jobs: a good recipe for Plasmodium vivax in French Guiana. Malar. J. 12, 90.

Bennett, K.L., Gomez Martinez, C., Almanza, A., Rovira, J.R., Mcmillan, W.O., Enriquez, V., Barraza, E., Diaz, M., Sanchez-Galan, J.E., Whiteman, A., Gittens, R.A., Loaiza, J.R., 2019. High infestation of invasive Aedes mosquitoes in used tires along the local transport network of Panama. Parasit. Vectors 12, 264.

Berry, A., Iriart, X., Wilhelm, N., Valentin, A., Cassaing, S., Witkowski, B., Benoit-Vical, F., Menard, S., Olagnier, D., Fillaux, J., Sire, S., Le Coustumier, A., Magnaval, J.F., 2011. Imported Plasmodium knowlesi malaria in a French tourist returning from Thailand. Am. J. Trop. Med. Hyg. 84, 535–538.

Bhattacharya, D., Bensaci, M., Luker, K.E., Luker, G., Wisdom, S., Telford, S.R., Hu, L.T., 2011. Development of a baited oral vaccine for use in reservoir-targeted strategies against Lyme disease. Vaccine 29, 7818–7825.

Bielby, J., Donnelly, C.A., Pope, L.C., Burke, T., Woodroffe, R., 2014. Badger responses to small-scale culling may compromise targeted control of bovine tuberculosis. Proc. Natl. Acad. Sci. U. S. A. 111, 9193–9198.

Bloomfield, L.S.P., McIntosh, T.L., Lambin, E.F., 2020. Habitat fragmentation, livelihood behaviours and contact between people and nonhuman primates in Africa. Landsc. Ecol. 35, 985–1000.

Boundenga, L., Ollomo, B., Rougeron, V., Mouele, L.Y., Mve-Ondo, B., Delicat-Loembet, L.M., Moukodoum, N.D., Okouga, A.P., Arnathau, C., Elguero, E., Durand, P., Liegeois, F., Boue, V., Motsch, P., Le Flohic, G., Ndoungouet, A., Paupy, C., Ba, C.T., Renaud, F., Prugnolle, F., 2015. Diversity of malaria parasites in great apes in Gabon. Malar. J. 14, 111.

Bousema, T., Youssef, R.M., Cook, J., Cox, J., Alegana, V.A., Amran, J., Noor, A.M., Snow, R.W., Drakeley, C., 2010. Serologic markers for detecting malaria in areas of low endemicity, Somalia, 2008. Emerg. Infect. Dis. 16, 392–399.

Bousema, T., Griffin, J.T., Sauerwein, R.W., Smith, D.L., Churcher, T.S., Takken, W., Ghani, A., Drakeley, C., Gosling, R., 2012. Hitting hotspots: spatial targeting of malaria for control and elimination. PLoS Med. 9, e1001165.

Braima, K.A., Sum, J.S., Ghazali, A.R., Muslimin, M., Jeffery, J., Lee, W.C., Shaker, M.R., Elamin, A.E., Jamaiah, I., Lau, Y.L., Rohela, M., Kamarulzaman, A., Sitam, F., Mohd-Noh, R., Abdul-Aziz, N.M., 2013. Is there a risk of suburban transmission of malaria in Selangor, Malaysia? PLoS One 8, e77924.

Brant, H.L., 2011. Changes in abundance, diversity and community composition of mosquitoes based on different land use in Sabah, Malaysia. Master of Science, Imperial College London.

Brant, H.L., Ewers, R.M., Vythilingam, I., Drakeley, C., Benedick, S., Mumford, J.D., 2016. Vertical stratification of adult mosquitoes (Diptera: Culicidae) within a tropical rainforest in Sabah, Malaysia. Malar. J. 15, 370.

Brasil, P., Zalis, M.G., De Pina-Costa, A., Siqueira, A.M., Junior, C.B., Silva, S., Areas, A.L.L., Pelajo-Machado, M., De Alvarenga, D.A.M., Da Silva Santelli, A.C.F., Albuquerque, H.G., Cravo, P., Santos De Abreu, F.V., Peterka, C.L., Zanini, G.M., Suarez Mutis, M.C., Pissinatti, A., Lourenco-De-Oliveira, R., de Brito, C.F.A., De Fatima Ferreira-Da-Cruz, M., Culleton, R., Daniel-Ribeiro, C.T., 2017. Outbreak of human malaria caused by Plasmodium simium in the Atlantic Forest in Rio de Janeiro: a molecular epidemiological investigation. Lancet Glob. Health 5, e1038–e1046.

Brock, P.M., fornace, K.M., Parmiter, M., Cox, J., Drakeley, C.J., Ferguson, H.M., Kao, R.R., 2016. Plasmodium knowlesi transmission: integrating quantitative approaches from epidemiology and ecology to understand malaria as a zoonosis. Parasitology 143, 389–400.

Brock, P.M., Fornace, K.M., Grigg, M.J., Anstey, N.M., William, T., Cox, J., Drakeley, C.J., Ferguson, H.M., Kao, R.R., 2019. Predictive analysis across spatial scales links zoonotic malaria to deforestation. Proc. R. Soc. B, 286.

Bronner, U., Divis, P.C., Farnert, A., Singh, B., 2009. Swedish traveller with Plasmodium knowlesi malaria after visiting Malaysian Borneo. Malar. J. 8, 15.

Brown, R., Chua, T.H., Fornace, K., Drakeley, C., Vythilingam, I., Ferguson, H.M., 2020. Human exposure to zoonotic malaria vectors in village, farm and forest habitats in Sabah, Malaysian Borneo. PLoS Negl. Trop. Dis. 14, e0008617.

Bruun, B., Aagaard-Hansen, J., 2008. The social context of schistosomiasis and its control: an introduction and annotated bibliography. World Health Organization, Geneva.

Bryan, J.E., Shearman, P.L., Asner, G.P., Knapp, D.E., Aoro, G., Lokes, B., 2013. Extreme differences in forest degradation in Borneo: comparing practices in Sarawak, Sabah, and Brunei. PLoS One 8, e69679.

Busch, J., Ferretti-Gallon, K., Engelmann, J., Wright, M., Austin, K.G., Stolle, F., Turubanova, S., Potapov, P.V., Margono, B., HANSEN, M.C., Baccini, A., 2015. Reductions in emissions from deforestation from Indonesia's moratorium on new oil palm, timber, and logging concessions. Proc. Natl. Acad. Sci. U. S. A. 112, 1328–1333.

Carrasco-Escobar, G., Castro, M.C., Barboza, J.L., Ruiz-Cabrejos, J., Llanos-Cuentas, A., Vinetz, J.M., Gamboa, D., 2019. Use of open mobile mapping tool to assess human mobility traceability in rural offline populations with contrasting malaria dynamics. PeerJ 7, e6298.

Carvalho, R.M., Nascimento, L.F., 2012. Spatial distribution of dengue in the city of Cruzeiro, Sao Paulo State, Brazil: use of geoprocessing tools. Rev. Inst. Med. Trop. Sao Paulo 54, 261–266.

Chapman, C.A., Gillespie, T.R., Speirs, M.L., 2005. Parasite prevalence and richness in sympatric colobines: effects of host density. Am. J. Primatol. 67, 259–266.

Chapman, C.A., Speirs, M.L., Gillespie, T.R., Holland, T., Austad, K.M., 2006. Life on the edge: gastrointestinal parasites from the forest edge and interior primate groups. Am. J. Primatol. 68, 397–409.

Chen, J., Franklin, J.F., Spies, T.A., 1995. Growing-season microclimatic gradients from clearcut edges into old-growth douglas-fir forests. Ecol. Appl. 5, 74–86.

Chen, J., Saunders, S.C., Crow, T.R., Naiman, R.J., Brosofske, K.D., Mroz, G.D., Brookshire, B.L., Franklin, J.F., 1999. Microclimate in forest ecosystem and landscape ecology: variations in local climate can be used to monitor and compare the effects of different management regimes. BioScience 49, 288–297.

Chin, W., Contacos, P.G., Coatney, G.R., Kimball, H.R., 1965. A naturally acquited quotidian-type malaria in man transferable to monkeys. Science 149, 865.

Chin, W., Contacos, P.G., Collins, W.E., Jeter, M.H., Alpert, E., 1968. Experimental mosquito-transmission of Plasmodium knowlesi to man and monkey. Am. J. Trop. Med. Hyg. 17, 355–358.

Chin, A.Z., Maluda, M.C.M., Jelip, J., Jeffree, M.S.B., Culleton, R., Ahmed, K., 2020. Malaria elimination in Malaysia and the rising threat of *Plasmodium knowlesi*. J. Physiol. Anthropol. 39, 36. https://doi.org/10.1186/s40101-020-00247-5.

Chinh, V.D., Masuda, G., Hung, V.V., Takagi, H., Kawai, S., Annoura, T., Maeno, Y., 2019. Prevalence of human and non-human primate Plasmodium parasites in anopheline mosquitoes: a cross-sectional epidemiological study in Southern Vietnam. Trop. Med. Health 47, 9.

Choisy, M., Rohani, P., 2006. Harvesting can increase severity of wildlife disease epidemics. Proc Biol Sci 273, 2025–2034.

Chua, T.H., Manin, B.O., Daim, S., Vythilingam, I., Drakeley, C., 2017. Phylogenetic analysis of simian Plasmodium spp. infecting Anopheles balabacensis Baisas in Sabah, Malaysia. PLoS Negl. Trop. Dis. 11, e0005991.

Clements, A.C., Reid, H.L., Kelly, G.C., Hay, S.I., 2013. Further shrinking the malaria map: how can geospatial science help to achieve malaria elimination? Lancet Infect. Dis. 13, 709–718.

Coatney, G.R., 1963. Simian malaria. Its importance to worldwide eradication of malaria. JAMA 184, 876–877.

Coatney, G.R., Chin, W., Contacos, P.G., King, H.K., 1966. Plasmodium inui, a quartan-type malaria parasite of Old World monkeys transmissible to man. J. Parasitol. 52, 660–663.

Coatney, G.R., Collins, W.E., Warren, M., Contacos, P.G., 1971. The Primate Malarias. The Division of Parasitic Diseases of the Centers for Disease Control and Prevention, Atlanta, GA.

Collinge, S.K., 1996. Ecological consequences of habitat fragmentation: implications for landscape architecture and planning. Landsc. Urban Plan. 36, 59–77.

Collins, W.E., Contacos, P.G., Guinn, E.G., 1967. Studies on the transmission of simian malarias. II. Transmission of the H strain of Plasmodium knowlesi by Anopheles balabacensis balabacensis. J. Parasitol. 53, 841–844.

Comte, S., Raton, V., Raoul, F., Hegglin, D., Giraudoux, P., Deplazes, P., Favier, S., Gottschek, D., Umhang, G., Boue, F., Combes, B., 2013. Fox baiting against Echinococcus multilocularis: Contrasted achievements among two medium size cities. Prev. Vet. Med. 111, 147–155.

Contacos, P.G., Elder, H.A., Coatney, G.R., 1962. Man to man transfer of two strains of plasmodium cynomolgi by mosquito bite. Am. J. Trop. Med. Hyg. 11, 186–193.

Cook, J., Reid, H., Iavro, J., Kuwahata, M., Taleo, G., Clements, A., McCarthy, J., Vallely, A., Drakeley, C., 2010. Using serological measures to monitor changes in malaria transmission in Vanuatu. Malar. J. 9, 169.

Cordina, C.J., Culleton, R., Jones, B.L., Smith, C.C., Macconnachie, A.A., Coyne, M.J., Alexander, C.L., 2014. Plasmodium knowlesi: clinical presentation and laboratory diagnosis of the first human case in a Scottish traveler. J. Travel Med. 21, 357–360.

Corran, P., Coleman, P., Riley, E., Drakeley, C., 2007. Serology: a robust indicator of malaria transmission intensity? Trends Parasitol. 23, 575–582.

Cotter, C., Sturrock, H.J., Hsiang, M.S., Liu, J., Phillips, A.A., Hwang, J., Gueye, C.S., Fullman, N., Gosling, R.D., Feachem, R.G., 2013. The changing epidemiology of malaria elimination: new strategies for new challenges. Lancet 382, 900–911.

Couto-Lima, D., Madec, Y., Bersot, M.I., Campos, S.S., Motta, M.A., Santos, F.B.D., Vazeille, M., Vasconcelos, P., Lourenco-De-Oliveira, R., Failloux, A.B., 2017. Potential risk of re-emergence of urban transmission of Yellow Fever virus in Brazil facilitated by competent Aedes populations. Sci. Rep. 7, 4848.

Coutrier, F.N., Tirta, Y.K., Cotter, C., Zarlinda, I., Gonzalez, I.J., Schwartz, A., Maneh, C., Marfurt, J., Murphy, M., Herdiana, H., Anstey, N.M., Greenhouse, B., Hsiang, M.S., Noviyanti, R., 2018. Laboratory challenges of Plasmodium species identification in Aceh Province, Indonesia, a malaria elimination setting with newly discovered P. knowlesi. PLoS Negl. Trop. Dis. 12, e0006924.

Cox-Singh, J., Singh, B., 2008. Knowlesi malaria: newly emergent and of public health importance? Trends Parasitol. 24, 406–410.

Cox-Singh, J., Davis, T.M., Lee, K.S., Shamsul, S.S., Matusop, A., Ratnam, S., Rahman, H.A., Conway, D.J., Singh, B., 2008. Plasmodium knowlesi malaria in humans is widely distributed and potentially life threatening. Clin. Infect. Dis. 46, 165–171.

Cross, M.L., Buddle, B.M., Aldwell, F.E., 2007. The potential of oral vaccines for disease control in wildlife species. Vet. J. 174, 472–480.

Crowl, T.A., Crist, T.O., Parmenter, R.R., Belovsky, G., Lugo, A.E., 2008. The spread of invasive species and infectious disease as drivers of ecosystem change. Front. Ecol. Environ. 6, 238–246.

Curtis, P.G., Slay, C.M., Harris, N.L., Tyukavina, A., Hansen, M.C., 2018. Classifying drivers of global forest loss. Science 361, 1108–1111.

Cushman, S.A., Macdonald, E.A., Landguth, E.L., Malhi, Y., Macdonald, D.W., 2017. Multiple-scale prediction of forest loss risk across Borneo. Landsc. Ecol. 32, 1581–1598.

Da Silva-Nunes, M., Codeco, C.T., Malafronte, R.S., Da Silva, N.S., Juncansen, C., Muniz, P.T., Ferreira, M.U., 2008. Malaria on the Amazonian frontier: transmission dynamics, risk factors, spatial distribution, and prospects for control. Am. J. Trop. Med. Hyg. 79, 624–635.

Daneshvar, C., Davis, T.M., Cox-Singh, J., Rafa'ee, M.Z., Zakaria, S.K., Divis, P.C., Singh, B., 2009. Clinical and laboratory features of human Plasmodium knowlesi infection. Clin. Infect. Dis. 49, 852–860.

Danylo, O., Pirker, J., Lemoine, J., Ceccherini, G., See, L., McCallum, I., Hadi, Kraxner, F., Achard, F., Fritz, S., 2021. A map of the extent and year of detection of oil palm plantations in Indonesia, Malaysia and Thailand. Scientific Data 8.

de Andrade, F.A., Gomes, M.N., Uieda, W., Begot, A.L., Ramos Ode, S., Fernandes, M.E., 2016. Geographical analysis for detecting high-risk areas for bovine/human rabies transmitted by the common hematophagous bat in the amazon region, Brazil. PLoS One 11, e0157332.

De Ang, J.X., Yaman, K., Kadir, K.A., Matusop, A., Singh, B., 2021. New vectors that are early feeders for Plasmodium knowlesi and other simian malaria parasites in Sarawak, Malaysian Borneo. Sci. Rep. 11, 7739.

De Canale, E., Sgarabotto, D., Marini, G., Menegotto, N., Masiero, S., Akkouche, W., Biasolo, M.A., Barzon, L., Palu, G., 2017. Plasmodium knowlesi malaria in a traveller returning from the Philippines to Italy, 2016. New Microbiol. 40, 291–294.

de Castro, M.C., Monte-Mor, R.L., Sawyer, D.O., Singer, B.H., 2006. Malaria risk on the Amazon frontier. Proc. Natl. Acad. Sci. U. S. A. 103, 2452–2457.

De Deyn, G.B., Cornelissen, J.H., Bardgett, R.D., 2008. Plant functional traits and soil carbon sequestration in contrasting biomes. Ecol. Lett. 11, 516–531.

Dearwent, S.M., Jacobs, R.R., Halbert, J.B., 2001. Locational uncertainty in georeferencing public health datasets. J. Expo. Anal. Environ. Epidemiol. 11, 329–334.

Desjeux, P., 2001. The increase in risk factors for leishmaniasis worldwide. Trans. R. Soc. Trop. Med. Hyg. 95, 239–243.

Despommier, D., Ellis, B.R., Wilcox, B.A., 2006. The role of ecotones in emerging infectious diseases. Ecohealth 3, 281–289.

Divis, P.C., SINGH, B., Anderios, F., Hisam, S., Matusop, A., Kocken, C.H., Assefa, S.A., Duffy, C.W., Conway, D.J., 2015. Admixture in humans of two divergent plasmodium knowlesi populations associated with different macaque host species. PLoS Pathog. 11, e1004888.

Dobson, A., 2004. Population dynamics of pathogens with multiple host species. Am. Nat. 164 (Suppl 5), S64–S78.

Donnelly, C.A., Woodroffe, R., 2015. Badger-cull targets unlikely to reduce TB. Nature 526, 640. https://doi.org/10.1038/526640c.

Douine, M., Lambert, Y., Musset, L., Hiwat, H., Blume, L.R., Marchesini, P., Moresco, G.G., Cox, H., Sanchez, J.F., Villegas, L., De Santi, V.P., Sanna, A., Vreden, S., Suarez-Mutis, M., 2020. Malaria in gold miners in the Guianas and the amazon: current knowledge and challenges. Curr. Trop. Med. Rep. 7, 37–47.

Drakeley, C.J., Corran, P.H., Coleman, P.G., Tongren, J.E., McDonald, S.L., Carneiro, I., Malima, R., Lusingu, J., Manjurano, A., Nkya, W.M., Lemnge, M.M., Cox, J., Reyburn, H., Riley, E.M., 2005. Estimating medium- and long-term trends in malaria transmission by using serological markers of malaria exposure. Proc. Natl. Acad. Sci. U. S. A. 102, 5108–5113.

Druetz, T., Stresman, G., Ashton, R.A., Van Den Hoogen, L.L., Joseph, V., Fayette, C., Monestime, F., Hamre, K.E., Chang, M.A., Lemoine, J.F., Drakeley, C., Eisele, T.P., 2020. Programmatic options for monitoring malaria in elimination settings: easy access group surveys to investigate Plasmodium falciparum epidemiology in two regions with differing endemicity in Haiti. BMC Med. 18, 141.

Dubey, S., Singh, R., Gupta, B., Patel, R., Soni, D., Dhakad, B.M.S., Reddy, B.M., Gupta, S., Sharma, N., 2021. Leptospira: An emerging zoonotic pathogen of climate change, global warming and unplanned urbanization: A review. J. Entomol. Zool. Stud. 9, 564–571.

Ducheyne, E., Mweempwa, C., de Pus, C., Vernieuwe, H., de Deken, R., Hendrickx, G., van den Bossche, P., 2009. The impact of habitat fragmentation on tsetse abundance on the plateau of eastern Zambia. Prev. Vet. Med. 91, 11–18.

Durnez, L., Mao, S., Denis, L., Roelants, P., Sochantha, T., Coosemans, M., 2013. Outdoor malaria transmission in forested villages of Cambodia. Malar. J. 12, 329.

Dutta, G.P., SINGH, P.P., Banyal, H.S., 1978. Macaca assamensis as a new host for experimental Plasmodium knowlesi infection. Indian J. Med. Res. 68, 923–926.

Edwards, H.M., Sriwichai, P., Kirabittir, K., Prachumsri, J., Chavez, I.F., Hii, J., 2019. Transmission risk beyond the village: entomological and human factors contributing to residual malaria transmission in an area approaching malaria elimination on the Thailand-Myanmar border. Malar. J. 18, 221.

Estoque, R.C., Ooba, M., Avitabile, V., Hijioka, Y., Dasgupta, R., Togawa, T., Murayama, Y., 2019. The future of Southeast Asia's forests. Nat. Commun. 10, 1829.

Eyles, D.E., Coatney, G.R., Getz, M.E., 1960. Vivax-type malaria parasite of macaques transmissible to man. Science 131, 1812–1813.

Eyles, D.E., Laing, A.B.G., Warren, M.W., Sandosham, A.A., 1962. Malaria parasites of Malayan leaf monkeys of the genus Presbytis. Med. J. Malaya 17, 85–86.

FAO, 2020. Global Forest Resources Assessment 2020: Main Report. Food and Agriculture Organization of the United Nations, Rome.

Feddema, J.J., Oleson, K.W., Bonan, G.B., Mearns, L.O., Buja, L.E., Meehl, G.A., Washington, W.M., 2005. The importance of land-cover change in simulating future climates. Science 310, 1674–1678.

Ferrari, M.J., Djibo, A., Grais, R.F., Bharti, N., Grenfell, B.T., Bjornstad, O.N., 2010. Rural-urban gradient in seasonal forcing of measles transmission in Niger. Proc Biol Sci 277, 2775–2782.

Ferrari, M.J., Perkins, S.E., Pomeroy, L.W., Bjornstad, O.N., 2011. Pathogens, social networks, and the paradox of transmission scaling. Interdiscip. Perspect. Infect. Dis. 2011, 267049.

Figtree, M., Lee, R., Bain, L., Kennedy, T., Mackertich, S., Urban, M., Cheng, Q., Hudson, B.J., 2010. Plasmodium knowlesi in human, Indonesian Borneo. Emerg. Infect. Dis. 16, 672–674.

Florentinus, S.R., Souverein, P.C., Griens, F.A., Groenewegen, P.P., Leufkens, H.G., Heerdink, E.R., 2006. Linking community pharmacy dispensing data to prescribing data of general practitioners. BMC Med. Inform. Decis. Mak. 6, 18.

Fooden, J., 1995. Systematic Review of Southeast Asian Longtail Macaques *Macaca fascicularis*. Fieldiana, vol. 81. Field Museum of Natural History.

Fornace, K.M., Abidin, T.R., Alex, E.R., Brock, P., Grigg, M.J., Murphy, A., William, T., Menon, J., Drakeley, C.J., Cox, J., 2016a. Association between landscape factors and spatial patterns of plasmodium knowlesi infections in Sabah, Malaysia. Emerg. Infect. Dis. 22, 201–208.

Fornace, K.M., Nuin, N.A., Betson, M., Grigg, M.J., William, T., Anstey, N.M., Yeo, T.W., Cox, J., Ying, L.T., Drakeley, C.J., 2016b. Asymptomatic and submicroscopic carriage of plasmodium knowlesi malaria in household and community members of clinical cases in Sabah, Malaysia. J. Infect. Dis. 213 (5), 784–787. https://doi.org/10.1093/infdis/jiv475.

Fornace, K.M., Herman, L.S., Abidin, T.R., Chua, T.H., Daim, S., Lorenzo, P.J., Grignard, L., Nuin, N.A., Ying, L.T., Grigg, M.J., William, T., Espino, F., Cox, J., Tetteh, K.K.A., Drakeley, C.J., 2018a. Exposure and infection to Plasmodium knowlesi in case study communities in Northern Sabah, Malaysia and Palawan, The Philippines. PLoS Negl. Trop. Dis. 12, e0006432.

Fornace, K.M., Surendra, H., Abidin, T.R., Reyes, R., Macalinao, M.L.M., Stresman, G., Luchavez, J., Ahmad, R.A., Supargiyono, S., Espino, F., Drakeley, C.J., Cook, J., 2018b. Use of mobile technology-based participatory mapping approaches to geolocate health facility attendees for disease surveillance in low resource settings. Int. J. Health Geogr. 17, 21.

Fornace, K.M., Alex, E.R., Abidin, T.R., Brock, P.M., Chua, T.H., Vythilingam, I., Ferguson, H.M., Manin, B.O., Wong, M.L., Ng, S.H., Cox, J., Drakeley, C., 2019a. Local human movement patterns and land use impact exposure to zoonotic malaria in Malaysian Borneo. Elife 8, 22.

Fornace, K.M., Brock, P.M., Abidin, T.R., Grignard, L., Herman, L.S., Chua, T.H., Daim, S., William, T., Patterson, C.L.E.B., Hall, T., Grigg, M.J., Anstey, N.M., Tetteh, K.K.A., Cox, J., Drakeley, C.J., 2019b. Environmental risk factors and exposure to the zoonotic malaria Plasmodium knowlesi across Northern Sabah, Malaysia: a cross-sectional survey. Lancet Planet Health 3, E179–E186.

Fornace, K.M., Reyes, R.A., Macalinao, M.L.M., Bareng, A.P.N., Luchavez, J.S., Hafalla, J.C., Espino, F.E., Drakeley, C.J., 2020. Disentangling fine-scale effects of environment on malaria detection and infection to design risk-based disease surveillance systems in changing landscapes. medRxiV. https://www.medrxiv.org/content/10.1101/2020.04.15.20065656v2.

Fornace, K.M., Diaz, A.V., Lines, J., Drakeley, C.J., 2021. Achieving global malaria eradication in changing landscapes. Malar. J. 20 (1), 69.

Foster, D., Cox-Singh, J., Mohamad, D.S., Krishna, S., Chin, P.P., Singh, B., 2014. Evaluation of three rapid diagnostic tests for the detection of human infections with Plasmodium knowlesi. Malar. J. 13, 60.

Fungfuang, W., Udom, C., Tongthainan, D., Kadir, K.A., Singh, B., 2020. Malaria parasites in macaques in Thailand: stump-tailed macaques (Macaca arctoides) are new natural hosts for Plasmodium knowlesi, Plasmodium inui, Plasmodium coatneyi and Plasmodium fieldi. Malar. J. 19, 350.

Gachelin, G., Opinel, A., 2011. Malaria epidemics in Europe after the First World War: the early stages of an international approach to the control of the disease. História, Ciências, Saúde-Manguinhos 18, 431–470.

Gamalo, L.E., Dimalibot, J., KADIR, K.A., SINGH, B., Paller, V.G., 2019. Plasmodium knowlesi and other malaria parasites in long-tailed macaques from the Philippines. Malar. J. 18, 147.

Gaveau, D.L., Sheil, D., Husnayaen, Salim, M.A., Arjasakusuma, S., Ancrenaz, M., Pacheco, P., Meijaard, E., 2016. Rapid conversions and avoided deforestation: examining four decades of industrial plantation expansion in Borneo. Sci. Rep. 6, 32017.

Gaveau, D.L., Locatelli, B., Salim, M.A., Husnayaen, Manurung, T., Descals, A., Angelsen, A., Meijaard, E., Sheil, D., 2021. Slowing deforestation in Indonesia follows declining oil palm expansion and lower oil prices. Research Square.

Ghinai, I., Cook, J., Hla, T.T., Htet, H.M., Hall, T., Lubis, I.N., Ghinai, R., Hesketh, T., Naung, Y., Lwin, M.M., Latt, T.S., Heymann, D.L., Sutherland, C.J., Drakeley, C., Field, N., 2017. Malaria epidemiology in central Myanmar: identification of a multi-species asymptomatic reservoir of infection. Malar. J. 16, 16.

Gibb, R., Moses, L.M., Redding, D.W., Jones, K.E., 2017. Understanding the cryptic nature of Lassa fever in West Africa. Pathog Glob. Health 111, 276–288.

Giles, J.R., Eby, P., Parry, H., Peel, A.J., Plowright, R.K., Westcott, D.A., McCallum, H., 2018. Environmental drivers of spatiotemporal foraging intensity in fruit bats and implications for Hendra virus ecology. Sci. Rep. 8, 9555.

Gillespie, T.R., Chapman, C.A., 2006. Prediction of parasite infection dynamics in primate metapopulations based on attributes of forest fragmentation. Conserv. Biol. 20, 441–448.

Gottdenker, N.L., Streicker, D.G., Faust, C.L., Carroll, C.R., 2014. Anthropogenic land use change and infectious diseases: a review of the evidence. Ecohealth 11, 619–632.

Grigg, M.J., William, T., Barber, B.E., Parameswaran, U., Bird, E., Piera, K., Aziz, A., Dhanaraj, P., Yeo, T.W., Anstey, N.M., 2014. Combining parasite lactate dehydrogenase-based and histidine-rich protein 2-based rapid tests to improve specificity for diagnosis of malaria Due to Plasmodium knowlesi and other Plasmodium species in Sabah, Malaysia. J. Clin. Microbiol. 52, 2053–2060.

Grigg, M.J., William, T., Menon, J., Dhanaraj, P., BARBER, B.E., Wilkes, C.S., Von Seidlein, L., Rajahram, G.S., Pasay, C., McCarthy, J.S., Price, R.N., Anstey, N.M., Yeo, T.W., 2016. Artesunate-mefloquine versus chloroquine for treatment of uncomplicated Plasmodium knowlesi malaria in Malaysia (ACT KNOW): an open-label, randomised controlled trial. Lancet Infect. Dis. 16, 180–188.

Grigg, M.J., Cox, J., William, T., Jelip, J., Fornace, K.M., Brock, P.M., Von Seidlein, L., Barber, B.E., Anstey, N.M., Yeo, T.W., Drakeley, C.J., 2017. Individual-level factors associated with the risk of acquiring human Plasmodium knowlesi malaria in Malaysia: a case control study. Lancet Planet. Health. 1, e97–104.

Grignard, L., Shah, S., Chua, T.H., William, T., Drakeley, C.J., Fornace, K.M., 2019. Natural Human Infections with Plasmodium cynomolgi and Other Malaria Species in an Elimination Setting in Sabah, Malaysia. J Infect Dis 220, 1946–1949.

Grogan, K., Pflugmacher, D., Hostert, P., Mertz, O., Fensholt, R., 2019. Unravelling the link between global rubber price and tropical deforestation in Cambodia. Nat. Plants 5, 47–53.

Gryseels, C., Durnez, L., Gerrets, R., Uk, S., Suon, S., Set, S., Phoeuk, P., Sluydts, V., Heng, S., Sochantha, T., Coosemans, M., Peeters Grietens, K., 2015. Re-imagining malaria: heterogeneity of human and mosquito behaviour in relation to residual malaria transmission in Cambodia. Malar. J. 14, 165.

Guerra, C.A., Snow, R.W., Hay, S.I., 2006. A global assessment of closed forests, deforestation and malaria risk. Ann. Trop. Med. Parasitol. 100, 189–204.

Guimaraes, L.O., Bajay, M.M., Wunderlich, G., Bueno, M.G., Rohe, F., Catao-Dias, J.L., Neves, A., Malafronte, R.S., Curado, I., Kirchgatter, K., 2012. The genetic diversity of Plasmodium malariae and Plasmodium brasilianum from human, simian and mosquito hosts in Brazil. Acta Trop. 124, 27–32.

Guivier, E., Galan, M., Chaval, Y., Xuereb, A., Ribas Salvador, A., Poulle, M.L., Voutilainen, L., Henttonen, H., Charbonnel, N., Cosson, J.F., 2011. Landscape genetics highlights the role of bank vole metapopulation dynamics in the epidemiology of Puumala hantavirus. Mol. Ecol. 20, 3569–3583.

Hahn, M.B., Gangnon, R.E., Barcellos, C., Asner, G.P., Patz, J.A., 2014. Influence of deforestation, logging, and fire on malaria in the Brazilian Amazon. PLoS One 9, e85725.

Halliday, F.W., Rohr, J.R., LAINE, A.L., 2020. Biodiversity loss underlies the dilution effect of biodiversity. Ecol. Lett. 23, 1611–1622.

Halsey, E.S., Miller, J.R., 2020. Maintenance of Borrelia burgdorferi among vertebrate hosts: a test of dilution effect mechanisms. Ecosphere 11.

Hambali, K.A., Ismail, A.H., Zulkifli, S.Y.Z., 2012. Human–macaque conflict and pest behaviors of Long-tailed macaques (Macaca fascicularis) in Kuala Selangor Nature Park. Trop. Nat. Hist. 12, 189–205.

Han, D., Bonner, M.R., Nie, J., Freudenheim, J.L., 2013. Assessing bias associated with geocoding of historical residence in epidemiology research. Geospat. Health 7, 369–374.

Hansen, M.C., Stehman, S.V., Potapov, P.V., Loveland, T.R., Townshend, J.R., Defries, R.S., Pittman, K.W., Arunarwati, B., Stolle, F., Steininger, M.K., Carroll, M., Dimiceli, C., 2008. Humid tropical forest clearing from 2000 to 2005 quantified by using multitemporal and multiresolution remotely sensed data. Proc. Natl. Acad. Sci. U. S. A. 105, 9439–9444.

Hansen, M.C., Potapov, P.V., Moore, R., Hancher, M., Turubanova, S.A., Tyukavina, A., Thau, D., Stehman, S.V., Goetz, S.J., Loveland, T.R., Kommareddy, A., Egorov, A., Chini, L., Justice, C.O., Townshend, J.R., 2013. High-resolution global maps of 21st-century forest cover change. Science 342, 850–853.

Hansen, M.C., Krylov, A., Tyukavina, A., Potapov, P.V., Turubanova, S., Zutta, B., Ifo, S., Margono, B.A., Stolle, F., Moore, R., 2016. Humid tropical forest disturbance alerts using Landsat data. Environ. Res. Lett. 11.

Hausermann, H., Tschakert, P., Smithwick, E.A.H., Ferring, D., Amankwah, R., Klutse, E., Hagarty, J., Kromel, K., 2012. Contours of risk: spatialising human behaviours to understand disease dynamics in changing landscapes. Ecohealth 9, 251–255.

Hawkes, F.M., Manin, B.O., Cooper, A., Daim, S., Homathevi, R., Jelip, J., Husin, T., Chua, T.H., 2019. Vector compositions change across forested to deforested ecotones in emerging areas of zoonotic malaria transmission in Malaysia. Sci. Rep. 9.

Hay, S.I., Battle, K.E., Pigott, D.M., Smith, D.L., Moyes, C.L., Bhatt, S., Brownstein, J.S., Collier, N., Myers, M.F., George, D.B., Gething, P.W., 2013. Global mapping of infectious disease. Philos. Trans. R. Soc. Lond. B Biol. Sci. 368, 20120250.

Herdiana, H., Cotter, C., Coutrier, F.N., Zarlinda, I., Zelman, B.W., Tirta, Y.K., Greenhouse, B., Gosling, R.D., Baker, P., Whittaker, M., Hsiang, M.S., 2016. Malaria risk factor assessment using active and passive surveillance data from Aceh Besar, Indonesia, a low endemic, malaria elimination setting with Plasmodium knowlesi, Plasmodium vivax, and Plasmodium falciparum. Malar. J. 15, 468.

Herdiana, H., Irnawati, I., Coutrier, F.N., Munthe, A., Mardiati, M., Yuniarti, T., Sariwati, E., Sumiwi, M.E., Noviyanti, R., Pronyk, P., Hawley, W.A., 2018. Two clusters of Plasmodium knowlesi cases in a malaria elimination area, Sabang Municipality, Aceh, Indonesia. Malar. J. 17, 186.

Herman, L.S., Fornace, K., Phelan, J., Grigg, M.J., Anstey, N.M., William, T., Moon, R.W., Blackman, M.J., Drakeley, C.J., Tetteh, K.K.A., 2018. Identification and validation of a novel panel of Plasmodium knowlesi biomarkers of serological exposure. PLoS Negl. Trop. Dis. 12, e0006457.

Herrera-Silveira, J.A., Ramirez-Ramirez, J., 1996. Effects of natural phenolic material (tannin) on phytoplankton growth. Limnol. Oceanogr. 41, 1018–1023.

Hii, J., 1985. Anopheles malaria vector in Malaysia with reference to Sabah. In: Harinasuta, R. (Ed.), Problems of malaria in endemic countries. Southeast Asian Medical Information Centre, Tokyo.

Hijioka, Y., Lin, E., Pereira, J.J., Corlett, R.T., Cui, X., Insarov, G.E., Lasco, R.D., Lindgren, E., Surjan, A., Barros, V.R., Field, C.B., Dokken, D.J., Mastrandrea, M.D., Mach, K.J., Bilir, T.E., Chatterjee, M., Ebi, K.L., Estrada, Y., Genova, R.C., Girma, B., Kissel, E.S., Levy, A.N., Maccracken, S., Mastrandrea, P.R., White, L., 2014. Asia. In: Climate Change 2014: Impacts, Adaptation and Vulnerability. Part B: Regional Aspects. Contribution of Working Group II to the Fifth Assessment Report of the Intergovernmental Panel on Climate Change. Cambridge University Press, Cambridge, UK and New York, USA.

Hoosen, A., Shaw, M.T., 2011. Plasmodium knowlesi in a traveller returning to New Zealand. Travel Med. Infect. Dis. 9, 144–148.

Imai, N., White, M.T., Ghani, A.C., DRAKELEY, C.J., 2014. Transmission and control of Plasmodium knowlesi: a mathematical modelling study. PLoS Negl. Trop. Dis. 8, e2978.

Imwong, M., Madmanee, W., Suwannasin, K., Kunasol, C., Peto, T.J., Tripura, R., von Seidlein, L., Nguon, C., Davoeung, C., Day, N.P.J., Dondorp, A.M., White, N.J., 2019. Asymptomatic natural human infections with the simian malaria parasites Plasmodium cynomolgi and Plasmodium knowlesi. J Infect Dis 219 (5), 695–702. https://doi.org/10.1093/infdis/jiy519.

Inada, R., Kitajima, K., Hardiwinoto, S., Kanzaki, M., 2017. The effect of logging and strip cutting on forest floor light condition and following change. Forests 8, 425.

Iwagami, M., Nakatsu, M., Khattignavong, P., Soundala, P., Lorphachan, L., Keomalaphet, S., Xangsayalath, P., Kawai, S., Hongvanthong, B., Brey, P.T., Kano, S., 2018. First case of human infection with Plasmodium knowlesi in Laos. PLoS Negl. Trop. Dis. 12, e0006244.

Jacquot, M., Abrial, D., Gasqui, P., Bord, S., Marsot, M., Masseglia, S., Pion, A., Poux, V., Zilliox, L., Chapuis, J.L., Vourc'H, G., Bailly, X., 2016. Multiple independent transmission cycles of a tick-borne pathogen within a local host community. Sci. Rep. 6, 31273.

Jiang, N., Chang, Q., Sun, X., Lu, H., Yin, J., Zhang, Z., Wahlgren, M., Chen, Q., 2010. Co-infections with Plasmodium knowlesi and other malaria parasites, Myanmar. Emerg. Infect. Dis. 16, 1476–1478.

Jones, B.A., Grace, D., Kock, R., Alonso, S., Rushton, J., Said, M.Y., Mckeever, D., Mutua, F., Young, J., McDermott, J., Pfeiffer, D.U., 2013. Zoonosis emergence linked to agricultural intensification and environmental change. Proc. Natl. Acad. Sci. U. S. A. 110, 8399–8404.

Jongwutiwes, S., Putaporntip, C., Iwasaki, T., Sata, T., Kanbara, H., 2004. Naturally acquired Plasmodium knowlesi malaria in human, Thailand. Emerg. Infect. Dis. 10, 2211–2213.

Jongwutiwes, S., Buppan, P., Kosuvin, R., Seethamchai, S., Pattanawong, U., Sirichaisinthop, J., Putaporntip, C., 2011. Plasmodium knowlesi Malaria in humans and macaques, Thailand. Emerg. Infect. Dis. 17, 1799–1806.

Joveen-Neoh, W.F., Chong, K.L., Wong, C.M., Lau, T.Y., 2011. Incidence of malaria in the interior division of sabah, malaysian borneo, based on nested PCR. J. Parasitol. Res. 2011, 104284.

Kahime, K., Boussaa, S., Bounoua, L., Fouad, O., Messouli, M., Boumezzough, A., 2014. Leishmaniasis in Morocco: diseases and vectors. Asian Pac. J. Trop. Dis. 4, 273–276.

Kalinga, A., Post, R.J., 2011. An apparent halt to the decline of Simulium woodi in the Usambara foci of onchocerciasis in Tanzania. Ann. Trop. Med. Parasitol. 105, 273–276.

Kantele, A., Jokiranta, T.S., 2011. Review of cases with the emerging fifth human malaria parasite, Plasmodium knowlesi. Clin. Infect. Dis. 52, 1356–1362.

Kantele, A., Marti, H., Felger, I., Muller, D., Jokiranta, T.S., 2008. Monkey malaria in a European traveler returning from Malaysia. Emerg. Infect. Dis. 14, 1434–1436.

Karesh, W.B., Noble, E., 2009. The bushmeat trade: increased opportunities for transmission of zoonotic disease. Mt. Sinai J. Med. 76, 429–434.

Keesing, F., Belden, L.K., Daszak, P., Dobson, A., Harvell, C.D., Holt, R.D., Hudson, P., Jolles, A., Jones, K.E., Mitchell, C.E., Myers, S.S., Bogich, T., Ostfeld, R.S., 2010. Impacts of biodiversity on the emergence and transmission of infectious diseases. Nature 468, 647–652.

Keiser, J., de Castro, M.C., Maltese, M.F., Bos, R., Tanner, M., Singer, B.H., Utzinger, J., 2005a. Effect of irrigation and large dams on the burden of malaria on a global and regional scale. Am. J. Trop. Med. Hyg. 72, 392–406.

Keiser, J., Maltese, M.F., Erlanger, T.E., Bos, R., Tanner, M., Singer, B.H., Utzinger, J., 2005b. Effect of irrigated rice agriculture on Japanese encephalitis, including challenges and opportunities for integrated vector management. Acta Trop. 95, 40–57.

Keiser, J., Singer, B.H., Utzinger, J., 2005c. Reducing the burden of malaria in different eco-epidemiological settings with environmental management: a systematic review. Lancet Infect. Dis. 5, 695–708.

Kettle, C., 2009. Ecological considerations for using dipterocarps for restoration of lowland rainforest in Southeast Asia. Biodivers. Conserv. 19, 1137–1151.

Khim, N., Siv, S., Kim, S., Mueller, T., Fleischmann, E., Singh, B., Divis, P.C., Steenkeste, N., Duval, L., Bouchier, C., Duong, S., Ariey, F., Menard, D., 2011. Plasmodium knowlesi infection in humans, Cambodia, 2007-2010. Emerg. Infect. Dis. 17, 1900–1902.

Kilpatrick, A.M., Randolph, S.E., 2012. Drivers, dynamics, and control of emerging vector-borne zoonotic diseases. Lancet 380, 1946–1955.

Knowles, R., Das Gupta, B.M., 1932. A study of monkey-malaria and its experimental transmission to man. Ind. Med. Gaz. 67, 301–320.

Kondgen, S., Schenk, S., Pauli, G., Boesch, C., Leendertz, F.H., 2010. Noninvasive monitoring of respiratory viruses in wild chimpanzees. Ecohealth 7, 332–341.

Kowalewski, M.M., Salzer, J.S., Deutsch, J.C., Rano, M., Kuhlenschmidt, M.S., Gillespie, T.R., 2011. Black and gold howler monkeys (Alouatta caraya) as sentinels of ecosystem health: patterns of zoonotic protozoa infection relative to degree of human-primate contact. Am. J. Primatol. 73, 75–83.

Kraemer, M.U.G., Faria, N.R., Reiner Jr., R.C., Golding, N., Nikolay, B., Stasse, S., Johansson, M.A., Salje, H., Faye, O., Wint, G.R.W., Niedrig, M., Shearer, F.M., Hill, S.C., Thompson, R.N., Bisanzio, D., Taveira, N., Nax, H.H., Pradelski, B.S.R., Nsoesie, E.O., Murphy, N.R., Bogoch II, Khan, K., Brownstein, J.S., Tatem, A.J., De Oliveira, T., Smith, D.L., Sall, A.A., Pybus, O.G., Hay, S.I., Cauchemez, S., 2017. Spread of yellow fever virus outbreak in Angola and the Democratic Republic of the Congo 2015–16: a modelling study. Lancet Infect. Dis. 17, 330–338.

Kweka, E.J., Kimaro, E.E., Munga, S., 2016. Effect of deforestation and land use changes on mosquito productivity and development in western kenya highlands: implication for Malaria Risk. Front. Public Health 4, 238.

Lacroix, C., Jolles, A., Seabloom, E.W., Power, A.G., Mitchell, C.E., Borer, E.T., 2014. Non-random biodiversity loss underlies predictable increases in viral disease prevalence. J. R. Soc. Interface 11, 20130947.

Lash, R.R., Carroll, D.S., Hughes, C.M., Nakazawa, Y., Karem, K., Damon, I.K., Peterson, A.T., 2012. Effects of georeferencing effort on mapping monkeypox case distributions and transmission risk. Int. J. Health Geogr. 11, 23.

Laurance, W.F., Yensen, E., 1991. Predicting the impacts of edge effects in fragmented habitats. Biol. Conserv. 55, 77–92.

Laurance, W.E., Croes, B.M., Tchignoumba, L., Lahm, S.A., Alonso, A., Lee, M.E., Campbell, P., Ondzeano, C., 2006. Impacts of roads and hunting on central African rainforest mammals. Conserv. Biol. 20, 1251–1261.

Laurance, W.F., Camargo, J.L.C., Fearnside, P.M., Lovejoy, T.E., Williamson, G.B., Mesquita, R.C.G., Meyer, C.F.J., Bobrowiec, P.E.D., Laurance, S.G.W., 2018. An Amazonian rainforest and its fragments as a laboratory of global change. Biol. Rev. Camb. Philos. Soc. 93, 223–247.

Lee, K.S., Cox-Singh, J., Brooke, G., Matusop, A., Singh, B., 2009a. Plasmodium knowlesi from archival blood films: further evidence that human infections are widely distributed and not newly emergent in Malaysian Borneo. Int. J. Parasitol. 39, 1125–1128.

Lee, K.S., Cox-Singh, J., Singh, B., 2009b. Morphological features and differential counts of Plasmodium knowlesi parasites in naturally acquired human infections. Malar. J. 8, 73.

Lee, Y.C., Tang, C.S., Ang, L.W., Han, H.K., James, L., Goh, K.T., 2009c. Epidemiological characteristics of imported and locally-acquired malaria in Singapore. Ann. Acad. Med. Singapore 38, 840–849.

Lee, K.S., Divis, P.C., Zakaria, S.K., Matusop, A., Julin, R.A., Conway, D.J., Cox-Singh, J., Singh, B., 2011. Plasmodium knowlesi: reservoir hosts and tracking the emergence in humans and macaques. PLoS Pathog. 7, e1002015.

Leonardo, L.R., Rivera, P.T., Crisostomo, B.A., Sarol, J.N., Bantayan, N.C., Tiu, W.U., Bergquist, N.R., 2005. A study of the environmental determinants of malaria and schistosomiasis in the Philippines using Remote Sensing and Geographic Information Systems. Parassitologia 47, 105–114.

Li, W., Fu, D., Su, F., Xiao, Y., 2020. Spatial–temporal evolution and analysis of the driving force of oil palm patterns in Malaysia from 2000 to 2018. ISPRS Int. J. Geo Inf. 9, 280.

Liew, J.W.K, Mohd Bukhari, F.D., Jeyaprakasam, N.K., Phang, W.K., Vythilingam, I., Lau, Y.L., 2021. Natural Plasmodium inui infections in humans and Anopheles cracens mosquito, Malaysia. Emerg. Infect. Dis. https://doi.org/10.3201/eid27010.210412.

Liu, W., Li, Y., Learn, G.H., Rudicell, R.S., Robertson, J.D., Keele, B.F., Ndjango, J.B., Sanz, C.M., Morgan, D.B., Locatelli, S., Gonder, M.K., Kranzusch, P.J., Walsh, P.D., Delaporte, E., Mpoudi-Ngole, E., Georgiev, A.V., Muller, M.N., Shaw, G.M., Peeters, M., Sharp, P.M., Rayner, J.C., Hahn, B.H., 2010. Origin of the human malaria parasite Plasmodium falciparum in gorillas. Nature 467, 420–425.

Loaiza, J.R., Dutari, L.C., Rovira, J.R., Sanjur, O.I., Laporta, G.Z., Pecor, J., Foley, D.H., Eastwood, G., Kramer, L.D., Radtke, M., Pongsiri, M., 2017. Disturbance and mosquito diversity in the lowland tropical rainforest of central Panama. Sci. Rep. 7, 7248.

Looi, L.M., Chua, K.B., 2007. Lessons from the Nipah virus outbreak in Malaysia. Malays. J. Pathol. 29, 63–67.

Lubis, I.N., Wijaya, H., Lubis, M., Lubis, C.P., Divis, P.C., Beshir, K.B., Sutherland, C.J., 2017. Contribution of Plasmodium knowlesi to multi-species human malaria infections in North Sumatera, Indonesia. J Infect Dis 215 (7), 1148–1155. https://doi.org/10.1093/infdis/jix091.

Luchavez, J., Espino, F., Curameng, P., Espina, R., Bell, D., Chiodini, P., Nolder, D., Sutherland, C., Lee, K.S., Singh, B., 2008. Human Infections with Plasmodium knowlesi, the Philippines. Emerg. Infect. Dis. 14, 811–813.

Luis, A.D., Kuenzi, A.J., Mills, J.N., 2018. Species diversity concurrently dilutes and amplifies transmission in a zoonotic host-pathogen system through competing mechanisms. Proc. Natl. Acad. Sci. U. S. A. 115, 7979–7984.

MacDonald, A.J., Mordecai, E.A., 2019. Amazon deforestation drives malaria transmission, and malaria burden reduces forest clearing. Proc. Natl. Acad. Sci. U. S. A. 116, 22212–22218.

Mackroth, M.S., Tappe, D., Tannich, E., Addo, M., Rothe, C., 2016. Rapid-antigen test negative Malaria in a traveler returning from Thailand, molecularly diagnosed as Plasmodium knowlesi. Open Forum Infect. Dis. 3. ofw039.

Madsen, H., Coulibaly, G., Furu, P., 1987. Distribution of freshwater snails in the river Niger basin in Mali with special reference to the intermediate hosts of schistosomes. Hydrobiologia 146, 77–88.

Maki, J., Guiot, A.L., Aubert, M., Brochier, B., Cliquet, F., Hanlon, C.A., King, R., Oertli, E.H., Rupprecht, C.E., Schumacher, C., Slate, D., Yakobson, B., Wohlers, A., Lankau, E.W., 2017. Oral vaccination of wildlife using a vaccinia-rabies-glycoprotein recombinant virus vaccine (RABORAL V-RG (R)): a global review. Vet. Res. 48, 26.

Manin, B.O., Ferguson, H.M., Vythilingam, I., Fornace, K., William, T., Torr, S.J., Drakeley, C., CHUA, T.H., 2016. Investigating the contribution of peri-domestic transmission to risk of zoonotic malaria infection in humans. PLoS Negl. Trop. Dis. 10, e0005064.

Mbora, D.N., Wieczkowski, J., Munene, E., 2009. Links between habitat degradation, and social group size, ranging, fecundity, and parasite prevalence in the Tana River mangabey (Cercocebus galeritus). Am. J. Phys. Anthropol. 140, 562–571.

McElwee, P., 2009. Reforesting "bare hills" in Vietnam: social and environmental consequences of the 5 million hectare reforestation program. Ambio 38, 325–333.

MESA Track 2021. Plasmodium knowlesi. In: Mesa Alliance, I. (ed.). Barcelona, Spain.

Moon, R.W., Hall, J., Rangkuti, F., Ho, Y.S., Almond, N., Mitchell, G.H., Pain, A., Holder, A.A., Blackman, M.J., 2013. Adaptation of the genetically tractable malaria pathogen Plasmodium knowlesi to continuous culture in human erythrocytes. Proc. Natl. Acad. Sci. U. S. A. 110, 531–536.

Moon, R.W., Sharaf, H., Hastings, C.H., Ho, Y.S., Nair, M.B., Rchiad, Z., Knuepfer, E., Ramaprasad, A., Mohring, F., Amir, A., Yusuf, N.A., Hall, J., Almond, N., Lau, Y.L., Pain, A., Blackman, M.J., Holder, A.A., 2016. Normocyte-binding protein required for human erythrocyte invasion by the zoonotic malaria parasite Plasmodium knowlesi. Proc. Natl. Acad. Sci. U. S. A. 113, 7231–7236.

Moyes, C.L., Henry, A.J., Golding, N., Huang, Z., Singh, B., Baird, J.K., Newton, P.N., Huffman, M., Duda, K.A., Drakeley, C.J., Elyazar, I.R., Anstey, N.M., Chen, Q., Zommers, Z., Bhatt, S., Gething, P.W., Hay, S.I., 2014. Defining the geographical range of the Plasmodium knowlesi reservoir. PLoS Negl. Trop. Dis. 8, e2780.

Moyes, C.L., Shearer, F.M., Huang, Z., Wiebe, A., Gibson, H.S., Nijman, V., Mohd-Azlan, J., Brodie, J.F., Malaivijitnond, S., Linkie, M., Samejima, H., O'brien, T.G., Trainor, C.R., Hamada, Y., Giordano, A.J., Kinnaird, M.F., ELYAZAR, I.R., Sinka, M.E., Vythilingam, I., Bangs, M.J., Pigott, D.M., Weiss, D.J., Golding, N., HAY, S.I., 2016. Predicting the geographical distributions of the macaque hosts and mosquito vectors of Plasmodium knowlesi malaria in forested and non-forested areas. Parasit. Vectors 9, 242.

Muro, A.I., Raybould, J.N., 1990. Population decline of Simulium woodi and reduced onchocerciasis transmission at Amani, Tanzania, in relation to deforestation. Acta Leiden. 59, 153–159.

Mweempwa, C., Marcotty, T., DE Pus, C., Penzhorn, B.L., Dicko, A.H., Bouyer, J., DE Deken, R., 2015. Impact of habitat fragmentation on tsetse populations and trypanosomosis risk in Eastern Zambia. Parasit. Vectors 8, 406.

Namkhan, M., Gale, G.A., Savini, T., Tantipisanuh, N., 2021. Loss and vulnerability of lowland forests in mainland Southeast Asia. Conserv. Biol. 35, 206–215.

Ng, L.S., Campos-Arceiz, A., Sloan, S., Hughes, A.C., Tiang, D.C.F., Li, B.V., Lechner, A.M., 2020. The scale of biodiversity impacts of the Belt and Road Initiative in Southeast Asia. Biol. Conserv. 248, 108691. https://doi.org/10.1016/j.biocon.2020.108691.

Ninan, T., Nalees, K., Newin, M., Sultan, Q., Than, M.M., Shinde, S., Habana, A.V.F., Mohd Yusof, N., 2012. Plasmodium knowlesi malaria infection in human. Brunei Int. Med. J. 8, 358–361.

Noor, A.M., Alegana, V.A., Gething, P.W., Snow, R.W., 2009. A spatial national health facility database for public health sector planning in Kenya in 2008. Int. J. Health Geogr. 8, 13.

Norris, D.E., 2004. Mosquito-borne diseases as a consequence of land use change. Ecohealth 1, 19–24.

Nowak, S.P., Zmora, P., Pielok, L., Kuszel, L., Kierzek, R., Stefaniak, J., Paul, M., 2019. Case of Plasmodium knowlesi Malaria in Poland linked to travel in southeast Asia. Emerg. Infect. Dis. 25, 1772–1773.

Nunn, C.L., Altizer, S., Jones, K.E., Sechrest, W., 2003. Comparative tests of parasite species richness in primates. Am. Nat. 162, 597–614.

Nunn, C.L., Brezine, C., Jolles, A.E., Ezenwa, V.O., 2014. Interactions between micro- and macroparasites predict microparasite species richness across primates. Am. Nat. 183, 494–505.

Oduro, A.R., Bojang, K.A., Conway, D.J., Corrah, T., Greenwood, B.M., Schellenberg, D., 2011. Health centre surveys as a potential tool for monitoring malaria epidemiology by area and over time. PLoS One 6, e26305.

Olivero, J., Fa, J.E., Real, R., Marquez, A.L., Farfan, M.A., Vargas, J.M., Gaveau, D., Salim, M.A., Park, D., Suter, J., King, S., Leendertz, S.A., Sheil, D., Nasi, R., 2017. Recent loss of closed forests is associated with Ebola virus disease outbreaks. Sci. Rep. 7, 14291.

Orth, H., Jensen, B.O., Holtfreter, M.C., Kocheril, S.J., Mallach, S., MacKenzie, C., Müller-Stöver, I., Henrich, B., Imwong, M., White, N.J., Häussinger, D., Richter, J., 2013. *Plasmodium knowlesi* infection imported to Germany, January 2013. Euro. Surveill. 18 (40), 20603. https://doi.org/10.2807/1560-7917.es2013.18.40.20603. PMID: 24128698.

Ozbilgin, A., Cavus, I., Yildirim, A., Gunduz, C., 2016. The first monkey malaria in Turkey: a case of Plasmodium knowlesi. Mikrobiyol. Bul. 50, 484–490.

Page, S.E., Hooijer, A., 2016. In the line of fire: the peatlands of Southeast Asia. Philos. Trans. R. Soc. Lond. B Biol. Sci. 371.

Parrish, C.R., Holmes, E.C., Morens, D.M., Park, E.C., Burke, D.S., Calisher, C.H., Laughlin, C.A., Saif, L.J., Daszak, P., 2008. Cross-species virus transmission and the emergence of new epidemic diseases. Microbiol. Mol. Biol. Rev. 72, 457–470.

Pearce, J.C., Learoyd, T.P., Langendorf, B.J., Logan, J.G., 2018. Japanese encephalitis: the vectors, ecology and potential for expansion. J. Travel Med. 25, S16–S26.

Phang, W.K., Hamid, M.H.A., Jelip, J., Mudin, R.N., Chuang, T.W., Lau, Y.L., Fong, M.Y., 2020. Spatial and Temporal Analysis of Plasmodium knowlesi Infection in Peninsular Malaysia, 2011 to 2018. Int. J. Environ. Res. Public Health 17, 11.

Pindolia, D.K., Garcia, A.J., Wesolowski, A., Smith, D.L., Buckee, C.O., Noor, A.M., Snow, R.W., Tatem, A.J., 2012. Human movement data for malaria control and elimination strategic planning. Malar. J. 11, 205. https://doi.org/10.1186/1475-2875-11-205.

Pindolia, D.K., Garcia, A.J., Huang, Z., Fik, T., Smith, D.L., Tatem, A.J., 2014. Quantifying cross-border movements and migrations for guiding the strategic planning of malaria control and elimination. Malar. J. 13, 169.

Plowright, R.K., Reaser, J.K., Locke, H., Woodley, S.J., Patz, J.A., Becker, D.J., Oppler, G., Hudson, P.J., Tabor, G.M., 2021. Land use-induced spillover: a call to action to safeguard environmental, animal, and human health. Lancet Planet Health 5, e237–e245.

Poulsen, J.R., Clark, C.J., Mavah, G., Elkan, P.W., 2009. Bushmeat supply and consumption in a tropical logging concession in northern Congo. Conserv. Biol. 23, 1597–1608.

Prist, P.R., Ps, D.A., Metzger, J.P., 2017. Landscape, Climate and Hantavirus Cardiopulmonary Syndrome Outbreaks. Ecohealth 14, 614–629.

Putaporntip, C., Hongsrimuang, T., Seethamchai, S., Kobasa, T., Limkittikul, K., Cui, L., Jongwutiwes, S., 2009. Differential prevalence of Plasmodium infections and cryptic Plasmodium knowlesi malaria in humans in Thailand. J Infect Dis 199, 1143–1150.

Putaporntip, C., Jongwutiwes, S., Thongaree, S., Seethamchai, S., Grynberg, P., Hughes, A.L., 2010. Ecology of malaria parasites infecting Southeast Asian macaques: evidence from cytochrome b sequences. Mol. Ecol. 19, 3466–3476.

Putz, F.E., Zuidema, P.A., Pinard, M.A., Boot, R.G., Sayer, J.A., Sheil, D., Sist, P., Elias, Vanclay, J.K., 2008. Improved tropical forest management for carbon retention. PLoS Biol. 6, e166.

Quesada, B., Arneth, A., De Noblet-Ducoudre, N., 2017. Atmospheric, radiative, and hydrologic effects of future land use and land cover changes: a global and multimodel climate picture. J. Geophys. Res. Atmos. 122, 5113–5131.

Rabinovich, R.N., Drakeley, C., Djimde, A.A., Hall, B.F., Hay, S.I., Hemingway, J., Kaslow, D.C., Noor, A., Okumu, F., Steketee, R., Tanner, M., Wells, T.N.C., Whittaker, M.A., Winzeler, E.A., Wirth, D.F., Whitfield, K., Alonso, P.L., 2017. malERA: An updated research agenda for malaria elimination and eradication. PLoS Med. 14, e1002456.

Raja, T.N., Hu, T.H., Kadir, K.A., Mohamad, D.S.A., Rosli, N., Wong, L.L., Hii, K.C., Simon Divis, P.C., Singh, B., 2020. Naturally acquired human plasmodium cynomolgi and P. knowlesi Infections, Malaysian Borneo. Emerg. Infect. Dis. 26, 1801–1809.

Rajahram, G.S., Barber, B.E., William, T., Menon, J., Anstey, N.M., Yeo, T.W., 2012. Deaths due to Plasmodium knowlesi malaria in Sabah, Malaysia: association with reporting as Plasmodium malariae and delayed parenteral artesunate. Malar. J. 11, 284.

Randolph, S.E., Dobson, A.D., 2012. Pangloss revisited: a critique of the dilution effect and the biodiversity-buffers-disease paradigm. Parasitology 139, 847–863.

Reaser, J.K., Witt, A., Tabor, G.M., Hudson, P.J., Plowright, R.K., 2021. Ecological countermeasures for preventing zoonotic disease outbreaks: when ecological restoration is a human health imperative. Restor. Ecol. https://doi.org/10.1111/rec.13357.

Reyes, R.A., Fornace, K.M., Macalinao, M.L.M., Boncayao, B.L., de la Fuente, E.S., Sabanal, H.M., Bareng, A.P.N., Medado, I.A.P., Mercado, E.S., Baquilod, M.S., Luchavez, J.S., Hafalla, J.C.R., Drakeley, C.J., Espino, F.E.J., 2021. Enhanced health facility surveys to support malaria control and elimination across different transmission settings in the Philippines. Am. J. Trop. Med. Hyg. 104 (3), 968–978.

Riley, E.P., 2008. Ranging patterns and habitat use of Sulawesi Tonkean macaques (Macaca tonkeana) in a human-modified habitat. Am. J. Primatol. 70, 670–679.

Roe, K., Thangarajan, A., Lilley, K., Dowd, S., Shanks, D., 2020. Plasmodium knowlesi infection in an Australian soldier following jungle warfare training in Malaysia. J. Mil. Veterans' Health 28, 53–56.

Rohani, A., Wan Najdah, W.M.A., Mohd Hanif, O., Aidil Azahary, A.R., Zurainee, M., Yu, K.X., Jelip, J., Husin, T., Lim, L.H., 2019. Characterization of the larval breeding sites of Anopheles balabacensis (Baisas), in Kudat, Sabah, Malaysia. Southeast Asian J. Trop. Med. Public Health 49, 566–579.

Roque, A.L., Xavier, S.C., da Rocha, M.G., Duarte, A.C., D'andrea, P.S., Jansen, A.M., 2008. Trypanosoma cruzi transmission cycle among wild and domestic mammals in three areas of orally transmitted Chagas disease outbreaks. Am. J. Trop. Med. Hyg. 79, 742–749.

Ruiz Cuenca, P., Key, S., Drakeley, C.J., Fornace, K.M., 2021. Evidence of human-mosquito-human transmission of the zoonotic malaria Plasmodium knowlesi: a systematic literature review. World Health Organization, Geneva.

Rulli, M.C., Santini, M., Hayman, D.T., D'odorico, P., 2017. The nexus between forest fragmentation in Africa and Ebola virus disease outbreaks. Sci. Rep. 7, 41613.

Sakkas, H., Bozidis, P., Franks, A., Papadopoulou, C., 2018. Oropouche fever: a review. Viruses 10.

Sallum, M.A.M., Peyton, E.L., Wilkerson, R.C., 2005. Six new species of the Anopheles leucosphyrus group, reinterpretation of An. elegans and vector implications. Med. Vet. Entomol. 19 (2), 158–199. https://doi.org/10.1111/j.0269-283X.2005.00551.x.

Satitvipawee, P., Wongkhang, W., Pattanasin, S., Hoithong, P., Bhumiratana, A., 2012. Predictors of malaria-association with rubber plantations in Thailand. BMC Public Health 12, 1115.

Sato, S., Tojo, B., Hoshi, T., Minsong, L.I.F., Kugan, O.K., Giloi, N., Ahmed, K., Jeffree, S.M., Moji, K., Kita, K., 2019. Recent incidence of human malaria caused by plasmodium knowlesi in the villages in Kudat Peninsula, Sabah, Malaysia: mapping of the infection risk using remote sensing data. Int. J. Environ. Res. Public Health 16, 16.

Schmidt, L.H., Greenl, R., Genther, C.S., 1961. The transmission of Plasmodium cynomolgi to man. Am. Demogr., 679–688.

Seethamchai, S., Putaporntip, C., Malaivijitnond, S., Cui, L., Jongwutiwes, S., 2008. Malaria and Hepatocystis species in wild macaques, southern Thailand. Am. J. Trop. Med. Hyg. 78, 646–653.

Seilmaier, M., Hartmann, W., Beissner, M., Fenzl, T., Haller, C., Guggemos, W., Hesse, J., Harle, A., Bretzel, G., Sack, S., Wendtner, C., Loscher, T., Berens-Riha, N., 2014. Severe Plasmodium knowlesi infection with multi-organ failure imported to Germany from Thailand/Myanmar. Malar. J. 13, 422.

Sermwittayawong, N., Singh, B., Nishibuchi, M., Sawangjaroen, N., Vuddhakul, V., 2012. Human Plasmodium knowlesi infection in Ranong province, southwestern border of Thailand. Malar. J. 11, 36.

Setiadi, W., Sudoyo, H., Trimarsanto, H., Sihite, B.A., Saragih, R.J., Juliawaty, R., Wangsamuda, S., Asih, P.B., Syafruddin, D., 2016. A zoonotic human infection with simian malaria, Plasmodium knowlesi, in Central Kalimantan, Indonesia. Malar. J. 15, 218.

Sharp, P.M., Hahn, B.H., 2011. Origins of HIV and the AIDS pandemic. Cold Spring Harb. Perspect. Med. 1, a006841.

Shearer, F.M., Huang, Z., Weiss, D.J., Wiebe, A., Gibson, H.S., Battle, K.E., Pigott, D.M., Brady, O.J., Putaporntip, C., Jongwutiwes, S., Lau, Y.L., Manske, M., Amato, R., Elyazar, I.R., Vythilingam, I., Bhatt, S., Gething, P.W., Singh, B., Golding, N., HAY, S.I., Moyes, C.L., 2016. Estimating geographical variation in the risk of zoonotic plasmodium knowlesi infection in countries eliminating malaria. PLoS Negl. Trop. Dis. 10, e0004915.

Shimizu, S., Chotirat, S., Dokkulab, N., Hongchad, I., Khowsroy, K., Kiattibutr, K., Maneechai, N., Manopwisedjaroen, K., Petchvijit, P., Phumchuea, K., Rachaphaew, N., Sripoorote, P., Suansomjit, C., Thongyod, W., Khamsiriwatchara, A., Lawpoolsri, S., Hanboonkunupakarn, B., Sattabongkot, J., Nguitragool, W., 2020. Malaria cross-sectional surveys identified asymptomatic infections of Plasmodium falciparum, Plasmodium vivax and Plasmodium knowlesi in Surat Thani, a southern province of Thailand. Int. J. Infect. Dis. 96, 445–451.

Siner, A., Liew, S.T., Kadir, K.A., Mohamad, D.S.A., Thomas, F.K., Zulkarnaen, M., Singh, B., 2017. Absence of Plasmodium inui and Plasmodium cynomolgi, but detection of Plasmodium knowlesi and Plasmodium vivax infections in asymptomatic humans in the Betong division of Sarawak, Malaysian Borneo. Malar. J. 16, 417.

Singh, B., Daneshvar, C., 2010. Plasmodium knowlesi malaria in Malaysia. Med. J. Malaysia 65, 166–172.

Singh, B., Daneshvar, C., 2013. Human infections and detection of Plasmodium knowlesi. Clin. Microbiol. Rev. 26, 165–184.

Singh, M., Kumara, H.N., Kumar, M.A., Sharma, A.K., 2001. Behavioural responses of lion-tailed macaques (Macaca silenus) to a changing habitat in a tropical rain forest fragment in the Western Ghats, India. Folia Primatol (Basel) 72, 278–291.

Singh, B., Kim Sung, L., Matusop, A., Radhakrishnan, A., Shamsul, S.S., Cox-Singh, J., Thomas, A., Conway, D.J., 2004. A large focus of naturally acquired Plasmodium knowlesi infections in human beings. Lancet 363, 1017–1024.

Siregar, J.E., Faust, C.L., Murdiyarso, L.S., Rosmanah, L., Saepuloh, U., Dobson, A.P., Iskandriati, D., 2015. Non-invasive surveillance for Plasmodium in reservoir macaque species. Malar. J. 14, 404.

Sloan, S., Locatelli, B., Wooster, M.J., Gaveau, D.L., 2017. Fire activity in Borneo driven by industrial land conversion and drought during El Nino periods, 1982–2010. Glob. Environ. Chang. 47, 95–109.

Sodhi, N.S., Posa, M.R.C., Lee, T.M., Bickford, D., Koh, L.P., Brook, B.W., 2010. The state and conservation of Southeast Asian biodiversity. Biodivers. Conserv. 19, 317–328.

Sokolow, S.H., Nova, N., Pepin, K.M., Peel, A.J., Pulliam, J.R.C., Manlove, K., Cross, P.C., Becker, D.J., Plowright, R.K., McCallum, H., De Leo, G.A., 2019. Ecological interventions to prevent and manage zoonotic pathogen spillover. Philos. Trans. R. Soc. Lond. B Biol. Sci. 374, 20180342.

Stark, D., Salgado-Lynn, M., 2014. Interim Report on Primatology Component. MONKEYBAR project.

Stark, D.J., Fornace, K.M., Brock, P.M., Abidin, T.R., Gilhooly, L., Jalius, C., Goossens, B., Drakeley, C.J., Salgado-Lynn, M., 2019. Long-Tailed Macaque Response to Deforestation in a Plasmodium knowlesi-Endemic Area. Ecohealth 16 (4), 638–646. https://doi.org/10.1007/s10393-019-01403-9. Epub 2019 Mar 29. PMID: 30927165; PMCID: PMC6910895.

Stevenson, J.C., Stresman, G.H., Gitonga, C.W., Gillig, J., Owaga, C., Marube, E., Odongo, W., Okoth, A., China, P., Oriango, R., Brooker, S.J., Bousema, T., Drakeley, C., Cox, J., 2013. Reliability of school surveys in estimating geographic variation in malaria transmission in the western Kenyan highlands. PLoS One 8, e77641.

Stibig, H.J., Achard, F., Carboni, S., Rasi, R., Miettinen, J., 2014. Change in tropical forest cover of Southeast Asia from 1990 to 2010. Biogeosciences 11, 247–258.

Stoddard, S.T., Morrison, A.C., Vazquez-Prokopec, G.M., Paz Soldan, V., Kochel, T.J., Kitron, U., Elder, J.P., Scott, T.W., 2009. The role of human movement in the transmission of vector-borne pathogens. PLoS Negl. Trop. Dis. 3, e481.

Streicker, D.G., Recuenco, S., Valderrama, W., Gomez Benavides, J., Vargas, I., Pacheco, V., Condori Condori, R.E., Montgomery, J., Rupprecht, C.E., Rohani, P., Altizer, S., 2012. Ecological and anthropogenic drivers of rabies exposure in vampire bats: implications for transmission and control. Proc Biol Sci 279, 3384–3392.

Stresman, G., Kobayashi, T., Kamanga, A., Thuma, P.E., Mharakurwa, S., Moss, W.J., Shiff, C., 2012. Malaria research challenges in low prevalence settings. Malar. J. 11, 353.

Stresman, G.H., Stevenson, J.C., Owaga, C., MARUBE, E., Anyango, C., Drakeley, C., Bousema, T., Cox, J., 2014. Validation of three geolocation strategies for health-facility attendees for research and public health surveillance in a rural setting in western Kenya. Epidemiol. Infect. 142, 1978–1989.

Sturrock, H.J., Hsiang, M.S., Cohen, J.M., Smith, D.L., Greenhouse, B., Bousema, T., Gosling, R.D., 2013. Targeting asymptomatic malaria infections: active surveillance in control and elimination. PLoS Med. 10, e1001467.

Sulistyaningsih, E., Fitri, L.E., Loscher, T., Berens-Riha, N., 2010. Diagnostic difficulties with Plasmodium knowlesi infection in humans. Emerg. Infect. Dis. 16, 1033–1034.

Sundararaman, S.A., Liu, W., Keele, B.F., Learn, G.H., Bittinger, K., Mouacha, F., Ahuka-Mundeke, S., Manske, M., Sherrill-Mix, S., Li, Y., Malenke, J.A., Delaporte, E., Laurent, C., Mpoudi Ngole, E., Kwiatkowski, D.P., Shaw, G.M., Rayner, J.C., Peeters, M., Sharp, P.M., Bushman, F.D., Hahn, B.H., 2013. Plasmodium falciparum-like parasites infecting wild apes in southern Cameroon do not represent a recurrent source of human malaria. Proc. Natl. Acad. Sci. U. S. A. 110, 7020–7025.

Surendra, H., Supargiyono, Ahmad, R.A., Kusumasari, R.A., Rahayujati, T.B., Damayanti, S.Y., Tetteh, K.K.A., Chitnis, C., Stresman, G., Cook, J., Drakeley, C., 2020. Using health facility-based serological surveillance to predict receptive areas at risk of malaria outbreaks in elimination areas. BMC Med. 18, 9.

Ta, T.T., Salas, A., Ali-Tammam, M., Martinez Mdel, C., Lanza, M., Arroyo, E., Rubio, J.M., 2010. First case of detection of Plasmodium knowlesi in Spain by Real Time PCR in a traveller from Southeast Asia. Malar. J. 9, 219.

Ta, T.H., Hisam, S., Lanza, M., Jiram, A.I., Ismail, N., Rubio, J.M., 2014. First case of a naturally acquired human infection with Plasmodium cynomolgi. Malar. J. 13, 68.

Takaya, S., Kutsuna, S., Suzuki, T., Komaki-Yasuda, K., Kano, S., Ohmagari, N., 2018. Case Report: Plasmodium knowlesi Infection with Rhabdomyolysis in a Japanese Traveler to Palawan, the Philippines. Am. J. Trop. Med. Hyg. 99, 967–969.

Tan, C.H., Vythilingam, I., Matusop, A., Chan, S.T., Singh, B., 2008. Bionomics of Anopheles latens in Kapit, Sarawak, Malaysian Borneo in relation to the transmission of zoonotic simian malaria parasite Plasmodium knowlesi. Malar. J. 7, 52.

Tangena, J.A., Thammavong, P., Wilson, A.L., Brey, P.T., Lindsay, S.W., 2016. Risk and control of mosquito-borne diseases in southeast asian rubber plantations. Trends Parasitol. 32, 402–415.

Tanizaki, R., Ujiie, M., Kato, Y., Iwagami, M., Hashimoto, A., Kutsuna, S., Takeshita, N., Hayakawa, K., Kanagawa, S., Kano, S., Ohmagari, N., 2013. First case of Plasmodium knowlesi infection in a Japanese traveller returning from Malaysia. Malar. J. 12, 128.

Tarafder, M.R., Balolong Jr., E., Carabin, H., Belisle, P., Tallo, V., Joseph, L., Alday, P., Gonzales, R.O., Riley, S., Olveda, R., Mcgarvey, S.T., 2006. A cross-sectional study of the prevalence of intensity of infection with Schistosoma japonicum in 50 irrigated and rain-fed villages in Samar Province, the Philippines. BMC Public Health 6, 61.

Taubert, F., Fischer, R., Groeneveld, J., Lehmann, S., Muller, M.S., Rodig, E., Wiegand, T., Huth, A., 2018. Global patterns of tropical forest fragmentation. Nature 554, 519–522.

Tchouassi, D.P., Torto, B., Sang, R., Riginos, C., Ezenwa, V.O., 2021. Large herbivore loss has complex effects on mosquito ecology and vector-borne disease risk. Transbound. Emerg. Dis. 68 (4), 2503–2513. https://doi.org/10.1111/tbed.13918.

Tuno, N., Okeka, W., Minakawa, N., Takagi, M., Yan, G., 2005. Survivorship of Anopheles gambiae sensu stricto (Diptera: Culicidae) larvae in western Kenya highland forest. J. Med. Entomol. 42, 270–277.

Tusting, L.S., Willey, B., Lucas, H., Thompson, J., Kafy, H.T., Smith, R., Lindsay, S.W., 2013. Socioeconomic development as an intervention against malaria: a systematic review and meta-analysis. Lancet 382, 963–972.

Tusting, L.S., Ippolito, M.M., Willey, B.A., Kleinschmidt, I., Dorsey, G., Gosling, R.D., Lindsay, S.W., 2015. The evidence for improving housing to reduce malaria: a systematic review and meta-analysis. Malar. J. 14, 209.

Tusting, L.S., Bottomley, C., Gibson, H., Kleinschmidt, I., Tatem, A.J., Lindsay, S.W., Gething, P.W., 2017. Housing Improvements and Malaria Risk in Sub-Saharan Africa: A Multi-Country Analysis of Survey Data. PLoS Med. 14, e1002234.

Tyagi, R.K., DAS, M.K., Singh, S.S., Sharma, Y.D., 2013. Discordance in drug resistance-associated mutation patterns in marker genes of Plasmodium falciparum and Plasmodium knowlesi during coinfections. J. Antimicrob. Chemother. 68, 1081–1088.

Tyagi, K., Gupta, D., Saini, E., Choudhary, S., Jamwal, A., Alam, M.S., Zeeshan, M., Tyagi, R.K., Sharma, Y.D., 2015. Recognition of human erythrocyte receptors by the tryptophan-rich antigens of monkey malaria parasite Plasmodium knowlesi. PLoS One 10, e0138691.

Umhang, G., Possenti, A., Colamesta, V., D'aguanno, S., la Torre, G., Boue, F., Casulli, A., 2019. A systematic review and meta-analysis on anthelmintic control programs for Echinococcus multilocularis in wild and domestic carnivores. Food Waterborne Parasitol. 15, e00042.

United Nations Department of Economic and Social Affairs Population Division, 2018. World Urbanization Prospects: The 2018 Revision. United Nations, Geneva.

Vadivelan, M., Dutta, T., 2014. Recent advances in the management of Plasmodium knowlesi infection. Tropenmed. Parasitol. 4, 31–34.

Valentine, M.J., Murdock, C.C., Kelly, P.J., 2019. Sylvatic cycles of arboviruses in non-human primates. Parasit. Vectors 12, 463.

Van den Bossche, P., Shumba, W., Makhambera, P., 2000. The distribution and epidemiology of bovine trypanosomosis in Malawi. Vet. Parasitol. 88, 163–176.

van den Eede, P., Van, H.N., van Overmeir, C., Vythilingam, I., Duc, T.N., Hung Le, X., Manh, H.N., Anne, J., D'alessandro, U., Erhart, A., 2009. Human Plasmodium knowlesi infections in young children in central Vietnam. Malar. J. 8, 249.

Vittor, A.Y., Pan, W., Gilman, R.H., Tielsch, J., Glass, G., Shields, T., Sanchez-Lozano, W., Pinedo, V.V., Salas-Cobos, E., Flores, S., Patz, J.A., 2009. Linking deforestation to malaria in the Amazon: characterization of the breeding habitat of the principal malaria vector, Anopheles darlingi. Am. J. Trop. Med. Hyg. 81, 5–12.

Vythilingam, I., TAN, C.H., Asmad, M., Chan, S.T., Lee, K.S., SINGH, B., 2006. Natural transmission of Plasmodium knowlesi to humans by Anopheles latens in Sarawak, Malaysia. Trans. R. Soc. Trop. Med. Hyg. 100, 1087–1088.

Vythilingam, I., Noorazian, Y.M., Huat, T.C., Jiram, A.I., Yusri, Y.M., Azahari, A.H., Norparina, I., Noorrain, A., Lokmanhakim, S., 2008. Plasmodium knowlesi in humans, macaques and mosquitoes in peninsular Malaysia. Parasit. Vectors 1, 26.

Wai, K.T., Kyaw, M.P., Oo, T., Zaw, P., Nyunt, M.H., Thida, M., Kyaw, T.T., 2014. Spatial distribution, work patterns, and perception towards malaria interventions among temporary mobile/migrant workers in artemisinin resistance containment zone. BMC Public Health 14, 463.

Walsh, J.F., Molyneux, D.H., Birley, M.H., 1993. Deforestation: effects on vector-borne disease. Parasitology 106 (Suppl), S55–S75.

Warren, M., Cheong, W.H., Fredericks, H.K., Coatney, G.R., 1970. Cycles of jungle malaria in West Malaysia. Am. J. Trop. Med. Hyg. 19, 383–393.

Weisse, M., Goldman, E.D., 2021. Primary rainforest destruction increased 12% from 2019 to 2020. World Resources Institute, Washington DC. Available: https://research.wri.org/gfr/forest-pulse?utm_medium=globalforests&utm_source=email&utm_campaign=globalforestreview. (Accessed).

Wesolowski, A., Eagle, N., Tatem, A.J., Smith, D.L., Noor, A.M., Snow, R.W., Buckee, C.O., 2012. Quantifying the impact of human mobility on malaria. Science 338, 267–270.

Wilcove, D.S., McLellan, C.H., Dobson, A.P., 1986. Habitat fragmentation in the temperate zone. Conserv. Biol. 6, 237–256.

Wilcox, B.A., Ellis, B., 2006. Forests and emerging infectious diseases of humans. UNASYLVA-FAO, p. 57.

Wilkinson, D.A., Marshall, J.C., French, N.P., Hayman, D.T.S., 2018. Habitat fragmentation, biodiversity loss and the risk of novel infectious disease emergence. J. R. Soc. Interface 15.

William, T., Menon, J., Rajahram, G., Chan, L., Ma, G., Donaldson, S., Khoo, S., Frederick, C., Jelip, J., Anstey, N.M., Yeo, T.W., 2011. Severe Plasmodium knowlesi malaria in a tertiary care hospital, Sabah, Malaysia. Emerg. Infect. Dis. 17, 1248–1255.

William, T., Rahman, H.A., Jelip, J., Ibrahim, M.Y., Menon, J., Grigg, M.J., Yeo, T.W., Anstey, N.M., Barber, B.E., 2013. Increasing incidence of Plasmodium knowlesi malaria following control of P. falciparum and P. vivax Malaria in Sabah, Malaysia. PLoS Negl. Trop. Dis. 7, e2026.

William, T., Jelip, J., Menon, J., Anderios, F., Mohammad, R., Awang Mohammad, T.A., Grigg, M.J., Yeo, T.W., Anstey, N.M., Barber, B.E., 2014. Changing epidemiology of malaria in Sabah, Malaysia: increasing incidence of Plasmodium knowlesi. Malar. J. 13, 390.

Wilson, S., Booth, M., Jones, F.M., Mwatha, J.K., Kimani, G., Kariuki, H.C., Vennervald, B.J., Ouma, J.H., Muchiri, E., Dunne, D.W., 2007. Age-adjusted Plasmodium falciparum antibody levels in school-aged children are a stable marker of microgeographical variations in exposure to Plasmodium infection. BMC Infect. Dis. 7, 67.

Wimberly, M.C., de Beurs, K.M., Loboda, T.V., PAN, W.K., 2021. Satellite observations and malaria: new opportunities for research and applications. Trends Parasitol. 37, 525–537.

Wolfe, N.D., Escalante, A.A., Karesh, W.B., Kilbourn, A., Spielman, A., Lal, A.A., 1998. Wild primate populations in emerging infectious disease research: the missing link? Emerg. Infect. Dis. 4, 149–158.

Wolfe, N.D., Daszak, P., Kilpatrick, A.M., Burke, D.S., 2005. Bushmeat hunting, deforestation, and prediction of zoonoses emergence. Emerg. Infect. Dis. 11, 1822–1827.

Wong, M.L., Chua, T.H., Leong, C.S., Khaw, L.T., Fornace, K., Wan-Sulaiman, W.Y., William, T., Drakeley, C., Ferguson, H.M., Vythilingam, I., 2015a. Seasonal and Spatial Dynamics of the Primary Vector of Plasmodium knowlesi within a Major Transmission Focus in Sabah, Malaysia. PLoS Negl. Trop. Dis. 9, e0004135.

Wong, M.L., Vythilingam, I., Leong, S.C., Chua, T.H., Loke, T.K., Fornace, K., Yussof, W., Torr, S., Drakeley, C.J., Ferguson, H., 2015b. Dynamics of Anopheles balabacensis on Banggi Island and Kudat, Sabah, Malaysia in relation to *Plasmodium knowlesi*.

Woolhouse, M.E., Dye, C., Etard, J.F., Smith, T., Charlwood, J.D., Garnett, G.P., Hagan, P., Hii, J.L., Ndhlovu, P.D., Quinnell, R.J., Watts, C.H., Chandiwana, S.K., Anderson, R.M., 1997. Heterogeneities in the transmission of infectious agents: implications for the design of control programs. Proc. Natl. Acad. Sci. U. S. A. 94, 338–342.

Workman, A., Blashki, G., Bowen, K.J., Karoly, D.J., Wiseman, J., 2018. The political economy of health co-benefits: embedding health in the climate change agenda. Int. J. Environ. Res. Public Health 15.

World Health Organisation, 2019. Meeting report of the WHO Evidence Review Group on assessment of malariogenic potential to inform elimination strategies and plans to prevent re-establishment of malaria. World Health Organization, Geneva.

World Health Organisation Regional Office for Western Pacific, 2017. Expert consultation on Plasmodium knowlesi malaria to guide malaria elimination strategies. World Health Organization, Manila, Philippines.

Yakob, L., Bonsall, M.B., Yan, G., 2010. Modelling knowlesi malaria transmission in humans: vector preference and host competence. Malar. J. 9, 329.

Yakob, L., Lloyd, A.L., Kao, R.R., Ferguson, H.M., Brock, P.M., Drakeley, C., Bonsall, M.B., 2018. Plasmodium knowlesi invasion following spread by infected mosquitoes, macaques and humans. Parasitology 145, 101–110.

Yasuoka, J., Levins, R., 2007. Impact of deforestation and agricultural development on anopheline ecology and malaria epidemiology. Am. J. Trop. Med. Hyg. 76, 450–460.

Young, H., Griffin, R.H., Wood, C.L., Nunn, C.L., 2013. Does habitat disturbance increase infectious disease risk for primates? Ecol. Lett. 16, 656–663.

Yusof, R., Lau, Y.L., Mahmud, R., Fong, M.Y., JELIP, J., Ngian, H.U., Mustakim, S., Hussin, H.M., Marzuki, N., Mohd Ali, M., 2014. High proportion of knowlesi malaria in recent malaria cases in Malaysia. Malar. J. 13, 168.

Zhou, X., Huang, J.L., Njuabe, M.T., Li, S.G., Chen, J.H., Zhou, X.N., 2014. A molecular survey of febrile cases in malaria-endemic areas along China-Myanmar border in Yunnan province, People's Republic of China. Parasite 21, 27.

Printed in the United States
by Baker & Taylor Publisher Services